HEALTH PROMOTION

A Practical Guide to Effective Communication

EDITED BY
Merryn McKinnon

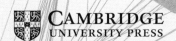

CAMBRIDGE
UNIVERSITY PRESS

CAMBRIDGE
UNIVERSITY PRESS

University Printing House, Cambridge CB2 8BS, United Kingdom

One Liberty Plaza, 20th Floor, New York, NY 10006, USA

477 Williamstown Road, Port Melbourne, VIC 3207, Australia

314–321, 3rd Floor, Plot 3, Splendor Forum, Jasola District Centre, New Delhi – 110025, India

79 Anson Road, #06–04/06, Singapore 079906

Cambridge University Press is part of the University of Cambridge.

It furthers the University's mission by disseminating knowledge in the pursuit of education, learning and research at the highest international levels of excellence.

www.cambridge.org
Information on this title: www.cambridge.org/9781108816045
© Cambridge University Press 2021

First published 2021

Cover designed by Marianna Berek-Lewis
Typeset by Integra Software Service Pvt. Ltd
Printed in Singapore by Markono Print Media Pte Ltd, March 2021

A catalogue record for this publication is available from the British Library

A catalogue record for this book is available from the National Library of Australia

ISBN 978-1-108-81604-5 Paperback

Additional resources for this publication at www.cambridge.org/highereducation/isbn/9781108816045/resources

HEALTH PROMOTION

A Practical
Guide to Effective
Communication

Health Promotion: A Practical Guide to Effective Communication introduces students to the fundamental principles and practices of health promotion in the Australian and international public health contexts. Combining the core principles and theories of health promotion with those of effective communication, the text guides readers through the practical steps of planning, implementing and evaluating programs that empower health consumers and facilitate improved and equitable health outcomes for individuals and communities.

The chapters consolidate and extend readers' understanding of key topics through case-study scenarios addressing the complexity of health promotion in practice, problem-based learning activities, revision questions and recommendations for further reading. The 'Elsewhere in the World' sections link the text to health promotion programs globally. The final chapter brings together key concepts and highlights initiatives in action through a selection of eight extended international case studies.

With contributions from academics and specialists across the public health, health promotion and science communication disciplines, this essential resource will equip students with the knowledge and tools to prepare them for practice across a range of health and policy settings.

Merryn McKinnon is a senior lecturer in the Centre for the Public Awareness of Science at the Australian National University.

Cambridge University Press acknowledges the Australian Aboriginal and Torres Strait Islander peoples of this nation. We acknowledge the traditional custodians of the lands on which our company is located and where we conduct our business. We pay our respects to ancestors and Elders, past and present. Cambridge University Press is committed to honouring Australian Aboriginal and Torres Strait Islander peoples' unique cultural and spiritual relationships to the land, waters and seas, and their rich contribution to society.

Contents

Part 3   Global health into the future

Case study boxes

About the authors

Editor

Merryn McKinnon is a senior lecturer in science communication at the Centre for the Public Awareness of Science at the Australian National University. She has worked in science communication nationally and internationally, in both academic and non-academic roles. Her teaching and research focus on helping the scientists, public health workers and policy makers of tomorrow to communicate clearly and with influence, and to identify ways of creating meaningful and genuinely inclusive public engagement.

Chapter contributors

Will J. Grant is a senior lecturer in science communication at the Centre for the Public Awareness of Science at the Australian National University. Will has been awarded for his public policy and outreach work, and has written dozens of works in scholarly and high-impact public facing outlets, focusing mostly on the interaction of science, politics and technology. He is co-founder of the researcher employment service PostAc and presents podcasts at The Wholesome Show and G'day Patriots.

Rod Lamberts is Deputy Director of the Centre for the Public Awareness of Science at the Australian National University (ANU). He has more than 20 years' experience as a science communication practitioner, researcher and consultant. Rod designed and delivered some of the first university science communication courses in the world and is a former chair of the ANU science and medicine ethics committee. His core research and practice interests lie in risk communication, science communication and public intellectualism and advocacy. He is a frequent public commentor and podcaster on science and science-related stories.

Linda Murray is a public health academic who researches maternal and child health, refugee and migrant health, violence as a social determinant of health, and the intersection between human health and the natural environment. She taught in the Master of Public Health program in the University of Tasmania's School of Medicine from 2013 to 2018. Linda coordinates the Master of Public Health and teaches health communication at Massey University, Aotearoa New Zealand.

Lindy A. Orthia is a senior lecturer in science communication at the Centre for the Public Awareness of Science at the Australian National University. She has received several awards for her science communication teaching, including the Vice-Chancellor's Award for Teaching Excellence. Her research interests include the history of science communication, science in popular fiction and the intersections of science with socio-political identifiers such as race, gender and sexual orientation.

Chapter 10 case study contributors

Biaowen Huang is an associate professor in the School of Language and Communication at Beijing Jiaotong University. He was awarded a PhD in communication by Renmin University of China in 2013. His research focuses on risk, health and environmental communication, specifically to explore public attitudes and behaviours toward scientific and health issues.

Josyula K. Lakshmi is a senior research fellow at The George Institute for Global Health at the University of New South Wales. Her research, advocacy and teaching interests include health promotion, disease and injury prevention, health system governance in a pluralistic medical society, planetary health, physical activity, ageing and research ethics.

Albert Lee is Clinical Professor of Public Health and Primary Care and Founding Director of the Centre for Health Education and Promotion at the Chinese University of Hong Kong. He is a pioneer in health settings research and has gained international recognition as an international member of the US National Academy of Medicine and has served as an adviser to the World Health Organization.

Lillibet Namakula is the Programs Manager and Co-Founder at Public Health Ambassadors Uganda (PHAU). With a Master's degree in Public Health from the University of the West of England (UWE) and experience in sexual and reproductive health and rights, advocacy, and health education and promotion in its many aspects, she is passionate about women and girl empowerment and improving young people's health.

Patrick Segawa is a Sexual and Reproductive Health Rights advocate, public health practitioner and social entrepreneur who strives to use information technology to improve the health of his community. He is the Founder and Team Leader of the Public Health Ambassadors Uganda (PHAU) where he works on youth and community empowerment projects. In 2018, he received the Impact to the Community Award for his outstanding contribution to the field of public health from Clarke International University. He is a finalist for a Master of Science in Public Health – Population and Reproductive Health at Uganda Martyrs University (UMU).

Christina Severinsen is a senior lecturer in the School of Health Sciences at Massey University, Aotearoa New Zealand. She has expertise in health promotion and community health, and her research maintains a critical public health lens to identify challenges, risks and determinants of health for communities to inform action.

Chloe Simpson is passionate about all things related to the promotion of reproductive health and rights. A health promotion specialist, she has been working for the past four years with local and international NGOs in Lebanon and Uganda. She holds a Master's in International Public Health, a BA and a Master's of Nursing from the University of Sydney. In between her international development work, she is based in Sydney, Australia, working as a qualified nurse.

Dennis Earnest Ssesanga is a public health technologist, youth advocate, published poet and social entrepreneur. He conducts health education and promotion activities, including edutainment – an informative performance arts approach to education. He mentors other youth in the use of information communication technology and creative arts as a means of educating young people about HIV/AIDS, STIs, family planning and unplanned teenage pregnancy. He is a global health corps alumni with a Master's of Science in Public Health from Clarke International University.

Mikihito Tanaka is an associate professor in the Graduate School of Political Science at Waseda University, Japan. He earned his PhD from the University of Tokyo and is also an experienced journalist. Mikihito researches public arguments about risk in mass media and social media, using both qualitative and quantitative methods.

Sudhir Raj Thout is a research fellow in the Food Policy Division at The George Institute for Global Health, India and a member of the International Network for Food and Obesity non-communicable diseases Research, Monitoring and Action Support (INFORMAS). His research focuses on dietary salt reduction and food policy to prevent diet-related, non-communicable diseases. Sudhir has experience across a broad range of international public health research and policy.

Andy Towers is an associate professor in the School of Health Sciences, Director of Teaching & Learning in the College of Health and co-leader of the Mental Health and Addiction Programme at Massey University, Aotearoa New Zealand. His research focuses on alcohol and other drug use, and healthy ageing.

Tehzeeb Zulfiqar is a clinician, public health specialist and medical epidemiologist. She is an assistant professor in the Department of Family Practice at the Health Services University in Pakistan. She has over 20 years of experience in primary health care, with an interest in maternal and child health care and preventive medicine. She was the national lead for the Third Party Evaluation of Lady Health Workers program, the largest community based primary health care program in South Asia, having over 100 000 female health workers working primarily in rural and remote Pakistan.

Acknowledgements

The editor and Cambridge University Press would like to acknowledge and thank the following contributors, who contributed case studies for this text: Shane Kawenata Bradbrook, Venkatesan Chakrapani, Daniel Craig, Amy R. Dobos, Matthew Dunn, Jasvir Kaur, Manmeet Kaur, Mitsuru Kudo, Rajesh Kumar, Albert Lee, Lindy A. Orthia, Shino Ouchi, Angelique Reweti, Christine Roseveare, Christina Severinsen and Andrea Waling.

The editor and Cambridge University Press would like to thank the following for permission to reproduce material in this book.

Figure 1.1: © 2017 The Australian Psychological Society. Reproduced with permission. **Figure 1.2**: reproduced from material © Australian Institute of Health and Welfare 2019. Reproduced under Creative Commons Attribution License CC BY 3.0: http://creativecommons .org/licenses/by/3.0/au/. **Figure 1.4**: © United Nations Sustainable Development Goals, https://www.un.org/sustainabledevelopment/. Reproduced with permission. The content of this publication has not been approved by the United Nations and does not reflect the views of the United Nations or its officials or Member States. **Figure 2.5**: reproduced from material © 2011, Springer Nature. Reproduced under Creative Commons Attribution License CC BY 2.0, https://creativecommons.org/licenses/by/2.0/. **Figure 3.2**: reproduced from material © World Health Organization. Reproduced with permission of the World Health Organization, https://www.who.int/nutrition/bfhi/bfhi-poster-A2.pdf. **Figure 3.3**: © Getty Images/PamelaJoe McFarlane. **Figure 5.1**: reproduced from data © Civiqs, Inc (civiqs.com). Reproduced with permission. **Figure 6.1**: © Amy Dobos 2012. Reproduced with permission. **Figure 7.1**: © 2020 Commonwealth of Australia as represented by the Department of Health. Reproduced with permission. **Figure 9.1**: © Getty Images/StockPlanets. **Figure 9.2**: reproduced from material © Commonwealth of Australia under a Creative Commons Attribution 3.0 Australia Licence. The Commonwealth of Australia does not necessarily endorse the content of this publication. **Figures 10.1** and **10.2**: © Beijing Tobacco Control Association, 2015. Reproduced from www .bjtca.org.cn with permission of the Beijing Tobacco Control Association.

Table 1.2: adapted from material © Australian Institute of Health and Welfare 2019. Reproduced under Creative Commons CC BY 3.0 licence: http://creativecommons.org/ licenses/by/3.0/au/. **Table 4.1**: adapted from material © 2013 Taylor & Francis. Reproduced with permission of The Licensor through PLSclear. **Table 4.2**: adapted from material © Cambridge University Press. **Table 9.1**: adapted from Global Health Estimates 2016: Deaths by Cause, Age, Sex, by Country and by Region, 2000–2016. © World Health Organization. Reproduced with permission: https://www.who.int/healthinfo/global_burden_disease/estimates/en/.

Case study 1.1: based on material © 2017, Oxford University Press. Reproduced with permission of Oxford University Press. **Case study 2.2**: based on material © Sage Publications. Reproduced under Creative Commons Attribution Licence CC BY 4.0, https://creative commons.org/licenses/by/4.0/. **Case study 8.2**: based on material © Kaur et al. Reproduced under Creative Commons CC BY 4.0 Licence: https://creativecommons.org/licenses/by/4.0/.

Every effort has been made to trace and acknowledge copyright. The publisher apologises for any accidental infringement and welcomes information that would redress this situation.

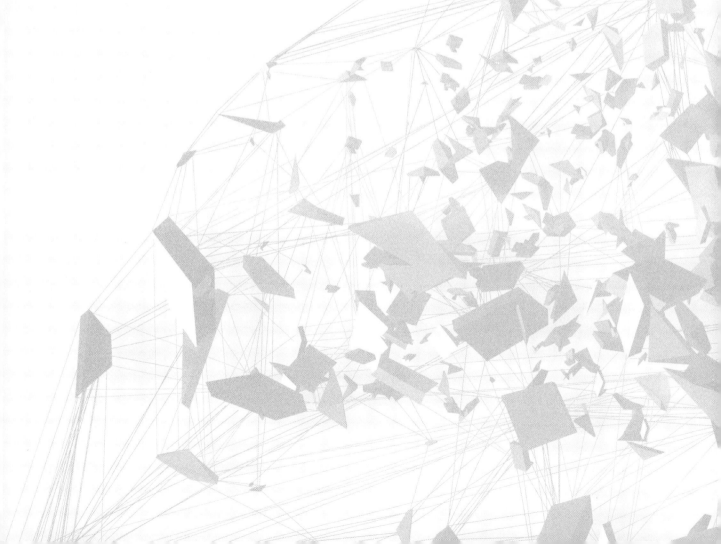

PART 1

Health promotion fundamentals

Influences on health

Merryn McKinnon

With contributions from Shane Kawenata Bradbrook, Angelique Reweti, Christine Roseveare and Christina Severinsen

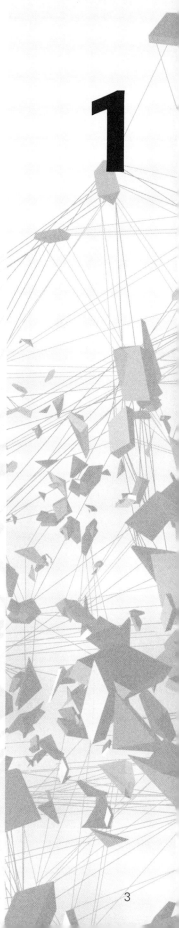

LEARNING OBJECTIVES

At the completion of the chapter, you will be able to:

- Describe the relationship between health promotion and public health.
- Define health and identify the different factors that influence health.
- Explain the different frameworks that guide health promotion and how these have evolved over time.
- Identify how communication can be implemented within health promotion frameworks.

Introduction

Health can be influenced by many different factors, some of which individuals can control and many of which they cannot. Individual health is not the result of simply eating well and exercising. These things are important, but they are a small part of a much larger system of influences in almost every aspect of our lives. Health promotion has a vital role in ensuring that people are able to take control of their health, and to advocate for health in places and policies. This means that a variety of opportunities and mechanisms are available for communication within this landscape.

This chapter begins with a brief overview of what constitutes health and how health can be influenced by contextual factors, using examples from within Australia. It then describes the guiding frameworks of health promotion and how these are applied to address health challenges. The chapter concludes with a preliminary exploration of how communication can support the achievement of desired health promotion goals.

What is health?

Health – 'a state of complete physical, mental and social wellbeing and not merely the absence of disease or infirmity' (WHO, 1948)

Health as a concept has been described since the times of ancient Greek, Indian and Chinese medicine (Svalastog et al., 2017). There are many different perspectives of health; however, most share similar elements, namely the absence of disease and physical and emotional wellbeing supported by the physical and social environments. The World Health Organization's (WHO) definition of **health** was articulated in 1948 and remains commonly accepted. It is a broad, all-encompassing definition that outlines the scope of areas in which health can be influenced, but it does have limitations. Sociologist Aaron Antonovsky (1979) explicitly rejected the WHO definition in his book *Health, Stress and Coping*, arguing that health and wellbeing are not the same thing; rather that health is part of wellbeing (Mittelmark & Bull, 2013). The European-influenced notions of mental health and mental illness, for example, can be too narrow to accurately reflect 'wellbeing' in some cultures (Dudgeon et al., 2017). In Australia, Aboriginal and Torres Strait Islander peoples consider health to be the physical, social, emotional and cultural wellbeing of the whole community. As each individual in the community achieves their full potential as a human, the wellbeing of their community is enhanced (National Aboriginal Community Controlled Health Organisation (NACCHO), 2011). Gee and colleagues (2014) developed the Social and Emotional Wellbeing framework to illustrate the factors that comprise Indigenous social and emotional wellbeing. There are seven interrelated and overlapping domains: body, mind and emotions, community, family and kinship, culture, Country and spirituality (Dudgeon et al., 2017). The relationship between these and the individual is shown in Figure 1.1. It is important to note here that the 'conception of self is grounded within a collectivist perspective that views the self as inseparable from, and embedded within, family and community' (Gee et al., 2014, p. 57). This is different from a Eurocentric perspective, which tends to be individualist and therefore focused on the goals and rights of the individual person. Culture and community are also intrinsic to Māori culture (see Case study 1.1).

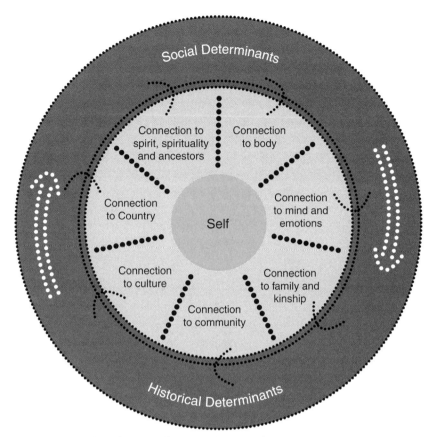

Figure 1.1   Domains of the Social and Emotional Wellbeing framework
Source: Dudgeon et al. (2017, p. 317).

CASE STUDY 1.1   Indigenous knowledge in Māori health promotion

Christina Severinsen and Angelique Reweti

Rangatahi Tū Rangatira – whānau led health promotion in Aotearoa New Zealand

Rangatahi Māori, the indigenous young people of Aotearoa New Zealand, is the fastest-growing population group in the country (Sokratov & O'Brien, 2014). However, research shows that *rangatahi* consistently experience significantly poorer health outcomes compared to *Pākehā*/non-Māori young people (Sokratov & O'Brien, 2014; Williams, Clark & Lewycka, 2018).

   Rangatahi Tū Rangatira (R2R) is a nationwide health promotion program that gives *rangatahi* and their *whānau* (wider family) opportunities to engage in physical activity while learning about *whakapapa* (ancestry) and their identity as Māori (Kōkiri Hauora,

(cont.)

(cont.)

2016). The program is based in *tikanga* Māori (values and practices) and aims to increase *rangatahi* participation in physical activity through *ngā taonga tākaro* (Māori ancestral games) (Severinsen & Reweti, 2019). Unique to the program is its emphasis on developing the total wellbeing of *rangatahi,* including strengthening *whānau* ties, developing leadership skills and promoting cultural awareness and pride in being Māori (Severinsen & Reweti, 2019).

Measuring the effect of R2R

The R2R program has been assessed using a *whānau ora* (holistic) framework, which includes the following outcome areas: *whānau* self-management, healthier lifestyles, increased community participation, increased resilience and increased participation in *te ao* Māori (the Māori world).

Whānau self-management is about *whānau* being able to build capacity to determine their own pathways (Durie et al., 2010; King et al., 2014; Te Puni Kōkiri, 2015). Although the focus of the R2R program is working with *rangatahi*, *whānau* are integral to the equation, with *whānau* participation reflected in *rangatahi* sharing what they have learned in their homes.

The evaluators found *rangatahi* were 'living more active lifestyles' with increased motivation and desire to succeed, not only in their physical pursuits but also outside of the program activities (Severinsen & Reweti, 2019). 'Increased community participation' is recognised as a crucial component in *whānau* wellbeing (Durie et al., 2010; Baker et al., 2012; King et al., 2014). This was demonstrated in *rangatahi* becoming more engaged in their local community through improved knowledge of different services and how to access them.

'Increased resilience' is reflected in how the R2R program helped to facilitate a sense of identity and belonging among participants. Developing *mana* (respect, control and intrinsic value) (Pere, 1997), spiritual vitality and self-esteem through engagement in sports, recreation and community events enhances *whānau* resilience, helping them to become proactive in overcoming adversity and challenges experienced in their day-to-day lives (Baker et al., 2012; Boulton & Gifford, 2014; King et al., 2014).

'Increased participation in *te ao* Māori' is reflected in how the program uses the Māori language and *tikanga* to empower *rangatahi* and *whānau*. Access to *te ao* Māori facilitates the building of a secure cultural identity, which is correlated with good health outcomes for *whānau* (Henwood, 2007; Durie et al., 2010; Irwin et al., 2011).

The importance of culture

Empowering *rangatahi* and *whānau* through the use of *tikanga* Māori and the normalisation of *te reo* Māori were important aspects in the overall success of the program. Communication methods used in the delivery of this program also recognised the importance of using *kaihapai* (program facilitators) from within the community in which the program is being delivered. This included tailoring the program to the specific area and providing opportunities for *rangatahi* to go out into their *rohe* (area) to learn about their *whakapapa* and their *iwi* (tribe).

Source: Adapted from Severinsen & Reweti (2019).

QUESTIONS

1. How can a *whānau*-centred approach improve outcomes for health promotion?

2. What wvould a program grounded in indigenous knowledge look like?

Regardless of the perspective or definition, the factors that influence health are many and complex, and there are some that are more important than others. The Ottawa Charter for Health Promotion, which is discussed later in this chapter, outlines the prerequisites for health – without the following basic prerequisites, improvements in health are not possible:

- peace
- shelter
- education
- food
- income
- a stable ecosystem
- sustainable resources
- social justice
- equity (WHO, 1986, p. 1).

Reading through this list, many of these factors transcend what would be considered the remit of a health department, as later sections in this chapter show. This is where other policy areas such as transport, environment, public works, education and finance can contribute. Policies and initiatives from a range of people, places and organisations can influence health. All of these work together within **public health**, and health promotion works to support the achievement of public-health goals by empowering and 'enabling people to increase control over, and to improve, their health' (WHO, 1986, p. 1).

Public health plays a vital role in assessing and monitoring the health of populations. Based on available information and evidence, public-health professionals develop responses and interventions to address the identified needs of communities. These responses and interventions can take a range of forms, but the primary focus of public health is that of prevention. Prevention can occur at three levels and may take a variety of forms. Primary prevention is focused on preventing disease or injury from occurring (Liamputtong, 2019). It can involve laws and regulations on the use of safety equipment, public awareness campaigns such as the risks of driving under the influence of alcohol or other drugs, and a combination of approaches (e.g. laws against drug driving that are reinforced by financial and/or criminal penalties). It can also include policies to ensure access to healthcare services and facilities. Secondary prevention is used to minimise negative outcomes when problems are detected (Liamputtong, 2019). This includes screening and testing programs to detect, for instance, cancers or scoliosis in at-risk

Public health – an interdisciplinary field that draws upon a range of knowledge to implement solutions to prevent disease and promote health in populations at the local, national and international levels

populations. Tertiary prevention aims to minimise the extent of the negative outcomes of disease or injury through medical care and rehabilitation services (Liamputtong, 2019). Health promotion is involved in each of these types of prevention in public health and can work with diverse stakeholders, as later chapters in this book will explore.

Public health policies and services may go completely unnoticed by society as they focus on preventing ill health; this makes their outcomes difficult to measure (Public Health Association Australia (PHAA), 2018a). Public health measures such as sanitation, water fluoridation and laws mandating the wearing of seat belts are commonplace in Australia. They are part of our day-to-day 'norm', so we may not recognise their effects on our health, or the policies may not appear to be health-related. For example, education is compulsory until at least the age of 15. This is actually a powerful public health policy that operates as a means of primary prevention. Research has shown that education has 'direct effects … on health outcomes and on the health behaviours that lead to health outcomes' (Feinstein et al., 2006, p. 174), a statement supported by evidence from around the world (Fonseca, Michaud & Zheng, 2019). For example, when girls complete their education they have increased job prospects, they delay having children and, if they do choose to have children, are better able to provide education and health care for them (World Bank, 2017). However, like most things related to health, education does not exist in a vacuum, and there are social, environmental and economic influences on health – known as 'determinants' – that cannot be ignored.

Determinants of health

Determinants – the factors that influence health, including social, cultural and structural factors, which can be found at the community, country and global levels

The Public Health Association of Australia (PHAA) describes **determinants** of health as 'the range of social, ecological, political, commercial and cultural factors that influence health status' (PHAA, 2018b, p. 1). Determinants can operate within a community, a country and, potentially, globally (Marmot, 2017). There are many different types of determinants: the social determinants tend to be the ones highlighted most frequently, likely because they 'are the conditions in which people are born, grow, work, live, and age, and the wider set of forces and systems shaping the conditions of daily life' (WHO, 2019a, para 1). The wider forces and systems include the other determinants listed in Table 1.1.

The relationship between social, ecological and cultural determinants is explored in greater detail in later chapters of this book. The political and commercial influences on health may seem more tangential, but they can be profound (see Case study 1.2). Policies and legislation can also have a potentially strong influence on people's ability to access care. For example, the International Covenant on Economic, Social and Cultural Rights outlines the 'right of everyone to the enjoyment of the highest attainable standard of physical and mental health' (United Nations, 1976, Article 12, p. 4) and identifies four steps needed to ensure the attainment of this goal, including reduction of still-births and infant mortality; provision of sanitation; prevention, treatment and control of all forms and sources of disease; and the creation of conditions providing everyone with access to medical services in the event of illness. Signatories to the covenant therefore agree to put these conditions

Table 1.1 Overview of the determinants of health

Determinant factor	Description	Examples
Social	Places, forces and systems that shape the conditions of everyday life and are the source of health inequities.	Housing Social support Employment Food
Ecological	Human survival relies on the diversity of other life forms and ecological systems. The environments we build should not come at the cost of the natural environment.	Clean water Oxygen Green spaces Fertile soil to grow crops for food Climate
Political	Legislation and policy can often determine the extent of the effects of the other determinants. Ideologies, competing powers and agendas all affect health within different political systems and processes.	Taxes Social security benefits Public services
Commercial	These are closely linked to the political determinants and relate to the rise in non-communicable diseases created by the private sector through promotion of products such as tobacco, alcohol and foods high in salt, fat and sugar.	Opposition to plain packaging, sugar reduction (sugar tax) Lobbying Social corporate responsibility programs that distract or deflect negative practices (see Case study 1.2)
Cultural	Factors that promote resilience, foster identity and good mental and physical health and wellbeing. Determinants are consistent with the UN Declaration on the Rights of Indigenous Peoples.	Ancestry Connection to land Kinship Protection and promotion of Traditional Knowledge Individual and collective rights

Source: Adapted from PHAA (2018b).

in place, with varying levels of progress and success within and between countries. In Australia, Queensland has taken the fourth step in the covenant further in its human rights legislation. Section 37 of the *Human Rights Act 2019* (Qld) states that every person has the right to access health services without discrimination and that no-one can be refused emergency medical treatment necessary to prevent death or serious impairment. This is the only legislation in Australia that protects the rights to health services (Queensland Human Rights Commission, 2019).

CASE STUDY 1.2 Foundation for a smoke-free world

Tobacco use kills over 7 million people around the world each year, with a further 1.2 million people dying from exposure to second-hand smoke (WHO, 2019c). In September 2017, one of the largest tobacco companies in the world – Philip Morris International (PMI) – announced the establishment of the Foundation for a Smoke-Free World (FSFW), with close to US $1 billion of funding. The FSFW is led by Derek Yach, the former head of the WHO's Tobacco Free Initiative.

FSFW's mission is 'to end smoking in this generation' (FSFW, 2019, para. 1) and it aims to do this by funding research and promoting innovation and collaboration to create initiatives to reduce death and disease caused by smoking.

There are three 'core work pillars' in FSFW:

- *Health, science and technology:* to develop effective tools to support smoking cessation or conversion to tobacco harm-reduction products such as e-cigarettes
- *Agriculture and livelihoods:* to diversify economies that rely on tobacco production, especially in developing countries
- *Industry transformation:* to deliver change across the tobacco industry globally, including actions taken by the industry to undermine progress towards a smoke-free world.

FSFW offers grants to support researchers and other partners in producing work in support of these pillars.

FSFW'S website states that the initial funding came from PMI but stresses that it 'must operate completely independently from PMI and cannot engage in activities designed to support PMI's interest' (FSFW, 2019, para. 7).

Credible or cunning?

The global health community is sceptical about the true intentions of the FSFW (Malone et al., 2017). Understanding how FSFW allocated its funds was not possible until the foundation filed its first tax return in 2018 (Legg et al., 2019). Those numbers tell an interesting story: of the US $80 million annual budget contributed by PMI, US $6.46 million went to research grants, with another $19 million or so allocated to approved grants, US $7.03 million spent on staffing and US $7.59 million on communications, mostly fees for engagement of public relations agencies (Legg et al., 2019). Approximately US $47 million dollars remains unspent, which may indicate that the FSFW is having trouble attracting independent researchers who are willing to conduct research using money from the tobacco industry (Legg et al., 2019).

FSFW uses many different forms of public communication, including a website, blog, newsletter, public events and social media. Any research centre wanting to address a global issue such as tobacco harm clearly needs to communicate information and research findings to a wide audience, so the use of a public relations agency to assist in such tasks is entirely conceivable. However, two of the main public relations agencies used by FSFW have worked with the tobacco industry for decades to promote tobacco use and to attempt to hide the harms caused by tobacco (Legg et al., 2019). In response to Legg and colleagues' (2019) article in *The Lancet*, Derek Yach, President of FSFW, argues that the foundation's 'communications and legal costs are commensurate with building a foundation from scratch' (Yach, 2019, p. 1008). He does not comment on the nature of the public relations agencies engaged to undertake this work.

PMI claims that the company wants to redirect its resources and influence towards products that can help people who are currently being harmed by the smoking of cigarettes (Igoe, 2019). Over the past few decades PMI has been attempting to rebrand itself as a socially responsible organisation; however, it also continues to market cigarettes to younger consumers, to create stronger products for some markets and to oppose policies that would genuinely limit tobacco use (Malone et al., 2017).

QUESTIONS

1. What are your thoughts after reading this case study?

2. The WHO Framework Convention on Tobacco Control prohibits industry interference in public health policy. This includes FSFW, as it is funded by PMI. Do you think this prohibition is warranted or is it acceptable for an industry funded foundation make a genuine contribution to health? Justify your response.

3. Based on the information presented here, do you believe that PMI is a socially responsible organisation? Use evidence to support your answer.

EXTENSION QUESTION

Look at the various prerequisites for health listed at the beginning of this chapter. Choose one, and conduct research to identify companies and industries that influence these prerequisites, positively or negatively (e.g. energy, defence, transport, food, beverage). Do these companies claim to be socially responsible? Are they? Justify your conclusions.

It can be strange to think that your personal health can be influenced by factors over which you have very little control. For example, the social and ecological determinants may include public transport, infrastructure, air-quality regulations, even access to green spaces and footpaths. As a citizen you may lobby your local (or even state or federal) government representatives, but these amenities are largely beyond your direct control. So much of our health can be influenced, positively and negatively, by our socio-economic status. The social determinants, in particular, can lead to high levels of inequity within and between countries (Marmot, 2017). This is especially pronounced in the structural factors of people's immediate lives, such as poor quality in physical, social and economic environments – these can be described as 'the causes of the causes' of diseases (King, 2006, p. 196). The compounding disadvantage of lower socio-economic status, which in turn influences the 'quality' of one's neighbourhood and access to education, food and health services, can create what Marmot (2017) describes as 'poverty in a sea of affluence' (p. 1312). These inequities are prevalent in any country or even community, including across Australia. Reflect on this as you complete Learning Activity 1.1. Consider the requisites for health you have in your life, and which may be missing or less secure. What do you think could happen to your health if one of these were taken away?

LEARNING ACTIVITY 1.1

Earlier in this chapter the prerequisites for health were listed as peace, shelter, education, food, income, a stable ecosystem, sustainable resources, social justice and equity. Write them down on one side of a page, leaving space in between each requisite.

1. How many of these requisites are present and stable in your life? (e.g. do you have ready access to clean drinking water? Schooling? A reliable supply of fresh food? A regular source of income?) Has this changed over the years? Think back, for example, to your childhood and compare 'then' to 'now'.

Now, across the top of the page, list each of the different categories of determinants of health.

2. For each requisite for health, using your own life experience, identify which determinants affect your health requisites, both positively and negatively, and give examples if appropriate.

3. Compare and combine your table with others in your group, and then with the class. Which determinants have the greatest positive and negative influences on:
   a. individuals
   b. your group/class
   c. your community or country?

Social determinants within Australia

The effects of social determinants within Australia can be seen in the statistics published by the Australian Institute of Health and Welfare (AIHW). At first glance, *Australia's health 2018: In brief* (AIHW, 2018) suggests that Australians' health is doing well: Australians are living longer, with life expectancies of over 80 years of age the population average; the number of people smoking decreased; and colon cancer survival third highest in the world, all of which place Australia in the best third of the 35 member countries of the Organisation for Economic Cooperation and Development (OECD) (AIHW, 2018). The leading causes of ill health are chronic conditions, many linked to lifestyle factors. Australia is in the worst third of OECD countries for obesity, and alcohol consumption is higher than the OECD average (AIHW, 2018). The country's leading causes of death differ by gender and age. People aged between 1 and 44 years are most likely to die by suicide or land transportation accidents (e.g. cars, bicycles, pedestrians) while those aged between 45 and 74 years are most likely to die from coronary heart disease or lung cancer (AIHW, 2018). Australian women are more likely to die from dementia and Alzheimer's disease; coronary heart disease continues to be a leading cause of death for those aged over 75 years, especially men (AIHW, 2018).

Socio-economic influences

The rate of people dying from coronary heart disease has decreased by 79 per cent since 1980 (AIHW, 2018), which illustrates the effectiveness of lifestyle-change messages and improvements in treatment and medical knowledge. However, these benefits are not shared equally. In a different report, AIHW examined the influence of social determinants on cardiovascular disease (which includes coronary heart disease), diabetes and chronic kidney disease. Men and women living in the lowest socio-economic areas of Australia had higher rates of heart attack, diabetes and chronic kidney disease and were 1.33 to 2.39 times more likely to die of these conditions than men and women in the highest socio-economic areas (AIHW, 2019c). Thus, Australians who have greater financial stability are likely to have better health outcomes. Socio-economic status is often beyond individual control; where you live or what you earn should not determine your health outcomes. Public health and health promotion attempt to address these disparities.

LEARNING ACTIVITY 1.2

Take a few minutes to think about the following questions, and then discuss your answers with the class:

- What has influenced your socio-economic standing?
- Have these influences been positive or negative?
- Have these influences been in your control?
- For each of these questions, also think about why or why not.

Geographic influences

Just as socio-economic status influences health, so too does where you live. Australians who live in outer-regional and remote areas of the country are likely to smoke and drink more and have a shorter life expectancy than those who live in inner-regional areas and major cities (Table 1.2; AIHW, 2019d). Those living in inner-regional areas are more

Table 1.2   Comparison of health status based on geographic location

Health factor	Outer regional and remote	Inner regional	Major cities
Daily smoking	19.6%	16.5%	12.8%
Overweight and obesity	70.1%	71%	65%
Alcohol	24%	19%	15%
Mental and behavioural conditions	22%	26%	21%
Asthma	13%	13%	11%
Life expectancy – males	76 years	79 years	81 years
Life expectancy – females	80 years	83 years	84 years

Source: Adapted from AIHW (2019d).

likely to have mental health and behavioural concerns, and overweight and obesity. Those who live in major cities tend to have the best health outcomes and life expectancies of all Australians (AIHW, 2019d). However, earlier results from the *Household, Income and Labour Dynamics in Australia Survey* showed that those who lived in major cities reported lower life satisfaction than people living in small towns and non-urban areas, but noted that this was counteracted by the socio-economic benefits, given that some of the least-disadvantaged areas tend to be in major cities (Wilkins, 2015).

Inequities between groups

Different groups have different health needs at different times, and sometimes can have little to no control over these needs, especially if they are driven or created by biological processes (e.g. puberty or menopause). This can be seen in both the (Australian) National Men's and National Women's Health Strategy 2020–2030 documents, which provide frameworks for gender-focused health care (Department of Health, 2019a) and 'acknowledge the different biological and societal factors that impact women's and men's health and wellbeing' (Department of Health, 2019b, p. 8). Both strategies identify priority population groups, many of whom are **vulnerable groups,** who are more likely to face poor health outcomes than others, as captured in Figure 1.2. The term 'vulnerable groups' is typically applied to children, people who are elderly, malnourished, pregnant, incarcerated, drug users, immigrants, refugees, or are ill or immunocompromised. These people are at higher risk of poor health outcomes than the general population due to factors beyond their control. A stark example of this in Australia is the disparity between Indigenous and non-Indigenous Australians.

Aboriginal and Torres Strait Islander people experience disadvantage from birth, and this is compounded throughout the life span, culminating in a life expectancy of around 8 years shorter than that of non-Indigenous people (Department of the Prime Minister and Cabinet, 2019). The AIHW estimates that 39 per cent of the gap in health outcomes between Indigenous and non-Indigenous Australians can be explained by social determinants. This includes housing circumstances (overcrowding or homelessness), lower levels of literacy and numeracy, and higher rates of unemployment and income in the lowest two quintiles (AIHW, 2017). Indigenous Australians are disproportionately represented (over 35 per cent) in the lowest decile of the Index of Relative Socio-Economic Advantage and Disadvantage. In comparison, less than 10 per cent of non-Indigenous Australians are in the same decile (AIHW, 2017). Since its inception in 2008, the Closing the Gap campaign has attempted to address the disparity in health outcomes, with limited success. The campaign aims to achieve the following seven targets, but by 2019 only two are were track:

1. Halve the gap in mortality rates by 2018 (not on track – Indigenous child mortality rates have declined by 10 per cent, but non-Indigenous child mortality rates have also declined and more quickly).
2. Have 95 per cent of Indigenous 4-year-olds enrolled in early childhood education by 2025 (achieved in 2017).
3. Close the gap in school attendance by 2018 (not on track – in 2018, 82 per cent of Indigenous children attended school, compared to 93 per cent of non-Indigenous students).

Vulnerable groups – the term is applied to groups of people who, through circumstances beyond their control, do not have the same benefits and opportunities as other groups; this may result in poor health outcomes

Vulnerable group	Key statistics
Children	In 2017–18, 22% (26 500) clients seeking specialist homelessness services as a result of family or domestic violence were aged 0–9.
Young women	In 2017, young women aged 15–34 accounted for more than half (53%, or 11 000) of all police-recorded female sexual assault victims.
Older people	In 2017–18, more than 10 900 calls were made to elder abuse helplines across Australia.
People with disability	People with disability were 1.8 times as likely to have experienced physical and/or sexual violence from a partner in the previous year, compared with people without disability.
People from culturally and linguistically diverse backgrounds	Between March 2013 and June 2016, the Australian Federal Police received 116 case referrals for forced marriage involving young females.
LGBTIQ+ people	In the last 5 years, workplace sexual harassment was higher among those identifying with diverse sexual orientation (52%) than among those identifying as straight or heterosexual (31%).
People in rural and remote Australia	People in *Remote* and *Very remote* Australia are more than 24 times as likely to be hospitalised for domestic violence as are people in *Major cities*.
People from socio-economically disadvantaged areas	People living in the most disadvantaged areas of Australia are 1.5 times as likely to experience partner violence as those living in areas of least disadvantage.
Indigenous Australians	Indigenous adults are 32 times as likely to be hospitalised for family violence as non-Indigenous adults.

Figure 1.2 Key Australian statistics illustrating the relationship between vulnerability and violence
Source: AIHW (2019a, viii–ix).

4. Close the gap in life expectancy by 2031 (not on track – there has been a small reduction in the gap but Indigenous peoples are still, on average, likely to live about 8 years less than non-Indigenous people).
5. Halve the gap in Year 12 attainment or equivalent by 2020 (not on track).
6. Halve the gap in reading and numeracy by 2018 (not on track).
7. Halve the gap in employment by 2018 (not on track) (Department of the Prime Minister and Cabinet, 2019, p. 10).

The 2019 Closing the Gap report acknowledges that success is most likely when Aboriginal and Torres Strait Islanders are involved in a true partnership and are able to guide funding and strategy decisions (Department of the Prime Minister and Cabinet, 2019). We return to a discussion of partnerships later in the chapter.

The relationship between determinants and health promotion

In 2003, Peter Howat and colleagues defined health promotion by combining the commonly used concepts of health promotion from the available international literature and national health promotion competencies and practice. They created what they termed a 'unified definition', which aimed to 'provid[e] guidance to the scope and nature of health promotion … [to] facilitate planning, implementing and evaluating interventions' (Howat et al., 2003, p. 82). At that time there was no consistent definition of health promotion, which Howat and colleagues argued constrained the profession of health promotion. Their definition is as follows:

> Health promotion can be regarded as a combination of educational, organisational, economic and political actions designed with consumer participation, to enable individuals, groups and whole communities to increase control over, and to improve their health through attitudinal, behavioural, social and environmental changes (Howat et al., 2003, p. 84).

The inclusion of terms such as 'organisational, economic and political actions' reflect the strategies identified by WHO as best practice in health promotion, whereas 'attitudinal, behavioural, social and environmental changes' incorporate the social determinants (Howat et al., 2003). The reference to consumer participation is also important, as it highlights the relevance of partnerships, which enable people and communities to increase control over their health, rather than health promotion simply being something that is 'done to' them.

LEARNING ACTIVITY 1.3

Read the case description and then answer the questions that follow.

Abdul is an undergraduate student with a full-time study load. He is living in self-catering accommodation on campus, away from home for the first time. He works at a restaurant three nights a week, is a member of the residential college soccer team and is also a peer tutor. Abdul is studying for a Bachelor of Public Policy and is very interested in working in the international context – in development or diplomacy.

He is very keen to finish off his degree with an internship so that he might gain valuable, real-world experience. The internship courses are highly competitive, so Abdul works hard to attend all his classes and submit all of his assignments to make sure his grades remian high.

Money is always a concern. Abdul tries to keep his costs down wherever he can. The nights he is at work he gets a meal at the restaurant. The nights when he is at home he tries to cook something cheap and quick – this often means he is consuming foods that are highly processed, like instant noodles. After soccer games and training the team generally goes to a local pub or café on campus to grab a meal together. Abdul might share a pizza with a mate or get hot chips or something cheap on the menu. He often skips breakfast, getting a bite to eat after his first lectures finish at 11.00 am.

With so much going on with uni, study and sport, Abdul is always busy. He can't afford not to work, even with the government student assistance he receives, and he wants to finish his degree as soon as he can so he can start to earn some money. He also wants to keep playing soccer because it is usually the only exercise he gets during the week, plus it allows him time to hang out with his friends. Abdul often feels tired and a bit burnt out. He is the eldest child in his family and the first one to go to university so he is determined to be self-sufficient and be an example to his younger brother and sisters.

QUESTIONS

1. What are the factors that may affect Abdul's health in positive and negative ways?

2. Imagine you are working at the health clinic at Abdul's university and he seeks help to manage his fatigue. What recommendations would you offer Abdul and why? Discuss in your group.

Guiding frameworks of health promotion

Ottawa Charter

In 1986, the WHO held the first international conference on health promotion in Ottawa, Canada. During this conference, the attendees developed the Ottawa Charter for Health Promotion, which 'was intended to promote a serious paradigm shift in the way in which public-health issues were conceptualised and addressed in the future' (Nutbeam, 2019, p. 706). The Ottawa Charter outlines three strategies for health promotion:

*   Advocate – health promotion should advocate for political, environmental, economic, social, cultural, behavioural and biological factors that support the attainment and retention of good health.
*   Enable – equip people with the skills, resources, information and opportunities they need to increase control over their health.
*   Mediate – health promotion must work across and beyond disciplinary boundaries to coordinate action across all groups, including government departments, non-government agencies, community organisations and groups, industry and media.

Each strategy relies on effective communication. Health promoters need to be able to talk to a range of different people, tailor information according to different interests and perspectives, and to educate and persuade. These actions all need to occur in the five key areas for action, which are:

1. Build healthy public policy – health promotion works to place health-supporting policies within all sectors, creating coordinated actions to support equity and health for all.
2. Create supportive environments – natural and built environments are fundamental influences on health. Our living, working and natural environments must be sustainably managed and maintained in order for them to support human health.
3. Strengthen community action – communities are empowered to take control of and improve their health through access to information, services and support.
4. Develop personal skills – personal and social development are attained and supported through lifelong education and enhancement of life skills to enable improved personal control and decision-making.
5. Re-orient health services – individual and community needs for health are supported by the health sector, in collaboration with individuals, community groups, government and private organisations. There is an increased focus on prevention rather than cure.

Equity – being fair or impartial; allocation of resources is determined by identified need

Equality – the state of being equal, including in status, rights and opportunities; for example, everyone gets the same amount of resources, irrespective of need

The use of the word **equity** in the Ottawa Charter, instead of **equality**, is important. While equality in health means everyone should have the same health outcomes – for example, in life expectancy – equity recognises that some groups need more assistance than others to attain that outcome. For instance, someone who lives in a remote area but is healthy, well-educated and enjoys a high socio-economic status will need less support to achieve good health outcomes than someone from the same remote area who identifies as a member of a vulnerable group, such as having left school at age 16, having low socio-economic status and living with a chronic disease. You could think of equity as being a necessary means of achieving equality.

Despite the focus on equity within the Ottawa Charter, its development was not equitable. The Charter was developed by a comparatively small number of countries – only 38 – and the focus was on the needs of industrialised countries (Nutbeam, 2019). Countries that likely had the greatest health needs were not part of the discussion; however, this has changed over time. Despite its initial shortcomings, the Ottawa Charter provided a solid foundation, which subsequent WHO-led international health promotion conferences have built upon and refined to better suit the needs of all countries, especially developing nations and those whose populations face poor health outcomes due to inequities (Figure 1.3).

Sustainable Development Goals

The United Nations (UN) 2030 Agenda for Sustainable Development was signed by all 193 member countries of the UN General Assembly and was adopted in 2015 (UN General Assembly, 2015). The Agenda sets out 17 Sustainable Development Goals (SDGs, see Figure 1.4), which call on all countries to work to eradicate poverty

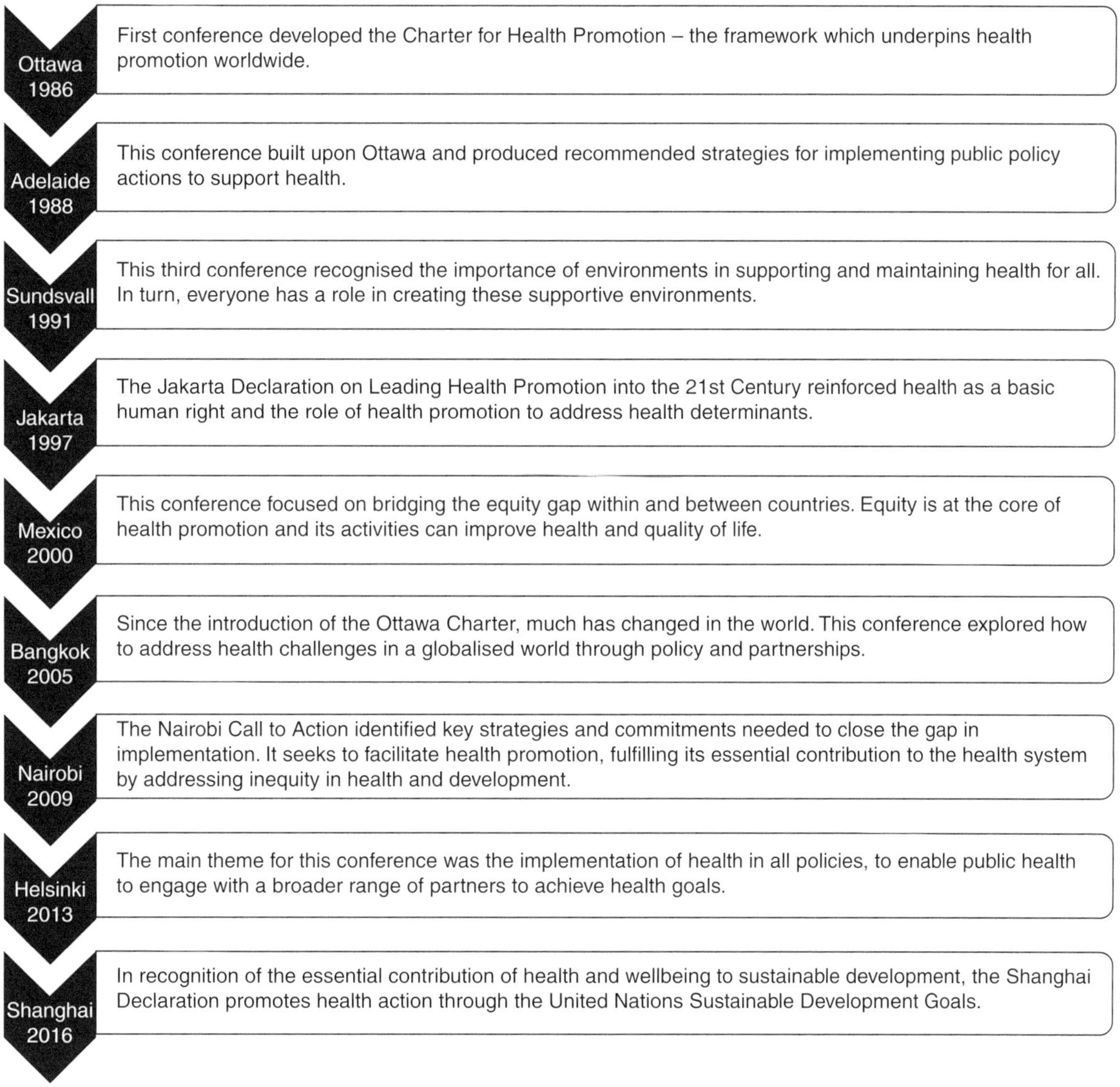

Ottawa 1986
First conference developed the Charter for Health Promotion – the framework which underpins health promotion worldwide.

Adelaide 1988
This conference built upon Ottawa and produced recommended strategies for implementing public policy actions to support health.

Sundsvall 1991
This third conference recognised the importance of environments in supporting and maintaining health for all. In turn, everyone has a role in creating these supportive environments.

Jakarta 1997
The Jakarta Declaration on Leading Health Promotion into the 21st Century reinforced health as a basic human right and the role of health promotion to address health determinants.

Mexico 2000
This conference focused on bridging the equity gap within and between countries. Equity is at the core of health promotion and its activities can improve health and quality of life.

Bangkok 2005
Since the introduction of the Ottawa Charter, much has changed in the world. This conference explored how to address health challenges in a globalised world through policy and partnerships.

Nairobi 2009
The Nairobi Call to Action identified key strategies and commitments needed to close the gap in implementation. It seeks to facilitate health promotion, fulfilling its essential contribution to the health system by addressing inequity in health and development.

Helsinki 2013
The main theme for this conference was the implementation of health in all policies, to enable public health to engage with a broader range of partners to achieve health goals.

Shanghai 2016
In recognition of the essential contribution of health and wellbeing to sustainable development, the Shanghai Declaration promotes health action through the United Nations Sustainable Development Goals.

Figure 1.3 Timeline of the Global Conference on Health Promotion, including the focus areas of the resulting declarations/charters

Source: Adapted from WHO (2020).

and inequality while preserving the planet. All 17 SDGs are interconnected, with SDG3 having a specific health focus. The 2016 Shanghai Global Conference on Health Promotion called for a re-framing of health promotion, positioning it at the centre of the 17 SDGs. The conference stated that 'promoting health is essential to responding to today's interconnected challenges and to delivering on the promise of sustainable development' (WHO, 2017, p. 1). The report outlines the importance of national actions to complement the local level implementation, requiring engagement of multiple stakeholders across different sectors. This requires multiple forms and techniques of communication.

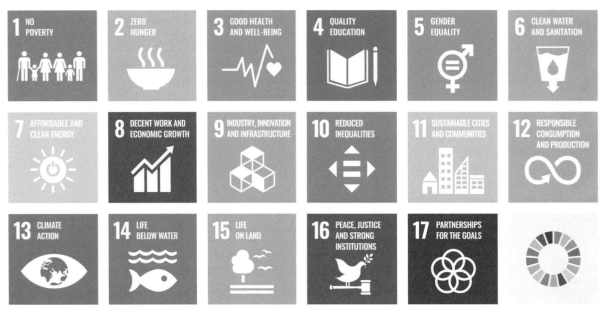

Figure 1.4   The Sustainable Development Goals
Source: United Nations (2019).

Communication and health promotion

Health communication – the study and use of communication tools and techniques to inform, educate and influence people's decisions and actions to improve health

The field of **health communication** aims to communicate health-promoting messages and to influence personal choices. However, there are many other communication fields (such as medical communication, science communication and public relations) that can and do these as well. In this text, the term 'communication' in general is used to refer to a set of skills, tools and strategies to influence, inform and empower an audience – be it an individual or a community.

Throughout this chapter we emphasise that the role of health promotion is to empower people to increase control over their health. This can be done through a variety of mechanisms, which are outlined in the Ottawa Charter (see page 17) under the headings 'Advocate', 'Enable' and 'Mediate'. 'Advocate' refers to the role of health promotion in supporting health within the context of all of the determinants. 'Enable' includes providing people with education, access to information and the knowledge needed to make informed decisions; it refers to equity between communities and genders. The importance of people being empowered to take control of their health, irrespective of their identity or circumstance, is embedded in this notion. 'Mediate' acknowledges the different contexts – social, cultural or economic – in which health promotion should adapt. It also defines the role of many different partners beyond the health sector who need to contribute in order to achieve health; everyone has a role to play.

This notion of partnerships, which has already been mentioned in this chapter, is a crucial element of communication within the health promotion context. To form successful partnerships, the people, groups and organisations involved need to understand what the problem is, why it is important to address and the desired outcome once the problem is 'fixed'. The expected outcome, or the 'vision', is often what convinces people to contribute or participate; it should align with the values and goals of the partners. Being able to clearly articulate that vision in a way that is understandable and relevant to your target audience is key. This text outlines the various steps you can take to ensure that your vision is as clear and compelling as possible. There are never any guarantees of success; communication does not happen in a vacuum and it is difficult to predict how the myriad influencing factors external to your communication activities will affect how your message is received. However, being aware of these factors and planning for them as best you can are important.

One vital partner in health promotion is the target individual or community you are supporting (see Case study 1.3). Acceptance of proposed changes to tobacco-control legislation could not have been achieved without the stories, submissions and the support of the Māori community. Even though progress towards effective tobacco control has not been as rapid as hoped, full participation of Māori people is seen as an essential means of accelerating progress (Ball et al., 2016). Your audiences are also your partners, so you need to understand them well in order to be effective in communication. This is explored in more detail in Chapter 6.

CASE STUDY 1.3 The Ottawa Charter in action

Shane Kawenata Bradbrook and Christine Roseveare

Finding a 'game changer' for tobacco control in Aotearoa New Zealand

Tobacco use is the leading cause of preventable death and disease in Aotearoa New Zealand, particularly among Māori and Pacific peoples. Māori smoking rates are significantly higher than the rest of the population in Aotearoa New Zealand. As director of anti-smoking organisation Te Reo Mārama Māori, Shane Bradbrook was frustrated by what he saw as lack of progress on tobacco control. He could see that decisive political action was needed on tobacco control. A meeting with a friend who was a local Member of Parliament (MP) gave him an idea of how to create the action needed.

During the meeting, the MP suggested using the Select Committee process to raise the issue in Parliament – in particular, the Māori Affairs Select Committee (MASC). Select Committees investigate and report to Parliament on topics of interest. Often, their focus is on legislation proposed by MPs, but the committees could also initiate inquiries of their own into 'significant topics'. The MASC had never been used

(cont.)

(cont.)

to investigate a health issue, but Bradbrook could see many advantages. The Select Committee process could shine a powerful spotlight on the effects of tobacco, the role of tobacco companies, and recommended legislative change. Being Māori-centred, the committee enquiry process would allow Bradbrook and his team to harness the power of indigenous communities and networks to which tobacco companies did not have access. Thus, Bradbrook and his small team began the hard work of gaining the necessary support for the idea of the Select Committee enquiry.

The power of networks

Drawing on their networks, the team arranged meeting after meeting to argue their case. An important milestone was gaining the support of deputy chair of the MASC, MP Hone Hariwira, followed by support from the Associate Minister for Health, Tariana Turia. After 18 months of effort, an inquiry into the actions of the tobacco industry to promote tobacco use among Māori, and the subsequent effects of tobacco use on the health of the Māori population, was announced in September 2009.

Once the inquiry began, Bradbrook remembers 'walking from one end of the country to the other', drawing on his connections with *iwi* (tribes), researchers, health providers and communities to generate written and oral submissions. He set up *hui* (meetings), developed submission templates and worked with the media to get coverage of the inquiry. The climax of the inquiry was when the MASC went 'on tour' around the country. Grassroots connections paid off, with some particularly moving and memorable stories shared with the MASC of the effects of tobacco. This included two children bringing a coffin made of cigarette packets as they talked about the death of their grandfather due to illness caused by long-term smoking. Another former smoker, who quit after receiving a heart transplant, brought his old, diseased heart – which had been removed after his fifth heart attack – to demonstrate the effects of smoking.

The power of people

After receiving more than 2000 submissions, in November 2010 the MASC reported to Parliament, including 42 recommendations. These included tax increases on the sale of tobacco, restrictions on smoking in public places, and mandating of plain packaging, with the goal of making Aotearoa New Zealand a smoke-free nation by 2025. Parliament voted overwhelmingly to accept the report.

QUESTIONS

1. Which parts of the Ottawa Charter do you see at work in this case study? Justify your answer using examples.

2. This is a large-scale example of policy change, but the way Bradbrook worked can be applied at a much smaller level. Identify a particular health issue relevant to your community. How could you work with your local council or community board to achieve a change in policy that might create an environment supportive of addressing this issue?

ELSEWHERE IN THE WORLD

Ethiopia: Parliament passing one of the strongest tobacco-control legislations in Africa

In February 2019, the Ethiopian parliament passed a strict new anti-tobacco law, one of the strongest in Africa. This followed the Ethiopian House of Peoples' Representatives receiving a WHO Award in 2014 for its significant contributions towards tobacco control through ratification of the WHO Framework Convention on Tobacco Control (WHO, 2019b), creation of a smoke-free work environment and assistance on tobacco control by the Ministry of Health and the Food, Medicine and Health Care Administration.

One final consideration of communication within health promotion, in relation to your target audience, is that of **health literacy**. The Shanghai Declaration, including excerpts from the keynote speakers, referred to the need for health literacy so that people can make informed decisions about their health; for the Declaration to be extended to policies as well as individuals; and for its identification as one of the 'three pillars of health promotion' by 'increasing knowledge and social skills to help people to make the healthiest choices and decisions for their families and themselves' (WHO, 2017, p.13). The Declaration further committed to supporting and developing health literacy throughout the life time of an individual as it 'empowers and drives equity' (WHO, 2017, p. 25). Nutbeam (2019) noted that while there are several different definitions and conceptions of health literacy, these are 'ultimately based on an observable set of skills that can be developed and improved through effective communication and education' (p. 708). Effective communication in health promotion, then, is more than a means for conveying a message: it contributes to the abilities of individuals, families and communities to make decisions about their own health and to advocate for better health policies that reduce inequity. If something is worth communicating, then it is worth communicating well – there is more at stake than might be assumed.

Health literacy – the capacity of an individual to locate and assess information in order to make an informed decision about their health; health literacy can apply from individual behaviours through to advocating for policy

Summary

The discipline of health promotion aims to support the overarching goals of public health and good health for everyone. However, the determinants of health, which are often beyond individuals' control, can make that inherently difficult. The role of health promotion, then, is to attempt to address these determinants through a variety of ways. The Ottawa Charter sets out a framework for how health promotion should function. This framework has been developed in the subsequent years in order to be more inclusive of global needs for the achievement of health.

Health is vitally important for sustainable development, of both people and planet. International health promotion conferences increasingly have recognised the role of health promotion in ensuring progress towards sustainable development goals. This includes advocating for health and equity in access to health. The roles of education and access to information are crucial, to enable people to make informed decisions about their health and that of their families. Effective communication in health promotion can provide information, convey solutions and build partnerships to continue to work towards the goal of 'health for all'.

REVISION QUESTIONS

1. What are common characteristics in the different definitions of health?
2. List the determinants that influence health and include an example of each.
3. Social determinants tend to gain the most attention from public health organisations and health promotion – why? Explain your answer with an example.
4. The Ottawa Charter was developed by the first WHO International Conference on Health Promotion. It provides a framework for health promotion and has been further developed over the past two decades. How has the focus of the outputs from the WHO international conferences on health promotion evolved over the years?
5. How can effective communication support the overarching goals of health promotion?

FURTHER READING

Government of South Australia & World Health Organization (2017). *Progressing the Sustainable Development Goals through Health in All Policies: Case studies from around the world*. Adelaide: Government of South Australia.

Liamputtong, P. (2019). *Public Health: Local and global perspectives* (2nd ed.). Melbourne: Cambridge University Press.

Nutbeam, D. (2019). Health education and health promotion revisited, *Health Education Journal*, 78(6), 705–9.

REFERENCES

Antonovsky, A. (1979). *Health, Stress and Coping*. San Francisco: Jossey-Bass.

Australian Institute of Health and Welfare (AIHW) (2017). *Aboriginal and Torres Strait Islander health performance framework 2017*: Supplementary online tables. Cat. no. WEB 170. Canberra: AIHW.

———(2018). *Australia's Health 2018: In brief*. Cat. no. AUS 222. Canberra: AIHW.

———(2019a). *Family, Domestic and Sexual Violence in Australia: Continuing the national story. In brief*. Cat. no. FDV 4. Canberra: AIHW, pp. viii–ix.

———(2019b). *The Health of Australia's Females*. Cat. no. PHE 240. Canberra: AIHW. Retrieved from: https://www.aihw.gov.au/reports/men-women/female-health

———(2019c). *Indicators of Socioeconomic Inequalities in Cardiovascular Disease, Diabetes and Chronic kidney disease*. Cat. no. CDK 12. Canberra: AIHW.

———(2019d). *Rural and Remote Health*. Cat. no. PHE 255. Canberra: AIHW. Retrieved from: https://www.aihw.gov.au/reports/rural-remote-australians/rural-remote-health

Baker, K., Williams, H. & Tuuta C. (2012). *Te pumautanga o te whānau: Tuhoe and South Auckland whānau*. Report No. 4/12. Wellington, Aotearoa New Zealand: Families Commission.

Ball, J., Edwards, R., Waa, A., Bradbrook, S.K., Gifford, H., Cunningham, C., Hoek, J., Blakely, T., Wilson, N., Thomson, G. & Taylor, S. (2016). Is the NZ Government responding adequately to the Māori Affairs Select Committee's 2010 recommendations on tobacco control? A brief review. *New Zealand Medical Journal*, 129(1428), 93–7.

Boulton, A. & Gifford H. (2014). Conceptualising the link between resilience and whānau ora, *MAI Journal*, 3(2), 111–25.

Department of Health (2019a). *National Men's Health Strategy 2020–2030*. Canberra: Department of Health.

———(2019b). *National Women's Health Strategy 2020–2030*. Canberra: Department of Health.

Department of the Prime Minister and Cabinet (2019). *Closing the Gap Report 2019: The annual report to Parliament on progress in Closing the Gap*. Canberra: Department of the Prime Minister and Cabinet.

Dudgeon, P., Bray, A., D'Costa, B. & Walker, R. (2017). Decolonising psychology: Validating social and emotional wellbeing, *Australian Psychologist*, 52(4), 316–25.

Durie, M., Cooper, R., Grennell, D., Snively, S. & Tuaine, N. (2010). *Whānau Ora: Report of the Taskforce on Whānau-Centred Initiatives*. Wellington, Aotearoa New Zealand: Ministry of Social Development.

Feinstein, L., Sabates, R., Anderson, T., Sorhaindo, A. & Hammond, C. (2006). *Measuring the Effects of Education on Health and Civic Engagement: Proceedings of the Copenhagen symposium*. OECD: Paris.

Fonseca, R., Michaud, P. & Zheng, Y. (2019). The effect of education on health: Evidence from national compulsory schooling reforms, *SERIEs – Journal of the Spanish Economic Association*, 11, 83–103.

Foundation for a Smoke-Free World (FSFW) (2019). Foundation for a smoke-free world: Our vision (Website). Retrieved from: https://www.smokefreeworld.org/our-vision/

Gee, G., Dudgeon, P., Schultz, C., Hart, A. & Kelly, K. (2014). Aboriginal and Torres Strait Islander social and emotional wellbeing. In P. Dudgeon, H. Milroy, & R. Walker (eds.), *Working Together: Aboriginal and Torres Strait Islander mental health and wellbeing principles and practice* (2nd ed., pp. 55–68). Canberra: Department of the Prime Minister and Cabinet.

Henwood, W. (2007). Māori knowledge: A key ingredient in nutrition and physical exercise health promotion programmes for Māori, *Social Policy Journal of New Zealand*, (32), 155–64.

Howat, P., Maycock, P., Cross, D., Collins, J., Jackson, L., Burns, S. & James, R. (2003). Towards a more unified definition of health promotion, *Health Promotion Journal of Australia*, 14(2), 82–5.

Igoe, M. (2019). Big tobacco, global health, and the limits of shared value, *Devex*, 25 May. Retrieved from: https://www.devex.com/news/big-tobacco-global-health-and-the-limits-of-shared-value-94263

Irwin, K., Davies, L., Werate, W., Tuuta, C., Rokx-Potae, H., Potaka, S. et al. (2011). *Whānau Yesterday, Today, Tomorrow: A Families Commission research report*, Report No. 1/11. Wellington, Aotearoa New Zealand:Families Commission.

King, L. (2006). The role of health promotion: Between global thinking and local action, *Health Promotion Journal of Australia*, 17(3), 196–9.

King, T.K., Durie, M., Durie, M., Cunningham, C., Borman, B. & Ellison-Loschman, L. (2014). *Te Puawaitanga o Nga Whānau: Six Markers of Flourishing Whānau:*

*A Discussion Document.*Palmerston North, Aotearoa New Zealand. *Office of the Assistant Vice Chancellor Māori & Pasifika.*

Kōkiri Hauora (2016). *Rangatahi Tu Rangatira* (Website). Retrieved from: https://www.r2r.org.nz/

Legg, T., Peeters, S., Chamberlain, P. & Gilmore, A.B. (2019). The Philip Morris-funded Foundation for a Smoke-Free World: Tax return sheds light on funding activities, *The Lancet*, 393(10190), 2487–8.

Liamputtong, P. (2019). *Public Health: Local and Global Perspectives* (2nd edn). Melbourne: Cambridge University Press.

Malone, R.E., Chapman, S., Gupta, P.C. Nakkash, R. et al. (2017). A 'Frank Statement' for the 21st century? *BMJ*, 26(6), 611–12. Retrieved from: https://tobaccocontrol.bmj.com/content/26/6/611

Marmot, M. (2017). The health gap: The challenge of an unequal world – The argument, *International Journal of Epidemiology*, 46(4), 1312–18.

Mittelmark, M.B. & Bull, T. (2013). The salutogenic model of health in health promotion research. *Global Health Promotion*, 20(2), 30–8.

National Aboriginal Community Controlled Health Organisation (NACCHO) (2011). *Constitution for the National Aboriginal Community Controlled Health Organisation.* Ratified, 15 November. Retrieved from: https://www.naccho.org.au/wp-content/uploads/NACCHO-CONSTITUTION-Ratified-Ver-151111-for-ASIC-.pdf

Nutbeam, D. (2019). Health education and health promotion revisited, *Health Education Journal*, 78(6), 705–9.

Pere, R.T. (1997). *Te wheke: A celebration of infinite wisdom.* Wairoa, Aotearoa New Zealand: Ao Ako Global Learning New Zealand with the assistance of Awareness Book Company.

Public Health Association Australia (PHAA) (2018a). *Fact sheet: What is public health?* Canberra: PHAA.

———(2018b). *Factsheet: What are the determinants of health?* Canberra: PHAA.

Queensland Human Rights Commission (2019). Right to health services (Website). Retrieved from: https://www.qhrc.qld.gov.au/your-rights/human-rights-law/right-to-health-services

Severinsen, C. & Reweti, A. (2019). Rangatahi Tū Rangatira: Innovative health promotion in Aotearoa New Zealand. *Health Promotion International*, 34(2), 291–9.

Sokratov, A. & O'Brien, J.M. (2014). *Hīkaka te manawa: Making a difference for rangatahi.* Wellington, NZ: Health and Disability Commissioner and Te Rau Matatini.

Svalastog, A.L., Donev, D., Jahren Kristoffersen, N. & Gajović, S. (2017). Concepts and definitions of health and health-related values in the knowledge landscapes of the digital society. *Croatian Medical Journal*, 58(6),431–5.

Te Puni Kokiri (2015). *Understanding Whānau–Centred Approaches: Analysis of phase one Whānau Ora research and monitoring results.* Wellington, Aotearoa New Zealand: Te Puni Kokiri.

UN General Assembly (2015). *Transforming Our World: The 2030 agenda for sustainable development, 21 October*, A/RES/70/1.

United Nations (1976). International Covenant on Economic, Social and Cultural Rights. United Nations Human Rights: Office of the High Commissioner. Retrieved from: https://www.ohchr.org/en/professionalinterest/pages/cescr.aspx

———(2019). *Sustainable Development Goals*. United Nations. Retrieved from: https:// www.un.org/sustainabledevelopment/wp-content/uploads/2019/01/SDG_ Guidelines_AUG_2019_Final.pdf

Wilkins, R. (2015). *The Household, Income and Labour Dynamics in Australia Survey: Selected findings from waves 1 to 12*. Melbourne: Applied Economic & Social Research, University of Melbourne.

Williams, A., Clark, T. & Lewycka, S. (2018). The associations between cultural identity and mental health outcomes for individual Māori youth in New Zealand, *Public Health*, 6, 319.

World Bank (2017). Girls' Education (Website). Retrieved from: https://www.worldbank .org/en/topic/girlseducation

World Health Organization (WHO) (1948). *Preamble to the Constitution of WHO*, as adopted by the International Health Conference, New York, 19 June–22 July 1946; signed on 22 July 1946 by the representatives of 61 States (Official Records of WHO, no. 2, p. 100) and entered into force on 7 April 1948.

———(1986). *The Ottawa Charter for Health Promotion*. Geneva: WHO.

———(2017). *Promoting Health in the SDGs. Report on the 9th global conference for health promotion, Shanghai, China, 21–24 November 2016: All for health, health for all*. Geneva: WHO.

———(2019a). *About social determinants of health*. Retrieved from: https://www.who .int/social_determinants/sdh_definition/en/

———(2019b). Ethiopia: Parliament passing one of the strongest tobacco control legislations in Africa, *Framework Convention on Tobacco Control*. Retrieved from: https://untobaccocontrol.org/impldb/ethiopia-parliament-passing-one-of-the- strongest-tobacco-control-legislations-in-africa/

———(2019c). *Fact Sheets: Tobacco*. Retrieved from: https://www.who.int/news-room/ fact-sheets/detail/tobacco

———(2020). *WHO Global Health Promotion Conferences*. Retrieved from: https://www .who.int/healthpromotion/conferences/en/

Yach, D. (2019). Foundation for a Smoke-Free World: Independent and making progress. *The Lancet*, 394(10203), 1008.

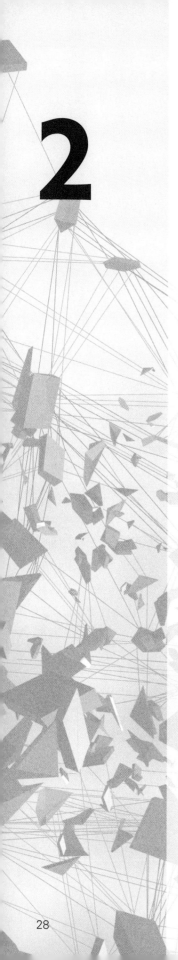

2

Health promotion theories and models

Merryn McKinnon

With contributions from Venkatesan Chakrapani,
Jasvir Kaur, Manmeet Kaur, Rajesh Kumar,
Angelique Reweti and Christina Severinsen

LEARNING OBJECTIVES

At the completion of the chapter, you will be able to:

- Identify key health promotion theories and models, applicable from individual to population levels.
- Understand the influence of audience, culture and context on theory/model choice.
- Apply health promotion theories and models to different scenarios by adapting communication approaches.
- Identify and apply the core components of health promotion program planning.

28

Introduction

There are many theories and models in health promotion. These models are also used in other disciplines, including psychology, environmental conservation and marketing. At their core, each of these health promotion theories and models is attempting to predict how people will act and what different approaches and interventions can be used to help 'move' them towards a desired outcome. This chapter does not examine all of these in great detail – there are many resources that already do this (see Further Reading). The aim of this chapter is to provide a brief overview of some of the main theories used in health promotion and how to incorporate the fundamentals of effective communication.

This chapter will begin by outlining theories and models aimed at individuals and progress through to community levels. The chapter ends with a brief overview of how to integrate theory and practice.

Theories and models in health promotion

Theories and **models** in health promotion are used to plan interventions. They are not blueprints or guarantees of success, but are useful tools in identifying appropriate ways to address health problems. Health is complex and there are many contributing factors; thus, one theory cannot be used to fit all situations. Rather, we draw from different disciplines to assess which theory or model best suits a particular issue. It is important to note that no one size fits all, and that there are some contexts in which none of the models or theories fit. This is where the fundamentals of effective science communication can assist. Who is our target audience? What is our goal? Understanding whom we are trying to reach – in as much detail as possible – is crucial to developing an effective health promotion strategy. The intended audience and the issue we are trying to address, not the theory or model, should be our primary concerns. Once we know whom we need to talk to, we can start to identify their context: who or what are the dominant influences on the health issue we want to influence? The more we understand about our audience, the better equipped we are to choose the theory or model that best suits our purpose.

Theories – A system of ideas intended to explain something, usually based on evidence and assumptions that are generalisable to a population

Models – A simplified description that can be used to predict something; models help us understand how structures, systems and/or interactions could work in the real world

Theories and models can be applied at different levels. Some focus on the individual, while others expand to include **populations**, but typically they all incorporate the different factors – internal and external – that influence the decision-making process. These influences are very important and should not be underestimated or ignored, especially those external to the individual. They also contribute to whether communications are accepted and/or are effective. This applies not only in health but also in science, marketing and advertising. In some ways we are 'selling' the health message, so thinking about what will make this message most relevant and interesting to our audience should help increase the likelihood of the message being successful in achieving the desired outcome.

Population – more than one individual, having at least one shared characteristic between them; a population can be defined by anything from demographics, such as age, gender identity, nationality or sexuality, by identity, such as being a parent, cyclist, vegetarian or smoker, through to personal values and beliefs, such as independence, justice, political ideology and religion.

It is very important to remember that a lack of information is rarely the determining factor in people deciding not to adopt desired behaviours. Simply giving people more information and expecting them to change is not enough. This is known as 'the deficit model', which posits that if people only knew all of the information they would surely change and do/accept the desired action or interventon. This considers people as 'empty vessels' who simply need to be filled with knowledge as motivation for change. We only need to look at the rates of non-communicable, preventable, lifestyle-related diseases to get the sense that this is not the case. Lack of information may be part of the problem, but rarely is it the defining factor. This is covered in greater detail in Chapter 5.

For most of the models presented in this chapter, a key feature is **self-efficacy**. Developed by psychologist Albert Bandura (1977), self-efficacy has been used in different kinds of research and is key to determining the actions and behaviours of people. If someone is not confident that a) they can make the desired change, or b) the desired change will have a positive outcome, then they are unlikely to act. For example, imagine someone who smokes. If they are not confident in their ability to quit – they may have tried before and failed – then this is a barrier to them taking action. If they also believe that not only are they unlikely to be able to quit, but also that quitting will not provide any benefits, then this makes changing the behaviour even harder to influence. And behavioural change cannot be influenced simply by giving people more information. Any kind of influence requires engagement with the individual's core values and beliefs.

Self-efficacy – the personal belief of an individual in their ability to achieve a desired result, and that the desired result will have a positive outcome

Individual level – intrapersonal

Individual or intrapersonal theories focus on the individual. To change the behaviour of a population, we need to understand how to influence a single person, at least as a start.

Health Belief Model

The Health Belief Model evolved from the United States Public Health Service, where it was first described in the 1950s through the work of Godfrey Hochbaum, S. Stephen Kegeles, Howard Leventhal and Irwin Rosenstock (Rosenstock, 1974). The premise of the Health Belief Model is that for an individual to change something – usually a behaviour – to prevent ill health they would need to have three key beliefs, that:

1. They are susceptible, or at risk (*perceived susceptibility*).
2. The health problem is serious (*perceived severity*).
3. The benefits of taking action outweigh the disadvantages of the health problem (*perceived benefits*).

This list explains why people take action, or not, but it does not explain the external influences. The model was expanded by various researchers to encompass three external factors, providing constructs that influence an individual's decision to act:

4. The belief that the effort/cost required to overcome perceived barriers is outweighed by the benefits (*perceived barriers*).
5. A cue to act is seen/received from another external source (e.g. mass media, reminder letter, illness of friend or family member) (*cues to action*).
6. The individual believes that they have the ability to successfully take the required action (*self-efficacy*).

The expanded list of constructs now incorporates some elements that are beyond the individual's control. For example, some of the perceived barriers may arise from some of the social and ecological determinants discussed in Chapter 1. Someone who wishes to improve their general health by eating better food and increasing their physical activity may find barriers to action due to a lack of green spaces, or the cost of fresh food may be prohibitive. The Health Belief Model can also be considered a list for people to weigh up the 'pros and cons' of taking action, or not. In order to act, people must believe that the negatives are outweighed by the benefits and that they are capable of achieving the desired outcome. As described in the previous section, a person's beliefs in their ability to succeed can also be very powerful. This is where the role of health promotion – to empower people to increase control over their health – is very important.

Communication focus

The Health Belief Model is suited for both short-term and long-term interventions, and can be used as a framework to guide communication tactics. At the individual level, we need to understand what the person values and how they perceive risk. Understanding what is most important to people can be used to help create that cue to action. Information needs to be personally relevant – we need to demonstrate the personal benefit for why they should act. We can then use our knowledge of the individual, and the population to which they belong, to develop other external cues to action, such as posters and social media campaigns in locations they frequent, physically and virtually. These cues can reinforce the benefits of taking action: they could help to develop self-efficacy by providing reinforcement, easy access to additional help and information, or by setting simple goals to help people take the first incremental step and achieve success early.

Transtheoretical model

First developed by Prochaska and DiClemente (1982), the transtheoretical model lists six different stages of preparedness for change. This model is useful in that it allows for planning with individuals at varying stages of 'readiness', and it recognises that failure can and does occur. The model encompasses six stages of change:

1. *Precontemplation* – the individual is not seeking to change; they may not realise that they need to change or are actively resistant to the idea.
2. *Contemplation* – the individual has recognised that they need to make a change.
3. *Preparation* – the individual begins to plan how best to make their intended change.
4. *Action* – the person actively attempts to make the desired change.
5. *Maintenance* – having made the attempted change, the individual is now actively working to maintain that change and avoid relapse.
6. *Termination* – the change has now become a habit and the individual does not have any desire to resume what they were doing before.

While the stages of change are presented here as a linear progression, the transtheoretical model is really a cycle (see Figure 2.1). Relapse can occur at any one of these stages and does not always means that the person will return to the previous stage (e.g. from maintenance to action). Should relapse occur, the person may relapse several stages to precontemplation ('It's too hard; I don't want to/can't do this') or it might lead them back to contemplation or preparation before they take action again. It is important to note that, for some health issues including addiction, termination (stopping the use of a substance) may never be reached. This

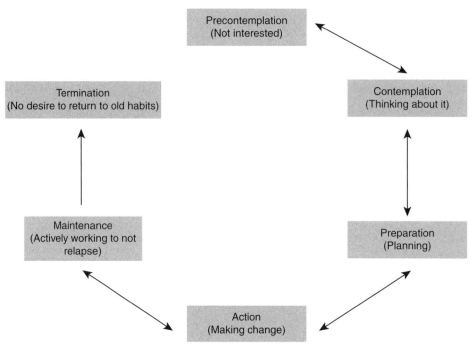

Figure 2.1 Cyclical nature of the transtheoretical (stages of change) model; the double arrows indicate potential for relapse at any stage

requires a realistic approach to the communication strategy, where perhaps action is the desired goal stage within the transtheoretical model rather than maintenance or cessation, to ensure that the individual's self-efficacy is not reduced to the point where they return to the first stage and remain there. It is also important to recognise the potential influence of the determinants of health here. If an individual wants to adopt a new behaviour but their external environment is not supportive (e.g. someone wishes to stop smoking, but all their friends and colleagues smoke) then this can make change – and maintaining that change – more difficult. Awareness of the individual's context can help to to mitigate some of the negative influences of the determinants of health.

Communication focus

Possibly the most important thing to do in the first instance is to listen to what the client is saying. This will help to identify where they are in the different stages of change and will help to tailor communication accordingly. Someone who is in the precontemplation stage is unlikely to be interested in strategies for action. Communication might focus on the benefits of the proposed change. Precontemplation and preparation stages might require the provision of materials outlining strategies for making change, where to find assistance and other information. Action and maintenance stages require communication tools that reinforce the efforts of the individual through mechanisms such as support groups, counsellors, online communities or additional information sources. Relapse communications should not blame or seek to punish the individual. Instead, they should recognise the progress the individual did make and help to support them to a point where they may wish to try again.

LEARNING ACTIVITY 2.1

This activity can be completed as a whole class or in a smaller group within your class.

Imagine you have a client who is at risk from heart disease. The client is a 46-year-old man who works in an office job. Although busy, he manages to keep his work hours mostly from 9.00 am to 5.00 pm. He tends to eat lunch at his desk and keeps working to ensure he can leave at 5.00 pm. Your client is married with two children aged 12 and 10 years. He does not exercise regularly, and is a non-smoker and social drinker, averaging about seven standard drinks per week. He does not really like fruit and does not eat wholegrains. The family eats fast food at least three times a week due to the children's various after-school commitments like sport and music.

1. What are the social determinants of health you can identify from this scenario that might contribute to your client's health outcomes?
2. Use the Health Belief Model to develop a strategy for your client.
3. Next, develop a strategy based on the transtheoretical model.
4. What kinds of actions do the models suggest you try? Which model is more useful in this case?

Interpersonal level

Social Cognitive Theory

Both the Health Belief Model and the transtheoretical model are intrapersonal – that is, they focus on the individual and their beliefs and perspectives. Social Cognitive Theory (SCT) is interpersonal; although still individually focused, it includes environmental and social influences on individual decision-making. Developed by Bandura (1986), SCT describes the interactions between an individual and their environment. A person's decision to act or not is determined by their beliefs about the world around them, including their own experiences, self-efficacy, observations of the actions of others and the perceived benefits of those actions. Beliefs are highly influential in terms of how people perceive and interpret situations and, ultimately, how they behave. Self-beliefs, self-efficacy and self-esteem are key influences on individual behaviour. People who have high self-esteem may be more likely to resist potentially negative influences, like peer pressure, than those with low self-esteem. This makes the SCT particularly useful in designing programs for school groups; for example, where teaching strategies for developing self-esteem may be particularly influential.

Self-efficacy is particularly important within SCT. Behaviours can be influenced by providing means of improving someone's self-efficacy. This can be done through what Bandura (1986) called mastery experiences, whereby a particular behaviour or skill is modelled and others learn by observing. For example, a cooking class or an exercise program could provide a mastery experience, with someone modelling the desired behaviour. Arguably, this method could be quite influential as participants can try the activity for themselves. Or it can serve as a practical use of role models, such as when a celebrity or someone 'famous' is used to model the desired behaviour. SCT also draws upon reciprocal determinism, which describes the two-way interactions between individuals and their environment. See, for example, Case study 2.1, which describes how posters and advertising a program to target drink driving were used in establishments serving alcohol. As already discussed in Chapter 1, the interactions between people and their contexts are key to understanding their behaviour. The SCT focuses on this interaction and enables identification of factors a program should address in order to create the desired change.

Communication focus

The SCT is commonly used as a model because it offers many different options for communicating with – and influencing – a target audience. At the individual level, communications should help build the confidence of individuals to achieve the desired behaviour, and to develop expectations of the benefits of the desired behaviour. This can be strengthened through strategies such as providing classes or workshops that allow observation of the desired behaviour. At a broader level, communications need to address the wider norms and beliefs of the group. Strategies to do this could include posters, group activities, goal-setting, incentives and reinforcement with prizes for engaging with the desired behaviour. Communication activities should be holistic, addressing internal and external factors to ensure individual changes are supported by the external group and environment, and vice versa.

CASE STUDY 2.1 Drink driving

In Australia, drink driving is the number one contributing factor to deaths on Australian roads, accounting for around 30 per cent of deaths (Australian Transport Council, 2011). Over one-quarter of all drivers and riders killed on Australian roads have a blood alcohol concentration above the legal limit of 0.05. In New South Wales, random breath testing was introduced in 1982 and by 2017 the number of fatal crashes involving alcohol had reduced from 40 to 15 per cent. However, drink driving remains one of the main causes of death and injury on New South Wales roads (Transport for NSW, 2019).

The Plan B campaign

In 2012, the New South Wales government launched the Plan B campaign, seeking to target drink driving. The main message of the campaign was 'If you are drinking, don't drive. Have a plan B to get home'. The program aimed to:

- reduce the overall road toll related to drink driving;
- change attitudes to drink driving by promoting alternatives to drink driving; and
- empower drivers to choose not to drink and drive.

The program also aimed to maintain awareness of random breath testing and the consequences (fines, potential loss of licence) of being caught driving above the legal limit. The intended audience of the campaign was all drivers, but especially men aged 17–25 years, a group over-represented in all alcohol-related road incidents.

The campaign took a positive and light-hearted approach to identifying practical means of getting home after a night out. Advertisements were shown in cinemas, on television and online, and some featured members of the New South Wales cricket team. Posters and other static advertisements were used on buses and taxis, and in licensed venues serving alcohol. A companion website provided links to apps and a travel planner to help users easily identify ways of getting home, including by taxi/rideshare or public transport.

Evaluation

Following the program's introduction in August 2012, campaign testing showed that nearly 75 per cent of the target audience recalled the key message 'if you're drinking, don't drive', with a similar percentage agreeing that the commercials helped people to consider alternative transport and that drinking and driving was not socially acceptable (Transport for NSW, 2017). Campaign testing also showed that over 80 per cent of young male drivers surveyed considered the campaign to be believable (Transport for NSW, 2017).

In 2018, alcohol was responsible for 18.4 per cent (64 people) of road fatalities and 6.8 per cent (354 people) of serious injuries on NSW roads. These indicate a slight decrease in alcohol-related serious injuries in road accidents from 2014 (7.3%) but an increase in the number of deaths (16.3% or 50 people) in 2014 – (Transport for NSW, 2019).

QUESTIONS

1. Based on the information provided, how did the Plan B campaign incorporate SCT? Justify your answer using examples.

2. About one-quarter of survey respondents did not agree with the statement that 'drinking and driving is socially unacceptable'. If you were working with Plan B, what other communication strategies would you employ to influence the 'social acceptability' of not drinking and driving?

ELSEWHERE IN THE WORLD

Bob the Designated Driver, Belgium

Originating in Belgium in 1995, Bob refers to a person who does not drink when they have to drive (VIAS Institute, 2019). Now used in other countries across the world, including Luxembourg, Germany and Taiwan (adapted to local cultural context), the persona of Bob, as designated driver, is always presented as the hero of the evening who provides a safe way home for their friends who want to drink.

Anti-Drink Driving Campaign, Singapore

This campaign uses the analogy of an alcoholic cocktail (Government of Singapore, 2020). The ingredients are the consequences of drink driving (fines, spattered blood, wreckage) with the key message 'Drinking & Driving is a Deadly Mix'.

Community level

Diffusion of innovations theory

The Diffusion of Innovations theory describes the typical adoption of new ideas, products, techniques and behaviours within a population. Developer Everett Rogers (1962) described diffusion as the process by which an innovation – defined as 'an idea perceived as new' (Rogers, 2004, p. 13) – is communicated through various channels and to a range of audiences over time. The factors that determine the rate at which an innovation is adopted are:

- *Relative advantage* – is the innovation better than what it is trying to replace?
- *Compatibility* – is the new innovation consistent with the needs, values and previous experiences of potential adopters?
- *Complexity* – how difficult is the innovation to understand and use?
- *Trialability* – does the innovation enable experimentation?
- *Observability* – are the results and/or benefits of the innovation visible to others?

Innovations that have greater relative advantage, compatibility, trialability and observability, and less complexity, are more likely to be quickly adopted. There are also different categories of people who are likely to adopt such innovations. Those most likely to adopt are considered *innovators*, typically representing around 2.5 per cent of a given population. *Early adopters* are the next likely to adopt an innovation, at 13.5 per cent of the population. Early adopters have 'the highest degree of opinion leadership', while the next category, *potential adopters*, is influenced by the information and advice of early adopters (Rogers, 2002, p. 991). The next categories are the *early majority* and the *late majority*, both comprising 34 per cent of a given population. *Laggards* are the final 16 per cent, who will accept the innovation themselves when everyone around them has adopted an innovation and is satisfied. It is important to note, however, that there will be some who may never accept or adopt the innovation.

Communication focus

Different communication mechanisms will work for different groups. Innovators act on the basis of knowledge about an innovation, and so communication activities should focus on getting information to them quickly. Awareness might trigger in the innovator group the desire to try the new innovation, which will then influence the early adopters, and so on. Probably the most valuable communication approach for this model – once you have those crucial innovators – is to focus on the early adopters. Marketing companies do this very well – the rise of the social media influencer and the use of celebrities in commercials are two examples of how early adopters are influenced. To do this for your own health promotion initiative, identify influential people within the audience you wish to influence. Invite these influencers to adopt the desired innovation and work with them to help spread the message. People are more likely to trust those they know, so engaging members of the audience you wish to influence should lead to the message being more readily accepted than someone external trying to impose a change. This strategy is consistent across the world, with large-scale international surveys such as the Edelman Trust Barometer showing that, while people do trust experts, 'someone like me' is consistently ranked one of the top three most trusted sources for information (Edelman, 2019).

The early and late majorities make up the largest numbers of the population, but many will need to know about the innovation and to see or experience the benefits before they will make the change. Consistency of messaging is key, using multiple **communication channels**; for example, radio and television advertisements supported by posters and social media, featuring the influential early adopter. Laggards are likely the most resistant to an innovation. Note that someone may be a laggard for one innovation but could be an innovator or early adopter for another – it all depends upon their interests, beliefs and values. To identify these, it is important to find out why this group has not adopted the innovation, rather than provide information about why they should. This can help you to identify barriers created by gaps in your communication strategy (e.g. lack of awareness, or fears), which you can then address. Or it may highlight that for some segments of the population this is simply something that they may be unwilling ever to consider. Consider what percentage of the population is a realistic target to achieve your aim.

> **Communication channels –** the various ways and means of getting information to an intended audience; channels include face-to-face communication and word of mouth; static advertisements such as posters, ads on public transport and road signs; print, electronic and social media; and events

Multidimensional models

Some models integrate many of the elements of the health promotion models described and seek to provide a holistic model of the influences on health. Individuals all exist within some larger context. The following models describe how these contextual factors can influence health.

Ecological model

The ecological model, also sometimes called the 'social ecological model', is a theory based framework that aims to focus attention in health promotion activities and interventions on both the individual and the social–environmental factors. In its original form, an illustration of the ecological model had individual factors nested at the core, then the interpersonal, institutional and community factors in concentric, connected circles and policy on the outside, as the external level. It is based on the assumption that if the social environment – including among others interpersonal, organisational and public policy factors – is changed then this will support the individual to change as well (McLeroy et al. 1988). The individual at the core of the model reflects this. The individual can also influence the environment, creating what McLeroy and colleagues called 'reciprocal causation'. People have the power to influence what others can do. For example, in the business context, consumers can ask cafés to provide healthier food choices, reusable cups or paper straws. If the business chooses not to, then individuals can opt to buy elsewhere, or not to buy at all. Businesses that do provide requested options will be supported by the individuals who continue to shop there. The business, in turn, supports the individual in their desire for options that support their health, philosophy or preferences. This example shows that successful implementation of social–environmental changes is essential for the support of individuals within the target population. In their seminal paper, McLeroy and colleagues outlined five factors that comprise the ecological model. These factors are summarised in Table 2.1 and represent what McLeroy et al. (1988) termed *multiple levels of influence*. Health promotion interventions can occur at any of these levels.

Table 2.1 Overview of the different levels of factors in the ecological model and examples of the different communication activities that could occur at each level

Factor	Example of factor	Example of communication activity
Individual (intrapersonal)	Individual characteristics such as knowledge, attitudes, beliefs, values and self-efficacy	Support group, one-on-one counselling, information resources (leaflets, posters)
Interpersonal	Relationships and external influences such as friends, family, colleagues who can provide external cues and reinforcement such as support and social identity including norms	Posters Group activities Mass media and social media campaign, potentially using a well-known member/s of that community as spokesperson, positively reinforcing desired behaviour
Institutional	Policies, regulations, formal and informal rules that govern acceptable behaviour	
Community	Norms and acceptable behavioural standards held by social networks, institutions and networks within defined boundaries	
Policy	Local, state/territory and federal legislation supporting and/or enforcing healthy behaviours	Advocacy

Source: Adapted from McLeroy et al. (1988); Rimer & Glanz (2005).

Influencing the health of individuals through policy and structure – the outer level of the ecological model – can be considered a means of affecting more people in a more equitable and efficient manner than other health promotion initiatives (Frieden, 2010). But this is not a simple task and success is not guaranteed (Golden et al., 2015). In 2015, in recognition of the challenges of change through policy and environments, Golden and colleagues (2015) proposed an 'inside-out' version of the social ecological model (see Figure 2.2). This version swaps the order of the original ecological model, placing policy and environment at the core, which are nested within the community, organisational, interpersonal and individual contexts. It illustrates the interrelated nature of these factors and their combined influence on the development of health-related policies and environments (Golden et al., 2015).

Communication focus

These multiple levels of influence provide many options for communication (see Case study 2.2). As described in the earlier models, communication strategies can target the individual's knowledge, attitudes and behaviours, and in turn these can be supported through communication activities that target social networks and workplaces. The actions and activities within these social networks and organisations can then provide external cues to reinforce and support the intrapersonal communication (see Table 2.1). For example, an individual wishing to become more active may get information and support from a gym or their doctor, but they still need to take action themselves. However, their workplace may offer a lunchtime activity, such as a yoga class or soccer

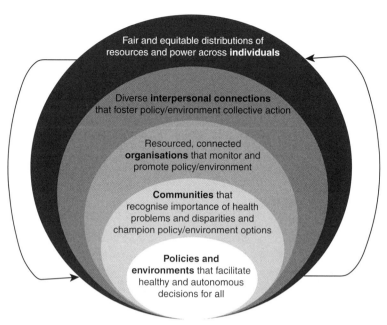

Figure 2.2   The inside-out social ecological model of policy and environmental change
Source: Golden et al. (2015, p. 10S).

competition and invite them to participate. Now they have the information as well as an easy means of engaging in physical activity, which is supported by their colleagues and their workplace.

It may be that all of the 'lower' levels in the ecological model are already in place, in which case communication can adopt a greater policy focus, potentially through advocacy or direct contribution to the policy development process if the opportunity exists. Changing policies as well as environmental factors are essential for improving health outcomes but doing so requires 'enormous individual efforts, research and advocacy … to implement' (Golden et al., 2015, p. 95). The inside-out ecological model has advocacy and policy at its core, supported and supplemented by individual, institutional and community efforts. Therefore, communication efforts that aimed to create policy change can be implemented at multiple levels and can work together.

CASE STUDY 2.2 Identifying influences on dietary behaviours in Chandigarh, India using the social ecological model

Jasvir Kaur, Manmeet Kaur, Venkatesan Chakrapani and Rajesh Kumar

Indian national dietary guidelines emphasise the need to limit consumption of fat, sugar and salt, and to increase consumption of fruits and vegetables. However, most Indians do not meet these guidelines. The prevalence of diet-related diseases is widespread, with one north Indian city – Chandigarh – showing high incidences of unhealthy dietary behaviours and associated disease, especially in urban areas.

(cont.)

(cont.)

Multi-level influences on dietary behaviours

To understand the influences on population consumption of fat, sugar, salt, fruits and vegetables, focus groups were held with adults from diverse socio-economic groups (low, middle and high income) in urban areas of Chandigarh. The study sought to identify the factors facilitating or hindering healthy dietary behaviours (Kaur et al. (2020)); these are summarised in Figure 2.3.

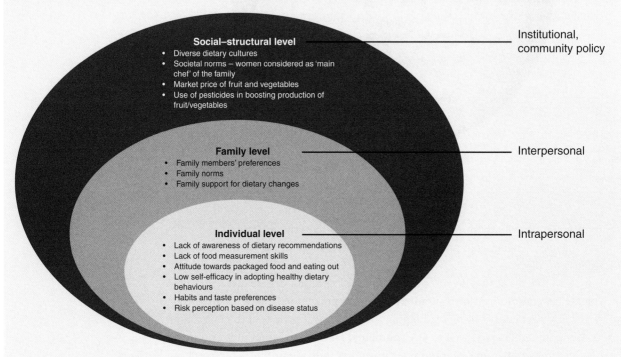

Figure 2.3   Multi-level influences on dietary behaviours related to fat, sugar, salt, fruit and vegetable consumption

Individual-level influences

Eating out, despite being perceived as 'not healthy', was frequently reported because of the need to attend social events and due to perceived time-saving and convenience.

Participants across all economic groups attributed taste preferences and habit to their consumption of high amounts of salt, sugar and oily foods. A cited barrier to initiating healthy eating in the home was difficulty in influencing family preferences – especially those of children – and behaviours.

Family-level influences

Family members play an important role in shaping dietary behaviour through motivation to adopt healthy behaviours or restrict unhealthy behaviours. A lack of support from family members was identified by some of the older adults as a major barrier to initiating healthy dietary behaviours. The prevalent family norm is not to proactively restrict fat and sugar intake. Rather than restrict consumption of fat, the use of *desi ghee* (clarified butter) was preferred as it was considered good for health due to being 'desi' (indigenous).

Social–structural influences

The influence of cultural practices on dietary behaviours was well reflected in the diverse population of Chandigarh. Sugar plays an indispensable role in Indian culture and customs through the practice of gifting and serving sweets at festivals, religious and social events. Diets rich in fat, sugar and salt are consumed on a routine basis. Social and cultural symbolism seemed to be another important influencer. The ability to use *desi ghee* was viewed as a status symbol by middle-income and high-income participants.

Most participants perceived fruit and vegetables to be expensive. This was especially the case for low-income participants, whose primary concern was the provision of food to meet the basic needs of their family. Unrestricted use of insecticides, pesticides and harmful chemicals to increase the production of fruit and vegetables was a major concern highlighted by all social classes.

Multi-level influences need multi-level interventions

The study's findings indicate that individuals alone may not be able to adopt healthy dietary behaviours without family support. Similarly, family food habits were found to be strongly influenced by the prevalent social norms and cultural practices regarding food consumption.

Overall, the findings indicate the need for a range of multi-level interventions that are more likely to promote and sustain healthy dietary behaviours by, for example, improving awareness about dietary recommendations (individual level); promoting positive family norms through involvement of family members (family level); or restrictive policies on the use of fat, sugar and salt in packaged food (structural level).

Source: Adapted from Kaur et al. (2020).

QUESTIONS

1. This case study shows how the social ecological model can be used to identify factors influencing behaviours. The authors suggest some interventions at different levels to address some of these factors. What other interventions – and associated communication activities – would you recommend?

2. Imagine you are responsible for developing an intervention in Chandigarh and you have limited resources. What audience/s would you focus on to achieve the greatest effect? Justify your choice.

Behaviour Change Wheel

A recent addition to the range of theories and models in health promotion is the Behaviour Change Wheel, developed by Michie and colleagues (2011). Using a systematic search and review of existing behaviour-change intervention frameworks, the Behaviour Change Wheel was developed with a core hub – a behaviour system – having three essential conditions of capability, opportunity and motivation (also called the 'COM-B system'):

- *Capability* – the physical and mental capacity of the individual to engage in the activity, including the knowledge and skills required
- *Opportunity* – all external factors that prompt or support the behaviour
- *Motivation* – all processes that 'energize and direct behaviour', including habits, emotional responses and analytical decision-making (Michie et al., 2011, p. 5).

The development of the Behaviour Change Wheel also identified the core categories of interventions – activities aimed at creating change – and policies that supported the interventions. Diagrammatically, potential interventions are placed around the outside of the COM-B hub, as these are the things that likely will influence behaviour. The potential policy categories are placed around the outside of these interventions because the policies will only influence behaviours through the interventions they support (see Figure 2.4). It is important to note that each of the categories within each layer can interact with each other. Within COM-B, capability and opportunity can influence motivation, which in turn will influence behaviour. Behaviour can also influence all three conditions. Likewise functions in the interventions layer can interact with each other, as can those within policy.

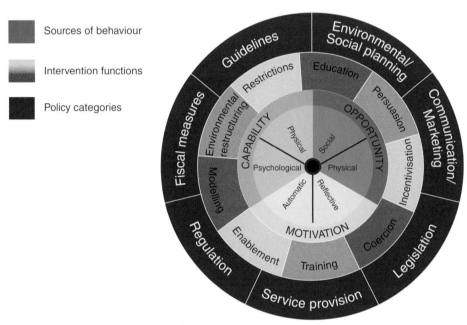

Figure 2.4   The Behaviour Change Wheel (the centre is the 'behaviour hub' from which interventions can be selected)

Source: Michie et al. (2011).

The nine intervention functions and seven policy categories are described here.

Intervention functions

1. *Education* – to improve knowledge and understanding
2. *Persuasion* – communication to encourage an emotional response and action
3. *Incentivisation* – rewards including prizes and giveaways
4. *Coercion* – penalties and disincentives (such as additional costs or fines)
5. *Training* – development or enhancement of skills
6. *Restriction* – rules to minimise or prevent engagement in undesirable behaviours (e.g. setting a legal age for consumption or purchase of certain items)
7. *Environmental restructuring* – changing the physical and/or social context (e.g. reminders for GPs to ask certain questions during a consultation)
8. *Modelling* – demonstration of the desired behaviour for people to emulate (e.g. using role models or popular television programs)
9. *Enablement* – increasing capability or opportunity to enhance skills training and restructuring environmental contexts (e.g. surgical intervention, medication, behavioural support).

Policy categories

1. *Communication/marketing* – using all forms of media
2. *Guidelines* – creating documents that set out recommended or mandated practices (e.g. treatment protocols or a recommended intake)
3. *Fiscal* – using mechanisms such as taxes to increase or decrease costs (e.g. on tobacco or alcohol products)
4. *Regulations* – rules or principles governing a behaviour or practice (such as plain packaging for cigarettes, or restriction of advertising to children)
5. *Legislation* – the creation or changing of laws
6. *Environmental/social planning* – environmental and social plans that support health (e.g. town planning that incorporates green spaces, footpaths and sanitation systems)
7. *Service provision* – delivery of services within a variety of contexts (e.g. workplaces, community groups) (Michie et al., 2011, p. 7).

Communication focus

Looking within the central COM-B hub, each source of behaviour can also be influenced through communication activities, which have been described within the earlier models presented in this chapter, and discussion of the paper by Michie and colleagues. It is interesting to note the position of communication or marketing at the policy level. The authors define communication and marketing policies as 'using print, electronic, telephonic or broadcast media' (Michie et al., 2011, p. 7). They also note the relevance of communication and marketing to education, persuasion, incentivisation, coercion and modelling. The role of media in presenting information and issues to a variety of audiences – and the positive, negative and unintended effects – are covered in greater detail in later chapters.

One element that does not appear to be incorporated explicitly within the Behaviour Change Wheel is culture. Arguably, it can be inferred that culture exists within the various elements of the COM-B hub; however, the influence and importance of culture in designing interventions and communication strategies for an audience cannot be understated. For some programs, such as the one presented in Case study 2.3, culture is the factor underpinning its relevance and success.

CASE STUDY 2.3 Health promotion through *waka ama* in Aotearoa New Zealand

Christina Severinsen and Angelique Reweti

Aotearoa New Zealand is experiencing a decreasing trend in levels of physical activity in the general population, which mirrors global patterns. Physical inactivity is a major contributor to the burden of disease and has a high economic cost. This case study looks at *waka ama*, outrigger canoeing, as effective in indigenous health promotion.

(cont.)

(cont.)

Waka ama is one of the fastest-growing sports in Aotearoa New Zealand and works as community development and settings-based health promotion, to strengthen community action and create supportive environments for health.

As well as the physical benefits for paddlers, *waka ama* also has strong *tikanga* (traditional values and practices) and encourages *te reo* Māori (Māori language) through *karakia* (prayer), *waiata* (song) and other activities associated with *waka ama*. *Waka ama* contributes to the health of paddlers, *whānau* (family) and communities. It is an exemplar of local engagement in physical activity and movement, and an effective means to improving health and wellbeing within communities. By maintaining broad and holistic understandings of health, it engages and empowers communities to control and improve their health.

Incorporating indigenous knowledge systems in health promotion

Waka ama is an example of positive Māori health promotion, using a framework of Māori values. This aligns with Te Pae Mahutonga, a health promotion framework developed by Sir Mason Durie. Te Pae Mahutonga is the constellation of stars popularly referred to as the Southern Cross; it was used by *tipuna* Māori (ancestors) as a navigational tool. The four central *whetu* (stars) represent the key tasks of health promotion: Mauriora, Toiora, Waiora and Te Oranga. These tasks are supported by the two pointer stars: Nga Manukura and Te Mana Whakahaere.

For example, in terms of Mauriora, *waka ama* provides access to Te Ao Māori, the Māori world, for both Māori and non-Māori paddlers. Culture works as a social determinant of health. In *waka ama*, paddlers gain increased access to cultural resources considered important to good health. The communication and practice of Māori *tikanga* creates a space for the promotion of secure cultural identity. Paddlers engage in *waiata*, *marae* (sacred meeting ground) stays, *karakia*, and *te reo* Māori on and off the water. *Waka ama* becomes an integrated and normalised space for cultural communication and expression, and where *tikanga* Māori is celebrated and facilitated. The promotion of healthy lifestyles, Toiora, is reflected in *waka ama*. By its very nature, *waka ama* engages paddlers in healthy behaviours and physical activity, reducing risk and promoting healthy lifestyles. Paddlers speak of communicating and learning alongside other paddlers. *Waka ama* has a positive, strength-based approach, and *rōpu* (groups) develop their collective aspirations and journeys to become healthier together. This allows them to realise their aspirations as a group; for some when competing at local, national and international levels.

Waiora acknowledges that people's health is linked to the environments in which they live; we are connected to the natural environment. *Waka ama* gives paddlers regular opportunities to experience the natural environment and gain spiritual connection and balance with the water. Beyond that, *rōpu* come together to value their environment in improving their own health, as well as the health of the rivers and seas upon which they paddle. Many paddlers engage in environmental protection, as *kaitiaki*, or guardians, of the rivers to ensure its health for future generations. Te Oranga is about participation in society, whereby paddlers become involved in their community. This extends beyond paddling on the water to roles in governance, organisation, learning, teaching and leadership. *Waka ama* provides many opportunities for paddlers to grow and develop skills, which strengthens the capacity of local people within the context of their communities.

Waka ama is an example of health promotion developed from within community, meaning that communication and action are consistent and responsive to local and cultural contexts. The broad foundation draws on Māori concepts of health, values and ways of working, communicating and providing spaces in which to improve health and social outcomes, so as to achieve sustainable and transformative change. This type of health promotion shows how we can shift the focus of promotion of physical activity from a deficit model of disease to one of health potential that is inherent in the social and environmental settings of everyday life.

QUESTIONS

1. Culture is central to this *waka ama* program. Identify other health promotion programs based in your community. What factors are central to this program?

2. Reflect on the role of grassroots health promotion action, as opposed to 'top-down interventions'.

LEARNING ACTIVITY 2.2

As an employee of your health department, you are designing posters to address a health issue. These posters will be displayed in public toilets.

1. Choose a health issue and design a poster using the constructs of one of the models described in this chapter.
2. Swap with another group and see if you can identify which model they used.
3. Share your poster with the rest of the class and justify your choice of health issue/model.

Putting theories and models into practice

You may have noticed similarities and overlap in the theories and models presented in this chapter. This is typically because the theories and models are building upon earlier ones, from expanding the Health Belief Model through to the Behaviour Change Wheel, which was created by integrating different frameworks. People, and their health, are complex; attempting to develop models that allow simple understanding of this complexity will always create overlaps, inconsistencies and challenges. So how do we ensure that we are doing the right thing? There is never a guarantee that we will get it 100 per cent right. What we can do is plan for success by knowing who the target audience is, what we want to achieve and then create a plan. Many different planning models are used within health promotion – refer to the resources listed under Further

Reading. For each of the planning models there are key steps or stages to follow. Each step is also relevant in planning the communication activities, as explored in more detail in Chapters 5–8.

Step 1: Conduct a needs assessment

The ability to conduct a needs assessment is considered a core competency of health promotion practitioners, and the ability to plan, implement and evaluate health promotion programs are the major skills required for those starting a health promotion career (AHPA, 2009). The needs assessment competencies (see box) show that health promoters need to be able to identify and analyse appropriate data, which might include speaking to stakeholders and other specialists, and making recommendations for action based on these analyses. Chapters 6 and 8 go into further detail about how to collect this data and engage with stakeholders.

Entry level skills in needs assessment

At the entry level, a health promotion practitioner must be able to demonstrate knowledge of how to:

- locate, conduct and critically analyse relevant literature – this includes peer-reviewed and grey literature, local, state and national strategic plans, and relevant area and organisational reports and policies;
- compile an epidemiological and socio-demographic overview of the geographical, community population or setting of interest;
- involve community members and stakeholders in the needs-assessment process;
- seek input from academic and practitioner specialists for the particular health issue or problem being assessed;
- determine priorities for health promotion action from available evidence, using local, state and national data and information;
- identify behavioural, environmental, social and organisational risk and contributory factors for the particular health issue or problem of concern;
- identify processes that are effective in setting priorities for health promotion action; and
- recommend specific actions based on the analysis of information.

Source: AHPA (2009, p. 3).

Start your needs assessment by asking questions: What is the problem you are trying to address? How do you know it is a problem? Creating a new program or initiative can be exciting but creating something new without looking at the needs of your target population can mean you have a solution in search of a problem! Before implementing anything new, take stock of what the problem is, the evidence that it is a problem and any existing program that could help address that problem. Evidence can be anything from incident reports, statistics, surveys, media coverage or submissions from members of the public. This evidence will help you to identify the need within the individual or community you are working with.

There are different types of need, described within a taxonomy of social need by Jonathan Bradshaw in 1972. Bradshaw (1972) identified four types of need:

- *Normative* – what expert opinion defines as a 'health need'. Can be influenced by the values of the expert.
- *Felt* – what communities say they need; however, taken in isolation, it is not an adequate measure of 'real' need. Can be influenced by the perception of individuals.
- *Expressed* – can be inferred by a community's use of services. If no applicable service exists, this need may not be identified.
- *Comparative* – using information from one population to determine the requirements of another similar population.

Once you have identified the need/s, dig deeper. Talk to people within relevant organisations, communities and groups. Examine the research, demographic data and other publications from as many sources as possible. Which part of the population is most affected or has the greatest need? What are the influences on health associated with this population? What can health promotion do to address these influences – if anything? Has anyone tried to address this problem before? If so, find out how and learn from their successes and mistakes.

Step 2: Set your goal and objectives

What does success look like? The goal is the big, long-term result you want to achieve. Objectives are the targets you set to make progress towards achieving your goal. Be as specific and realistic as possible when setting your objectives, and use the SMART mnemonic (derived from Doran, 1981):

Specific – who, what, where, when?
Measurable – a quantifiable measure of progress towards achievement of the objective
Achievable – be realistic
Relevant – is the objective related to your overarching goal?
Time specific – when will the program and the expected changes occur?

We will return to SMART objectives many times in this text. They are useful (necessary!) in your health promotion program as well as your communication activities. Knowing what you want to achieve, with whom, how and by when makes planning and implementing activities much easier and potentially more effective. It is easier to hit a target when you know what you are aiming for.

Step 3: Plan your program

Now that you know what the problem is and what you want to achieve, how are you going to address it? Here, knowing who you want to talk to and what you want to achieve is critical. In step 1 you should have identified who your intervention will target. Now you can start to plan what kind of intervention will be most effective. This may give you some insight into what kind of behaviour change theory you may be able to use to guide your planning. Do you need to influence the individual's beliefs or self-efficacy? Can this be reinforced using social (norms, role models/influencers) or structural (policy) actions? How and where will you provide these influences and reinforcements? Select the most appropriate behaviour change model for your audience and what you need to influence, to achieve your objective.

Step 4: Implement your program

This is the fun part, where you see your ideas go into action. Be prepared to make changes if you see things are not going in the right direction. This is formative evaluation and enables you to 'course correct' if an element of your intervention is not working in the way you intended.

Step 5: Evaluate your program

This is one of the most valuable steps, yet it is often overlooked – or worse, the evaluation is done but the data sits in a file somewhere and is never used to inform other activities. If things did start to go off course in step 4, you have already done some evaluation. At the end of the program you can do more evaluation to find out what worked, for whom and why. Knowing what works, as well as what does not, can help guide future needs assessments and program planning (your own and others) and potentially save time and money. Chapter 8 looks at evaluation in much more detail.

Regardless of the issue, the audience or the objective, these key steps should be followed every time you develop a new health promotion initiative. These steps are also very useful in helping to guide communication activities to support your health promotion initiative. We look at this in more detail in later chapters in this book.

LEARNING ACTIVITY 2.3

Choose a health issue that interests you, remembering the many different components of health described in Chapter 1. Work through the program planning process by answering the following questions:

1. Why is the health issue you have chosen a problem – how do you know?
2. Who could you contact to get more information?
3. Has anyone tried to address the issue through health promotion? What did they do and what can you learn from their experience?
4. What audience would you target and why?
5. What would be your objective?
6. Based on your answers to 4 and 5, choose the most appropriate behaviour change model to help guide your program development. Justify your choice of model.
7. What are some communication activities you could do to support your chosen model in addressing the identified needs? Justify your choices.

Summary

Health promotion can work from the individual to the population level. Influencing or empowering people to act requires more than simply providing information: their beliefs, values and context should be recognised. There are many factors, both within and external to the individual, that can influence behaviour, and while this adds complexity it also offers multiple opportunities for communication. By understanding as much as possible about the audience we are trying to influence, we are able to adapt our interventions to best suit their specific context and needs. In turn, this enables us to target communications appropriately, to support our achievement of the desired objectives.

REVISION QUESTIONS

1. Why is self-efficacy such an important concept for many behaviour change theories?
2. What are the key differences between the Health Belief Model and Social Cognitive Theory?
3. Give an example of reciprocal causation in your local community.
4. Describe the four different types of social need, and give an example of each.

FURTHER READING

Egger, G., Spark, R. & Donovan, R. (2013). *Health Promotion Strategies and Methods* (3rd ed.). North Ryde: McGraw Hill.

Nutbeam, D., Harris, E. & Wise, M. (2010). *Theory in a Nutshell: A practical guide to health promotion theories* (3rd ed.). North Ryde: McGraw Hill.

Rimer, B.K. & Glanz, K. (2005). *Theory at a Glance: A guide for health promotion practice*. Bethesda, MD: US Department of Health and Human Services, National Institutes of Health, National Cancer Institute.

REFERENCES

Australian Health Promotion Association (AHPA) (2009). *Core Competencies for Health Promotion Practitioners*. Australian Health Promotion Association. Retrieved from: https://www.healthpromotion.org.au/images/docs/core_competencies_for_hp_practitioners.pdf

Australian Transport Council (2011). *National Road Safety Strategy 2011–2020*. Retrieved from: https://www.roadsafety.gov.au/nrss/files/NRSS_2011_2020.pdf

Bandura, A. (1977). Self-efficacy: Toward a unifying theory of behavioral change, *Psychological Review*, 84(2), 191–215.

———(1986). *Social Foundations of Thought and Action: A social cognitive theory*. Englewood Cliffs, NJ: Prentice-Hall, Inc.

Bradshaw, J. (1972). Taxonomy of social need. In G. McLachlan (ed.), *Problems and Progress in Medical Care: Essays on current research*, 7th series. London: Oxford University Press, pp. 71–82.

Doran, G.T. (1981). There's a S.M.A.R.T. way to write management's goals and objectives, *Management Review*, 70(11), 35–6.

Edelman (2019). *Edelman Trust Barometer*. Retrieved from: https://www.edelman.com/trust-barometer

Frieden, T.R. (2010). A framework for public health action: The health impact pyramid. *American Journal of Public Health*, 100(4), 590–5.

Golden, S.D., McLeroy, K.R., Green, L.W., Earp, J.A.L. & Lieberman, L.D. (2015). Upending the social ecological model to guide health promotion efforts toward policy and environmental change, *Health Education & Behavior*, 42(1_suppl), 8S–14S.

Government of Singapore (2020). *Road Safety Campaigns.* Retrieved from: https://www .police.gov.sg/Advisories/Traffic/Road-Safety-Campaigns

Kaur, M., Kaur, M., Chakrapani, V. & Kumar, R. (2020). Multilevel influences on fat, sugar, salt, fruit, and vegetable consumption behaviors among urban indians: Application of the social ecological model, *SAGE Open*. Retrieved from: https:// doi.org/10.1177/2158244020919526

McLeroy, K.R., Bibeau, D., Steckler, A. & Glanz, K. (1988). An ecological perspective on health promotion programs, *Health Education Quarterly*, 15(4), 351–77.

Michie, S., van Stralen, M.M. & West, R. (2011). The behaviour change wheel: A new method for characterising and designing behaviour change interventions, *Implementation Science*, 6(1), 1–11.

Prochaska, J.O. & DiClemente, C.C. (1982). Transtheoretical therapy: Toward a more integrative model of change, *Psychotherapy: Theory, Research and Practice*, 19(3), 276–78.

Rimer, B.K. & Glanz, K. (2005). *Theory at a Glance: A guide for health promotion practice*. Bethesda, MD: US Department of Health and Human Services, National Institutes of Health, National Cancer Institute.

Rogers, E.M. (1962). *Diffusion of Innovations.* New York: Free Press.

———(2002). Diffusion of preventive innovations, *Addictive Behaviours*, 27(6), 989–93.

———(2004). A prospective and retrospective look at the diffusion model, *Journal of Health Communication*, 9(S1), 13–19.

Rosenstock, I.M. (1974). Historical origins of the health belief model, *Health Education Monographs*, 2(4), 328–35.

Transport for New South Wales (2017). *'Plan B'*, Centre for Road Safety. Retrieved from: https://roadsafety.transport.nsw.gov.au/campaigns/plan-b/index.html

———(2019). Crash and casualty statistics – NSW general view, Centre for Road Safety. Retrieved from: https://roadsafety.transport.nsw.gov.au/statistics/ interactivecrashstats/nsw.html?tabnsw=5

VIAS Institute (2019). *BOB: The designated driver*. Retrieved from: https://www.bob.be/

Communication in health settings

3

Linda Murray and Merryn McKinnon

With contributions from Matthew Dunn and Andrea Waling

LEARNING OBJECTIVES

At the completion of the chapter, you will be able to:

- Define the settings approach to health.
- Distinguish the health promotion needs of different audiences.
- Describe and compare traditional and non-traditional health settings.
- Identify communication activities typically used in a range of settings.
- Propose appropriate setting choices for different audiences.

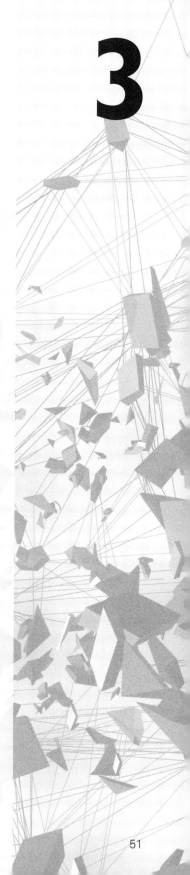

Introduction

Health promotion can take place in a range of different settings, both physical and virtual. There are many resources available that explore health settings in detail. The purpose of this chapter is to provide you with an overview of the main settings that are typically used to engage different audiences and to highlight some non-traditional settings that can be helpful in extending the reach of communication activities.

The first section of this chapter outlines the life-span approach to health promotion, identifying specific audiences for consideration. Each of these audiences can be found in different settings at different life stages, so understanding the needs of these audiences can help to identify appropriate settings in which to engage them. The following section outlines the settings that are typically used in health promotion activities and the kinds of communication activities that are usually conducted in those settings. It is highly likely that you may have experienced some of these types of activities in your own life. The final section explores the use of non-traditional settings: places where you may not expect to find health promotion activities. The chapter also looks at some non-typical uses of traditional settings that aim to drive audience engagement.

The settings approach to health promotion

Settings-based health promotion – a framework used to explore the influences of the interrelationships and interactions between people, places, programs and policies on health (after Dooris, 2006)

The environments in which people live, work and interact with each other all influence health. **Settings-based health promotion**, also called 'the settings approach', uses a socio-ecological model approach to understanding how the people, structural and systemic factors that exist within a given setting can influence health, positively or negatively. It tends to use a systems perspective both to understand how settings contribute to public health overall and how to create change to generate opportunities that maximise the contribution of settings (Dooris, 2006).

Health promotion across the life span

Life span – the total time between the birth and death of a person, which is influenced by environmental, biological and social factors

Where and when health promotion occurs can vary. Ideally, all members of a given population will be participants in health promotion activities or, at the very least, are the recipients of health promotion messages at some point in their lives. In health, it is common to take a **life-span** approach to describing the health needs of a population. This recognises that at different stages of life people will have different health concerns and needs. Typically, this is considered according to age group, which is a simple framework for identifying different audiences. It is important to note that age is only one variable. Other factors, such as biological stages of development, legally defined ages of consent or responsibility, and socially and culturally significant milestones can also be used as frameworks for understanding the different life stages of an individual and as a means of identifying the types of health information and support they may need.

Health span – the total extent of time a person is considered to be healthy, not just alive

An increasingly common term used in conjunction with – or instead of – life span is '**health span**'. Health span can be a useful term as it enables us to think of health as something measurable on a continuous and variable spectrum, but it is problematic as it can position health as dichotomous – simply being either 'good' or 'bad' (Kaeberlein, 2018). Health is subjective and it varies from individual to individual; what feels like 'good' health for one person might be considered 'bad' for another person, and vice versa.

For the purposes of this book, we focus on the settings available across the life span, recognising that social, environmental and biological factors all influence life span, and the health span that falls within it.

Audiences and their settings

If you are reading this book sequentially, you will know this first step well already: identify the audience! Who are they, specifically? Should you target them directly or does another audience have more influence over what they do? For example, if you wanted to target school children, then the audience with the most influence over them would be parents/guardians, caregivers, teachers and peers. Likewise, older adults may have adult children involved in providing or facilitating their care, so their carers will need information, too. Engaging both your target audience and their influencers using slightly different messages and tactics may be important. Children can have significant 'pester power' that influence the behaviours of their parents and guardians.

Once you have identified your audience, consider where they 'hang out', physically and virtually. Where can you find them to get information to them? Focus on that setting. Once you know where to find your target audience you can plan how you will engage them with your message. Some settings, like medical clinics and hospitals, set clear expectations that health information is available inside. Others may be surprising and unexpected, and this can help to make the message more memorable. Use whatever settings, or combination of settings, are needed to best reach your identified audience. Table 3.1 provides an overview of the typical settings for each age group; further details about other potential settings and audiences are provided for each age group below.

Table 3.1 Common health settings for each age group

Typical health settings	Population group					
	Infants and small children	Pre-teens and teenagers	Young adults	Adults 31–49 years	Adults 50–69 years	Older adults
Hospital	✓	✓	✓	✓	✓	✓
Dentist	✓	✓	✓	✓	✓	✓
Pharmacy	✓	✓	✓	✓	✓	✓
Medical clinic/ doctor's surgery	✓	✓	✓	✓	✓	✓
Maternal and child health services	✓		✓	✓		

Table 3.1 (cont.)

Typical health settings	Population group					
	Infants and small children	Pre-teens and teenagers	Young adults	Adults 31–49 years	Adults 50–69 years	Older adults
Early childcare	✓					
School	✓	✓				
University			✓	✓	✓	
Workplace		✓	✓	✓	✓	
Aged-care facility				✓	✓	✓

Infants and small children
Health needs and influences

Infants and small children are at a naturally vulnerable age, and health promotion for this group focuses on nutrition (breastfeeding promotion and complimentary feeding), prevention of common childhood illnesses (promotion of immunisation and notification of disease outbreaks) and, more recently, nurturing care and opportunities for learning to stimulate cognitive development (WHO, 2020a).

Issues specific to this audience

The crucial thing to note about health promotion activities for infants and young children is that the target audience is their parents/guardians and caregivers, which in many cultures may include extended family such as grandparents and older siblings.

Typical health settings for this audience

Maternal and child health clinics, medical practices, pharmacies, early childhood education centres, kindergartens and schools.

Other audiences to consider in communication activities

Educators of young children are also important health promoters for this age group.
   Workplaces and health services are other settings and potential audiences to consider, as these often require education and capacity building to be baby friendly (i.e. promoting how to assist workers to continue breastfeeding).

Pre-teens and teenagers
Health needs and influences

Pre-teens and teenagers are still growing, so the typical health promotion topics of good nutrition and physical activity continue to be crucial. Other topics including sexual health (including consent and positive relationships) as well as risky use of alcohol and other substances are also relevant, as is information about mental health and tolerance (anti-bullying).

Issues specific to this audience

Young people – teenagers and young adults – are generally capable of participating in health promotion activities and receiving health message themselves. However, caregivers remain important influencers, especially for pre-teens. Young people may be embarrassed to talk about sensitive topics such as puberty and sexuality, and cultural norms can also influence how and where they seek information.

Typical health settings for this audience

Medical clinics, hospitals, pharmacies and schools are common health settings. It is important that information is presented in a way that can be accessed confidentially by young people (e.g. online) and promoted in public settings so the information is normalised rather than associated with stigma.

Other audiences to consider in communication activities

Educators at schools, vocational institutions and extra-curricular activities (e.g. sports clubs, music, art and dance schools) can all contribute to health promotion and have particular roles to play in anti-bullying campaigns and mental health promotion. For example, the Australian Football League (AFL) has included some star players in the campaign 'I have your back', which targets racist bullying in Victorian schools (Victoria State Government, 2019). Celebrities (musicians, actors), 'YouTubers' and other social media influencers may also be worth considering to engage these audiences.

Young adults

Health needs and influences

Young adulthood can be a time of newfound autonomy and experimentation for many people. They may also experience some major life milestones such as graduating from school and university, moving out of the family home, going into full-time work, marriage/partnership and having children.

Issues specific to this audience

Gender identity, sexuality and sexual and reproductive health are all issues of importance to this audience, as are mental health and substance use. This includes the use of illicit substances, as well as the much more common issues of 'safe' drinking and the use of tobacco/nicotine (including vaping). Additional information about healthy relationships, including bodily autonomy, consent and family/domestic violence, is also pertinent.

Typical health settings for this audience

Medical clinics, hospitals, pharmacies, workplaces and higher education institutions (universities and technical colleges) are common health settings. Young adults may be engaged in study or vocational training, or may be employed part-time or full-time. Some members of this group may also experience marginalisation if they are unable to work or study, for example, due to a disability. Once they reach the legal age (typically 18 years), young adults are able to consume alcohol in licensed venues and clubs, which often display health messages, especially in relation to responsible alcohol use, drink driving and sexual consent.

Other audiences to consider in communication activities

Other than places of work or study, the family, peers and romantic partners of young adults are likely to be influential in their lives. Peers will continue to be important sources of information and guidance, especially online. Celebrities and online influencers as well as traditional media may also continue to be relevant.

Adults 31–49 years old
Health needs and influences

While people in this age group are generally thought of as 'productive working adults', they are also in an age group where their lifestyle can affect their risk of chronic disease further into adulthood. Perhaps surprisingly, loneliness can be an issue for this age group if they are new parents or full-time workers, especially those who relocate. The demands on the time of this age group can result in less time for participation in social and recreational activities such as the arts and sport, which can be protective for both mental and physical health.

Issues specific to this audience

This age group continues to have a focus on sexual health, family planning and fertility, and mental health. In particular, some cancers (testicular, ovarian, cervical cancer) associated with reproductive health emerge within this age group. Social connectedness and the needs of those facing difficulties in accessing services are important.

Typical health settings for this audience

Workplaces, universities/technical colleges, pharmacies, hospitals, medical clinics. This age group may also become parents, and thus need health information provided through maternal and child health, and parenting services. This age group may also need to start caring for their own parents, so some may start to visit aged-care facilities.

Other audiences to consider in communication activities

Family and friends, broader peer networks, including sporting clubs, media, special interest groups, working with social settings such as restaurants, food courts and bars, and institutions such as libraries and museums, may all provide means of engaging with this age group.

Adults 50–69 years old
Health needs and influences

Adults in this age group experience, or need to manage the progression of, chronic illness, and thus need information on diet and staying physically active. They may also be working less or planning to retire, which brings major lifestyle adjustments.

Issues specific to this audience

Working less may bring with it mental and emotional adjustments, especially for those who have gained much life meaning and satisfaction from their work. Those with reduced incomes may also face difficulties maintaining secure housing and having resources for adequate nutrition and access to health care.

Typical health settings for this audience

Workplaces, hospitals, medical clinics and pharmacies are common health settings. This age group may also be likely to frequent aged-care facilities – for their own parents or if their personal health or that of loved ones degenerates quickly.

Other audiences to consider in communication activities

Family, including grandchildren, will likely be a big influence. Special interest and community groups, volunteer organisations and community centres/clubs may also become more influential as this age group transitions from working to retirement.

Older adults

Health needs and influences

Older adults often experience progression in chronic diseases they may have acquired earlier in their life. They may also experience the death of a spouse or other loved one, and may become less independent in managing their health and activities of daily living.

Issues specific to this audience

Older adults may be managing one or more chronic diseases, and may also experience impairment or decrease in the use, or loss, of their senses (e.g. hearing, sight). Mental health (anxiety/depression) and other issues such as Alzheimer's disease and dementia are also important considerations in this population.

Typical health settings for this audience

Hospitals, medical practices, pharmacies and aged-care facilities are typical health settings for older adults. They may also receive information from health professionals visiting their home (e.g. community nursing and social work). Older adults living in the community may have more time to volunteer or be part of community organisations than other age groups, and these are good contexts for health promotion. Some may also live in institutional settings that aim to promote health and wellbeing.

Other audiences to consider in communication activities

Older adults may have other carers involved in some or all of their health care and decisions. It is important to involve caregivers and families in communication activities for them. Community clubs, special interest groups, libraries and museums may all be additional settings that can be used to engage with this audience.

Intersectionality in populations

Within each of the groups described above, there will be some members of populations for whom the challenges associated with establishing and maintaining good health are a little more difficult. '**Intersectionality**' means that certain groups are more disadvantaged than others from the outset, as their identities may compound their experience of structural forms of disadvantage or discrimination. First defined by Kimberle Crenshaw (1989), intersectionality recognises that the health issues of a white, middle-class person with regular employment are likely to be very different

Intersectionality – a theoretical framework for understanding how social identities, such as culture, race, gender, sexuality and class may combine to create compounding modes of discrimination and/or disadvantage

from those of someone who is, for example, from a different cultural background with English as a second or third language who works in a low-paid or casual job. Aside from the challenges of maintaining good health, finding health promotion interventions that are adequate for their needs may also be difficult. Here are a few more examples:

- A worker who lives in a remote Australian town may have trouble accessing a health service due to their distance from a major urban centre (geographic location is a recognised social determinant of health). However, this disadvantage may be further compounded if they are unemployed (cannot afford transport). An Aboriginal and Torres Strait Islander person from the same town would face the same structural disadvantage in terms of distance, but the health service itself may not be culturally safe, and therefore the barriers to care are further compounded.

- University students from rural and remote locations who have had to move major urban centres to study may feel socially isolated in a completely new city and institution. This isolation may be even more acute for those who have to move and are also neurodiverse, or who have a disability and face difficulty physically accessing classes and events on campus.

- Many women and children who experience homelessness do so because they are fleeing family violence. Immigrant women in some visa categories may not be eligible for emergency or family welfare payments, so they are further vulnerable to poverty in terms of affording food and rent. They may also require interpreters to help them seek assistance from police or shelter services, thereby compounding the difficulty of seeking help in a crisis.

CASE STUDY 3.1 Collective health literacy among Bhutanese–Nepali refugees in Australia

Linda Murray

Tasmania (Australia) is home to approximately 2000 Bhutanese–Nepali refugees who arrived after an extended period living as stateless persons in refugee camps in Nepal (Australian Bureau of Statistics (ABS), 2015). Most people in this community speak Nepali, which is the third-most commonly spoken language in Tasmania after English (ABS, 2017). Through their journey as refugees, many members of this population were denied opportunities for education, secure nutrition and health care. This has resulted in low literacy in any language, and increased risk of chronic illnesses requiring medication (Lamsal, 2014; Ethnic Communities Council of Victoria, 2012). In 2014, the author (LM) was part of a research team who worked with a general practitioner (GP) concerned about how many of her Bhutanese patients were having trouble adhering to their medication plans.

Could recording GP consultations help?

After considering the problem, the research team piloted a communication intervention whereby individual patients were given small MP3 recorders to take along to consultations with their GP. It was anticipated that this would improve communication by allowing patients to capture GP consultations, with interpreters present (with consent), and keep the audio recording for future reference. The intervention was based on research suggesting that recording consultations help patients to increase their recollection of management plans, empower patients to share information with others (Benson & Nanan, 2016; Elwyn, Barr & Grande, 2015) and reduce reliance on written materials (Murray, Elmer & Elkhair, 2018). Over a six-month period, a small number of community members who took at least one medication for a chronic illness were enrolled in the intervention and given a recorder. It was explained how audio recordings could assist as a prompt to listen to at home or when visiting the pharmacy, or for discussing health decisions with others. However, it soon became obvious that the recorders were not being used, despite participants demonstrating they could operate them.

After further community consultation, it became apparent that many of the participants were not individually managing their medications (i.e. storing prescriptions, buying and dispensing medication). The researchers re-framed the enquiry to consider the perspective of families rather than individuals. Then it was discovered that one or two family members (often a daughter-in-law or other family member working in health care) were collectively managing the medications for older relatives or an entire household, meaning that instructions for safety and use of medication were not being heard by the person giving the medication to the patient.

Context is crucial

This discovery demonstrated that the researchers had not understood the community context on a number of levels. First, the target audience for the intervention was too narrow, as only individual patients had been included, not collective family units. Second, the main message needed to be modified to focus on medication safety for households and families, not just improving how individuals follow doctor's instructions. Third, the channel for delivering the message needed to be reconsidered. While the decision not to rely on written material was correct, a format was needed that could be shared more easily than an MP3 recording accessed by an individual. A series of videos were created and published on YouTube, as these could be easily watched and shared using a smartphone, and even shown to patients by their GPs. The videos focused on household medication safety and navigating the Australian health system as a family. They were narrated in Bhutanese–Nepali using local community members as actors. The resulting communication materials (videos) were now owned by the community, and were more inclusive and accessible than the original intervention.

(cont.)

(cont.)

QUESTIONS

1. If you were to design a health communication campaign for a refugee community, what are some things you would need to consider about your target audience and the channel of communication?

2. If the target audience of your campaign was GPs rather than refugee patients, what message/s would you give them about how to promote medication safety among refugee communities?

ELSEWHERE IN THE WORLD

Let's talk about medicines

Devised by Wisconsin Health Literacy (2017), 'Let's Talk About Medicines' was a program designed specifically for refugee and immigrant populations. The program provided workbooks and face-to-face workshops for 13 different refugee and immigrant organisations, with participants from at least 10 language groups. Through running the workshops, the facilitators learned that even standard terms such as 'pharmacy' and 'prescription' needed to be defined, and that the differences between the roles of doctors and pharmacists needed to be explained. Information about herbal supplements, plants and other traditional cures was also included.

Different audiences can have both overlapping and distinct health information needs. The common theme between all of these groups is that at some stage they will all need to find health information.

Common settings for health promotion

The types of settings in which health promotion and health communication activities occur has widened over the past few decades. Health promotion's roots in health psychology and related fields mean it was originally focused on changing individual behaviour and therefore did not recognise social, environmental or structural influences on health (Baum & Fisher, 2014). With the Declaration of Alma Ata (WHO, 1978) and the Ottawa Charter for Health Promotion (WHO 1986), health promotion began to extend beyond the level of the individual to include dimensions such as supportive environments, community action and orientation of **health services** to the pursuit of health (rather than just treatment) (Whitelaw et al., 2001). It makes sense for health promotion work to be based largely in a particular geographical setting, be it a school, suburb, or an entire state or province. Therefore, terms such as 'settings-based health promotion', 'health promoting environments', 'community development for health' and 'health promoting arenas' are found throughout the health promotion literature (Whitelaw et al., 2001).

Health service – an institution or service that provides health care to people within a particular area, country or group, such as a hospital, primary care clinic and institutions such as aged-care facilities.

For ease of understanding, health promotion and health communication work are explained as occurring within three 'levels' (Figure 3.1). First, much health promotion continues to be aimed at the level of the individual, or the 'micro' level, which is concerned with messages about personal behavioural change (Baum & Fisher, 2014). The 'meso', or community level, refers to health promotion activities that may occur within a specific geographic community or health service; for example, within a local school or at a district hospital. Above this is the 'macro' level, which refers to health promotion that occurs at higher levels of governance; for example, enacting policy or structural change across an entire health system.

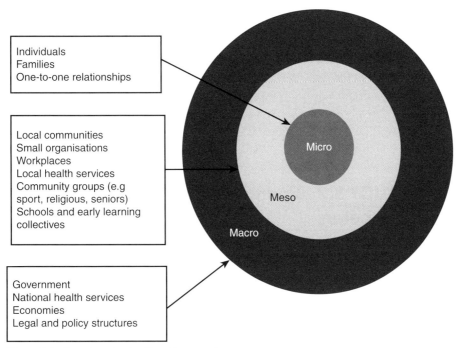

Figure 3.1   The three levels of health promotion

Health promotion in community based settings

There are many community based settings for health promotion. 'Community' can be defined in many ways, but in general it is used to describe groups of people who are related through webs of social connection. A community may be tied to a particular geographical place (see example below), or it may encompass groups of people that have similar interests (e.g. sports or craft groups), life experiences (seniors' groups or support groups for particular illnesses) or identities (e.g. LGBTIQ+). Community health promotion may occur in settings in which people gather, such as workplaces, markets, homes or community centres (see Case study 3.2). One interesting example of community based health promotion is the Healthy Islands initiative (WHO, 2015). At the macro (structural) level, this initiative provided national representatives from small-island states in Melanesia and the Pacific with information about emerging health threats, such as non-communicable diseases and climate change, and tools for designing interventions to tackle them. When evaluated, Healthy Islands was perceived by decision-makers as a 'brand' with recognisable language and frameworks that could be adapted to facilitate health promotion work in a range of settings (WHO, 2015).

Religious settings as sites for prevention of violence against women

Religious settings have traditionally been places in which communities of people regularly meet, making them ideal sites for dissemination of health messages. Religious organisations are also usually inherently concerned with social and family relationships so they are well placed to facilitate prevention of family violence. A recent survey in one town in Aotearoa New Zealand found that one in 10 people would go to their faith leader if they were experiencing family violence (New Zealand Government, 2020). This illustrates the need to train religious leaders to provide preventive education and be aware of local referral services for family violence. In order for this to occur, strong links need to be established between health promotion agencies and religious organisations and leaders, which the health promoter could have a key role in developing. It should also be noted that while many religious organisations seek to actively address family violence, others may stigmatise or even ostracise victims who speak out about it. Hence, a more appropriate starting point might be to develop sensitive and culturally appropriate messages that de-stigmatise talking about family violence (or simply to enhance awareness).

CASE STUDY 3.2 Ageing men, masculinity and social wellbeing

Andrea Waling

Threats to the health and wellbeing of older men

Older men in Australia are considered an at-risk group for physical health ailments and mental health concerns such as depression, anxiety and suicidal ideation. In 2018, men over the age of 85 had the highest rate (32.9 per 100 000) of suicide completions, and men between the ages of 45 and 54 years showed the highest increase in suicide completions (431 deaths) compared to 2017 (424 deaths) (ABS, 2018).

Loneliness and lack of connection and community are major contributing factors to decreases in older men's social, mental and physical wellbeing (Courtenay, 2000; 2010). Men's Sheds programs have been established to help older men (generally over the age of 60 years, though may include men in their 40s and 50s) who may be retired, retrenched, unemployed or living with illnesses and/or disabilities that prevent them from engaging in full-time or part-time work (Golding, 2015). They facilitate semi-structured or unstructured time in which such men may come together to build friendships (thereby reducing social isolation) and work on projects such as woodworking, arts and crafts, restoring furniture or bicycles, and building items such as benches and cubby houses for other community organisations (Wilson et al., 2015). While perceptions of masculinity are changing, older men in their 40s, 50s, and 60s may continue to hold onto notions of stoicism as a desirable masculine trait (O'Brien et al., 2005). Getting men to seek support for concerns such as physical health ailments associated with ageing, or to reach out if they are experiencing emotional or mental health distress can be challenging, as these practices have been previously believed to be contrary to performing 'appropriate' masculinity (Courtenay, 2000; O'Brien et al., 2005).

A Men's Shed in regional New South Wales

A Men's Shed program in regional New South Wales is focused on supporting older men from diverse cultural and linguistic communities (Waling & Fildes, 2017). Many of the men who attend this program have been retrenched from a now-closed steel mill, and are unable to find employment. In this shed, a semi-structured morning program of woodworking enable the men to work on small or large projects with support and guidance from facilitators. In these settings, the men are also given access to health promotion activities in which nurses or health educators teach them about certain health ailments such as prostate canceer, or offer onsite examinations and testing of blood pressure. An evaluation of the program found that, since attending the shed, participants noted improvements in their social connectedness, decreases in experiences of loneliness and greater awareness about taking care of physical and mental health ailments, such as getting tested and treated for prostate cancer, diabetes, depression and anxiety (Waling & Fildes, 2017).

Men's Sheds programs provide effective settings for health promotion communication as they rely on an established setting that is safe, comfortable and accessible for men who can take in important messaging while they engage in enjoyable and familiar activities. The non-medical and traditionally masculine setting enables the men to feel comfortable with onsite nurses or educators. Engagement with hands-on activities such as woodworking creates a comfortable space in which the men can speak with each other about sensitive topics such as the loss of a partner or how to cope with a life-threatening health concern.

QUESTIONS

1. Why might it be useful or helpful to rely on outdated ideas about gender identity to support a particular group of people when trying to improve physical, mental, and social wellbeing?

2. Would a Men's Shed format be applicable for men across all ages, cultures and identities? Why or why not?

ELSEWHERE IN THE WORLD

International Men's Sheds organisation

Men's Sheds (www.menshed.com) operate in Australia, Aotearoa New Zealand, Canada, Denmark, Ireland, Scotland, the United Kingdom and Wales. Visit the website to read further about the organisation's operations elsewhere in the world.

Institutional settings

Institutional settings can be located in both the meso and the macro levels of health promotion. Institutions can take many forms, and can develop where people learn, work or live. Traditionally, educational settings have been important sites for health promotion activities, with school-based health promotion usually conducted in collaboration with stakeholders such as teachers, parents/carers and local organisations and businesses such as sporting clubs and cafés (Bergeron et al., 2019). This creates opportunities for relationships to be built within and around the school community that can promote health and wellbeing. One critique of school-based health promotion is that its results cannot always be evaluated in a linear fashion, as its focus is usually on creating the conditions for health and wellbeing for the school community (Bergeron et al. 2019).

Health promotion in universities is often about ensuring that young adults have access to services that they need. There may be groups of students, such as international students, students with disabilities and LGBTIQ+ students who have specific health needs that may not be met in that context (see Case study 3.3). There is some evidence that many students find accessing student health services difficult for sensitive issues such as testing for sexually transmissible infections (STIs) due to the service opening hours or discomfort about interacting with health professionals (Cassidy et al., 2018). To overcome some of these difficulties, one study in the United States explored the use of an app to assist college students to manage their sexual health by tracking menstrual periods, providing reminders to renew prescriptions for birth control and offering information about symptoms of STIs and unplanned pregnancy (Richman et al., 2014). It was found that women, and students engaging in sexual activity, were interested in using the app as a way to maintain healthy sexuality. However, an app, or 'Dr Google', cannot and should not ever replace consultation with a health professional. It should act as a nudge or a trigger to seek professional medical advice.

CASE STUDY 3.3 Sexual health challenges for international students in Australia

Matthew Dunn

International students studying in Australia make up 25 per cent of all higher education enrolments (Department of Education and Training, 2014), and these students experience challenges additional to their shift away from their home cultures (Rosenthal et al., 2008). Previous studies have found that international students may have lower literacy in sexual health and higher notification levels of chlamydia than their Australian-born counterparts (Rosenthal et al., 2008; Simpson et al., 2015).

Understanding international students' sexual health needs

In order to understand how university events promoting sexual health could better reach international students, a survey was distributed by email to a random sample of students from a large Australian university. In the survey, students were asked to provide basic demographic information before answering questions on their prior sexual experiences, sexual-health testing and preferences, and their experiences of events promoting sexual health.

Unlike the overwhelming majority of Australian-born students, over 40 per cent of international students reported that they had not received any sexual health education in high school. Despite this, international students were even less likely to have attended a sexual health promotion event at university than their domestic counterparts, and those that did were less likely to find it relevant. In addition, while the top two preferences of domestic students were aligned with the event types on offer, international students' top two preferences (sexual-health testing and relevant movies) were the least likely options to occur. From this it was deduced that university based sexual health promotions were not meeting the needs of international students.

International students' high level of support for sexual-health testing may have derived from the fact that they were significantly less likely to have previously tested for STIs, when compared to their domestic counterparts, or due to cost or privacy concerns. Although all international students in Australia are required to purchase overseas student health insurance (Department of Health, 2017), students may be unsure what this covers or may be unwilling to claim for an expense that continues to be deeply stigmatised.

Potential ways to engage

International students also reported different incentives and motivations to attend events promoting sexual health, being significantly less in favour than their domestic counterparts of using alcohol as an incentive and strategies that involve combining sexual health events with a social element. This is likely due to differing attitudes about alcohol consumption, based on cultural and religious reasons, and greater stigma related to sexual health for culturally and linguistically diverse (CALD) youth populations in Australia (Newton et al., 2013). The two motivations that were significantly more likely to be selected by international students were events that were 'sensitive to my culture' and 'presented in my first language (if other than English)'.

QUESTIONS

1. Given the identified needs of international students, what kinds of communication activities could be implemented on campus?

2. What groups, individuals or resources could be useful when planning these activities?

3. What strategies could be used to ensure that activities meet the needs of the target audience?

4. If you wanted to run a similar survey related to sexual health, what challenges would you anticipate, and how would you address them?

ELSEWHERE IN THE WORLD

Demystifying sex and societal norms at an international college in Canada

Fraser International College in British Columbia runs a semester-long course about adapting to and understanding life in Canada, including a focus on consent, sexual health and gender identity. A recent survey found that around 85 per cent of participants reported the sexual health component as the most meaningful part of the program (Reid, 2019).

Workplaces are diverse and can include factories, call centres and traditional 'white collar' workplaces such as law firms. In addition to creating a safe work environment (e.g. complying with occupational health and safety regulations), workplaces are often good places in which to promote the health and wellbeing of their workers. Well-designed communications for workplaces can improve knowledge and prompt action about health issues (e.g. mental health), demonstrate health promoting skills (e.g. how to wear personal protective equipment) and increase demand for workplace health programs and services (Centers for Disease Control, 2018).

Institutions such as hospitals and prisons are also workplaces. Due to their highly institutional nature, prisons largely adopt health promotion involving policies to promote a healthy prison environment rather than deliver programs that individuals can opt into. Prison health promotion may also take an advocacy or human rights approach if there is under-funding for basic resources for nutrition and sanitation (WHO, 2020d). Many prisons provide a range of health promotion materials in their health clinics, and some even employ health promotion officers to run face-to-face activities. Prisoners can be helpful in raising awareness of particular health issues (e.g. fitness, hepatitis C and smoking) by becoming peer educators or health champions who can influence and support others. However, such programs are rarely standardised or delivered consistently between prisons (Woodall & Freeman, 2019).

Healthcare settings

While health services are often sites of treatment for disease, they can also serve health promotion functions. This may include providing materials such as posters and brochures in waiting rooms, interpersonal communication between health practitioner and patient, or through specific programs and initiatives. For example, hospitals might promote maternal and child health through the Baby Friendly Hospital Initiative (BFHI), a global movement started by the WHO in 1991 to encourage all hospitals to create environments optimal for breastfeeding women. The BFHI is now implemented in more than 152 countries worldwide (WHO, 2020b). The initiative has many dimensions, including requiring hospitals to have appropriate places for women (patients and staff) to breastfeed and express and store milk. In terms of communication, baby friendly hospitals often display signage (e.g. 'breastfeeding is welcome here' and posters outlining the benefits of breastfeeding, see Figure 3.2) in the

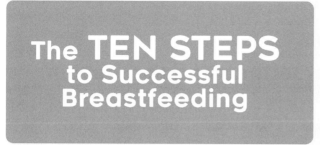

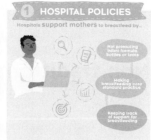

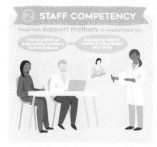

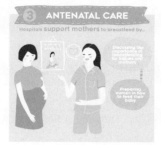

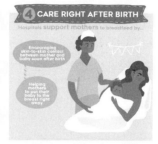

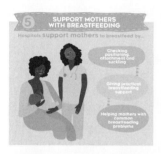

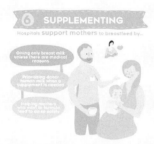

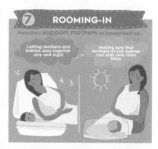

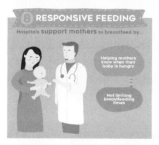

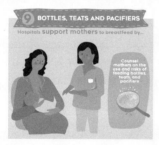

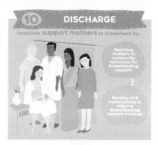

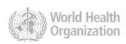

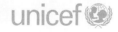

Figure 3.2   The ten steps to successful breastfeeding
Source: WHO (2020c).

clinical environment as well as in waiting rooms and other areas. Additionally, staff working in these hospitals must undergo training on how to promote the benefits of breastfeeding to women in an appropriate and sensitive way, thus encouraging clinical staff to also be health promoters. Other types of institutions, such as residential aged-care facilities, provide environments in which to promote not just the physical, but also the psychological and social dimensions of health. Examples of interventions to improve social connectedness in this age group are identified further below (see the section 'Unexpected partnerships').

Non-traditional settings and approaches

Health information does not always have to be presented in a traditional 'health' setting. It is always a challenge to figure out how to 'engage the unengaged' – people who are either not interested in, or face barriers to, accessing health information are unlikely to be found in the places where health information is commonly provided. This means that we need to be creative and think about where this information can be displayed, and how that information is presented to help get the message across. Sometimes it feels a bit like trying to achieve 'health by stealth'! But this process can also be fun and creative; an opportunity to adapt something that already 'works' to see if it can help achieve the desired objectives. This section outlines some alternative settings to think about. It describes some approaches that can be adopted to fit within a range of different settings, physical or virtual.

Different approaches

Story telling

Entertainment-education or 'edutainment' is the purposeful design and implementation of a message in a format that both entertains and educates, with the intent of positively influencing audience awareness, attitudes and behaviours to enact social change (Singhal & Rogers, 1999). It has long been used in health promotion, especially in relation to HIV/AIDS, human rights, family planning and environmental health (Storey & Sood, 2013). Edutainment can take a range of formats and might employ mass media, film, comic books and social media; however, its roots are in the oral and performing arts traditions, which include story telling. Story telling has the capacity to create behavioural change (Storey & Sood, 2013). It relies on narrative to convey its message and, if a narrative is compelling enough, by capturing attention and using imagery and feelings, an audience might perceive the narrative as being 'more real', which may in turn create stronger feelings towards the characters. Ultimately, this has potential to change beliefs (Green & Brock, 2000). It is important to ensure that, when using story telling in health promotion, the story we tell draws upon the local cultural context. If the intended audience cannot relate to the story then it limits its effectiveness as a communication tool (Petraglia, 2007).

Gaming and incentives

Wearable technologies such as pedometers, and the more advanced fitness tracker watches and movement trackers in smartphones, have been very useful tools for health agencies to increase awareness of the importance of physical activity. In Singapore, for example, 2020 signals the fifth year of the 'National Steps Campaign', which is an incentive-based national program to encourage Singaporeans to be more active (Ministry of Health Singapore, 2020). Participants download an app to their smartphone, which tracks their activity, or the Health Promotion Board provides a fitness tracker to people who do not have a smartphone. After registering, the trackers record their daily steps and physical activities. These are calculated and the number of steps or minutes spent doing moderate to vigorous physical activity allows the user to accrue points and the chance to win prizes in the 'Grand Draw', which includes airfares, cruise vouchers and household goods. Reward tiers also provide incentives in the form of shopping, food or beverage vouchers (Ministry of Health, 2020). Workplaces and community groups can also compete as a collective, with their own targets and rewards. In 2019, the National Steps Challenge had more than 800 000 participants, with many of these returning from previous seasons (Health Promotion Board, 2019).

Fitness trackers make measuring physical activity easy by encouraging people to monitor how much they move during a day, with 10 000 steps a readily identifiable and widely used target (Lee et al., 2019). However, the daily goal of 10 000 steps is not derived from hard evidence; rather, it is thought to be a marketing gimmick from 1965, when a Japanese company was selling a pedometer called *Manpo-kei*, which literally translates as '10 000-steps-per-metre' (Lee et al., 2019). As a communication outcome, the recognition and recall of the message is fantastic. But although step challenges are good to get people moving, if their focus is just on the number of steps rather than on the intensity of the walking or exercise, then it's not really contributing to overall health. This is why in its fourth season the National Steps Challenge introduced an exercise-intensity target as well as steps (Health Promotion Board, 2019), and why many other fitness challenges focus on different workouts of different intensities designed to achieve results in a certain number of days or weeks. The quality of the movement is just as important as the quantity.

Pokémon GO was a surprise success in terms of increasing physical activity. The augmented reality game app is downloaded onto smartphones and players are encouraged to 'catch' Pokémon (little monsters) that appeared virtually in real places (Figure 3.3). After launching in 2016, Pokémon GO continues to be popular, with 147 million active users in May 2018 (Tassi, 2018). The game seems to have had unintended

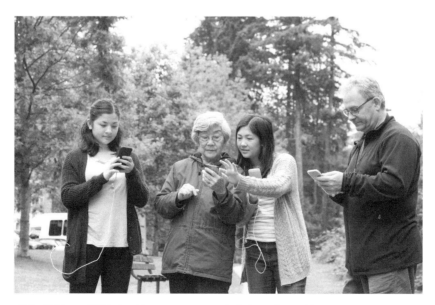

Figure 3.3   Pokémon GO helped to encourage people to be active outdoors

health benefits as players walk more, spend more time with their families outdoors and increase social interaction, which in turn could also improve mental health (Freeman et al., 2017). A systematic review found that Pokémon GO did appear to increase physical activity in players, but how long that increased activity was maintained is still unknown (Khamzina et al., 2019). It is also difficult to retain the engagement of participants once the novelty wears off (Khamzina et al., 2019), which arguably is applicable to any 'new' health promotion activity.

A meta-analysis of game-based interventions found that when narratives – or stories – are combined with games, they can improve health knowledge, self-efficacy and behaviours, making them powerful tools for health promotion (Zhou et al., 2020). The same study found that narrative games played by groups were also more effective in positively changing behaviours than those played by single players, and adults were more likely to show increased self-efficacy than children. The findings of this study suggest that combining elements into programs may be more effective than using either a game or a storytelling approach in isolation. Why not experiment with this in your own initiatives?

Most of these fitness challenges and new games are shared on the internet and social media. It is an easy way to get information to an audience quickly, so long as planning ensures the information finds the target audience.

The power of social media

As we discuss in more detail in later chapters, social media is a double-edged sword for health promotion. Social media enables experimentation with different ideas, comparatively cheaply and easily (Freeman et al., 2015). There are many different ways in which social media can be used to engage different audiences. The trick is to ensure that you use the right **engagement** strategy on the right platform to connect with the right audience. We discuss needs assessments and environmental scans in Chapter 6, and how to develop a communication strategy in Chapter 7. One crucial thing to remember is that not all social media platforms are equally useful in engaging audiences. In a study of the social media activity of fitness tracker brands Fitbit™ and Garmin™, the researchers found Instagram posts showed 30–200 times more engagement than those on Facebook and Twitter (Edney et al., 2018). The researchers also noted that companies used different creative approaches, depending upon the social media platform used, which indicates that companies are targeting their engagement strategies to the needs of their target markets as well. From lone health promotion professionals through to large, multinational corporations, 'know your audience' is a universal first step!

One of the great things that social media can provide is a groundswell of activity through a 'call to action'. This can be useful in getting people to sign up to participate in a campaign and to help maintain momentum (Freeman et al., 2015). One example of this is Movember, a global initiative to raise funds for research on prostate and testicular cancer, mental health and suicide prevention in men. Movember began as an idea of 30 men who decided to try to make the moustache fashionable again, in a way that contributed funds to a worthy cause (Movember, 2015). Within three years they had formally partnered with the Prostate Cancer Foundation of Australia and raised

Engagement – a multifaceted concept that can be influenced internally (e.g. motivation) or externally (e.g. context), and can change

$1.2 million. It now operates in over 20 countries and has over 5 million supporters internationally (Movember, 2015). Movember uses social media to facilitate ease of participation and, crucially, the making of donations. People who sign up to participate are provided with an online platform from which they can share the suggested links and pre-written posts to their fundraising pages, using their own social media accounts. It enables participants to feel like they are part of a community of 'Mo Bros' and 'Mo Sistas', which helps to drive participant engagement (Freeman et al., 2015). Movember is also an example of how social media settings can support work conducted in other settings. Aside from contributing to medical research, the funds raised by Movember provide support for diverse programs in locations around the world that offer local services and networks to support men's health. This includes surfing programs, which aim to build better mental health and wellbeing (WOW Sand n Surf, Australia), and programs for people to find employment, build relationships and social connection following incarceration (Ex-cell UK).

LEARNING ACTIVITY 3.1

Go online and find a health promotion activity or program, in any country and on any topic.

1. Find all the places where information about that activity is shared by the organisers – websites, social media accounts, YouTube channels etc.
2. Do the different online settings support and reinforce each other and, if so, how? Support your answer with examples.
3. Do the different platforms used seem to target different audiences and, if so, how can you tell? Give evidence to support your answer.
4. Are the online settings supporting programs in any other, non-online settings?

EXTENSION QUESTION

Reflect on the settings and audiences used in the program you chose. Are there any audiences or settings that have not been targeted that could be? Describe who, where and how.

Unexpected partnerships

In 2013, Australia's health and cultural ministers developed the National Arts and Health Framework, 'to enhance the profile of arts and health in Australia and to promote greater integration of arts and health practice and approaches into health promotion, services, settings and facilities' (Department of Communication and the Arts, 2013, p. 1). This framework recognises that all forms of art can contribute to the development and maintenance of health and wellbeing in numerous ways. One example is the use of dance with people diagnosed with dementia and Alzheimer's disease. Studies have shown that dance can improve the physical and mental abilities of patients, as well as their quality of life and that of their caregivers (Ruiz-Muelle & López-Rodríguez, 2019).

Museums are not necessarily the first places that spring to mind when you think about health promotion, but exhibits – especially interactive ones – can be a great way to get people thinking about health issues, sometimes without even realising it. Museums and science centres can make very large objects, such as giant inflatable organs that look like lungs. They can also reveal the world of microbes in meaningful ways. Whatever the size, museum exhibits can make the invisible visible. And explorable! This can help to create conversations and awareness, and potentially communicate complex ideas about health in simple ways. For example, a simple hands-on exhibit prototype was shown to successfully communicate the influence of the social determinants on health outcomes in a way that was engaging and easy to understand, for children as well as adults (Phiddian et al., 2019).

The effects and effectiveness of exhibits can differ depending upon what else is provided to the audience. Two different studies examined the effectiveness of a giant, inflatable walk-through 'colon' (with sections showing healthy tissue, polyps and colorectal cancer) for increasing knowledge about colorectal cancer and screening in underserved populations. One study compared the knowledge of visitors before and after a health fair, with half of the visitors receiving information during a short guided tour of the colon and the other half from a standard table display of information and materials (Briant et al., 2015b). Immediately after the visit, those who had gone through the colon had greater knowledge about colorectal cancer, but the difference was not significant. One month after the health fair, neither group remembered virtually any of the information from the health fair (Briant et al., 2015b). Compare this to a study, which used the same inflatable colon and tour, but this time also provided free testing kits to visitors aged over 50 years. Of the 300 kits distributed, just over 75 per cent of participants used the kits to get screened for colorectal cancer, indicating that combining education with access to a service is likely to increase compliance with health screenings (Briant et al., 2015a). Therefore, while choice of setting is important, it is only part of what you need to consider. Wherever you choose to set your event or program, you should also be actively attempting to remove barriers to participation and empowering your target audience to make informed decisions about what they do with your information.

LEARNING ACTIVITY 3.2

Imagine you are employed by a sexual health and family planning clinic that is responsible for serving the needs of your whole community. You have been asked to come up with a program about 'respectful relationships' for the major audience groups within your community.

1. List the key audiences in your community. (How would you find out who your key audiences were; what information source could you use?)
2. For each audience you wrote down in question 1:
   a. Describe how you would define and present the concept of 'respectful relationships' for that group. Justify your choices.
   b. Outline the intended goal of the program for each group. (What change do you want to see? What does success look like?)

> **c.** Identify the different settings that could be used to engage these audiences.
>
> **d.** Describe what else you could offer within or additional to that setting to reinforce the desired outcome you describe in b.
>
> ### EXTENSION QUESTION
> Reflect on one of the key audiences you identified. Are there any settings that could be counterproductive for achieving a desired outcome for this audience? Why or why not?

Summary

This chapter has described the different health needs of different audiences and how these needs can differ over time, even within groups. There are some settings in which people expect to receive health information and to which they will actively go to seek out health information. Some of these are common across all audience groups, while others have specific demographic groups they support. A particular challenge is engaging those who do not actively seek health information, which is where partnerships between health services and various settings – both typical and atypical – can be a useful means of ensuring you reach different audiences. While the interactions between audience and setting are important considerations, they are rarely enough to determine an outcome. You need to think about how you can support what happens in those settings with other resources and approaches, to ensure that the message is not only received but also acted upon.

REVISION QUESTIONS

1. What is the settings approach to health promotion?
2. Describe how health information needs can change across a life span.
3. What are some of the commonly used settings for health promotion, and what audiences do each of these usually serve?
4. Describe some different settings and approaches that can be used to engage audiences in health promotion programs and activities.

FURTHER READING

Dooris, M., Poland, B., Kolbe, L., de Leeuw, E., McCall, D.S. & Wharf-Higgins, J. (2007). Healthy settings. In D.V. McQueen & C.M. Jones (eds.), *Global Perspectives on Health Promotion Effectiveness*. New York: Springer.

Iedema, R., Piper, D. & Manidis, M. (2015). *Communicating Quality and Safety in Health Care*. Melbourne: Cambridge University Press.

Scriven, A. & Hodgins, M. (eds.) (2012). *Health Promotion Settings: Principles and practice*. Cornwall, UK: Sage.

REFERENCES

Australian Bureau of Statistics (ABS) (2015). *3101.0 – Australian Demographic Statistics, Dec 2015*. Canberra, ACT: Australian Bureau of Statistics. Retrieved from: https://www.abs.gov.au/ausstats/abs@.nsf/lookup/3101.0Media%20Release1Dec%202015

———(2017, June 27). *One in every five Tasmanians aged 65 years and over* [Media release]. Canberra: ABS. Retrieved from: https://www.abs.gov.au/ausstats/abs@.nsf/mediareleasesbyReleaseDate/7F1A862B6F8B6BA0CA258148000A41AC?OpenDocument

———(2018). *3303.0 – Causes of Death, Australia, 2018: Intentional Self Harm-Key Characteristics*. Canberra: ABS.

Baum, F. & Fisher, M. (2014). Why behavioural health promotion endures despite its failure to reduce health inequities, *Sociology of Health & Illness*, 36(2), 213–25.

Benson, K. & Nanan, R. (2016). Recording consultations: A win–win situation for physicians and patients, *Medical Journal of Australia*, 204(5),175–6.

Bergeron, D.A., Talbot, L.R. & Gaboury, I. (2019). Context and the mechanisms in intersectoral school-based health promotion interventions: A critical interpretative synthesis, *Health Education Journal*, 78(7),713–27.

Briant, K.J., Espinoza, N., Galvan, A., Carosso, E., Marchello, N., Linde, S., Copeland, W. & Thompson, B. (2015a). An innovative strategy to reach the underserved for colorectal cancer screening, *Journal of Cancer Education*, 30(2), 237–43.

Briant, K.J., Wang, L., Holte, S., Ramos, A., Marchello, N. & Thompson, B. (2015b). Understanding the impact of colorectal cancer education: A randomized trial of health fairs, *BMC Public Health*, 30(15),1196.

Cassidy, C., Bishop, A., Steenbeek, A., Langille, D., Martin-Misener, R. & Curran, J. (2018). Barriers and enablers to sexual health service use among university students: A qualitative descriptive study using the Theoretical Domains Framework and COM-B model, *BMC Health Services Research*, 18(1), 581.

Centers for Disease Control (2018). Workplace Health Promotion: Communications. Retrieved from: https://www.cdc.gov/workplacehealthpromotion/planning/communications.html

Courtenay, W.H. (2000). Constructions of masculinity and their influence on men's well-being: a theory of gender and health, *Social Science & Medicine*, 50(10),1385–401.

———(2010). Constructions of masculinity and their influence on men's well-being: A theory of gender and health. In S.R. Harper & F. Harris III (eds.), *College Men and Masculinities: Theory, research, and implications for practice* (p. 307–36). Jossey-Bass/Wiley.

Crenshaw, K. (1989). Demarginalizing the intersection of race and sex: A black feminist critique of antidiscrimination doctrine, feminist theory and antiracist politics. *University of Chicago Legal Forum*, 1989(1), Article 8. Retrieved from: http://chicagounbound.uchicago.edu/uclf/vol1989/iss1/8

Department of Communication and the Arts (2013). *National Arts and Health Framework*. Canberra: Department of Communication and the Arts.

Department of Education and Training (2014). *Selected Higher Education Statistics – 2013 Student Data, 2013 Student Summary*. Canberra: Department of Education and Training.

Department of Health (2017). *Overseas Student Health Cover – Frequently Asked Questions.* Canberra: Department of Health.

Dooris, M. (2006). Healthy settings: Challenges to generating evidence of effectiveness, *Health Promotion International*, 21(1), 55–65.

Edney, S., Bogomolova, S., Ryan, J., Olds, T., Sanders, I. & Maher, C. (2018). Creating engaging health promotion campaigns on social media: Observations and lessons from Fitbit and Garmin, *Journal of Medical Internet Research*, 20(12), e10911.

Elwyn, G., Barr, P.J. & Grande, S.W. (2015). Patients recording clinical encounters: A path to empowerment? Assessment by mixed methods, *BMJ Open*, 5: e008566.

Ethnic Communities Council of Victoria (2012). An Investment Not An Expense: Enhancing health literacy in culturally and linguistically diverse communities. Retrieved from: http://www.eccv.org.au/library/An_Investment_Not_an_Expense_ECCV_Health_Literacy_Paper_FINAL.pdf

Freeman, B., Potente, S,. Rock, V. & McIver, J. (2015). Social media campaigns that make a difference: What can public health learn from the corporate sector and other social change marketers? *Public Health Research & Practice*, 25(2), e2521517.

Freeman, B., Chau, J. & Mihrshahi, S. (2017). Why the public health sector couldn't create Pokémon GO, *Public Health Research & Practice*, 27(3), e2731724.

Golding, B. (2015). *The Men's Shed movement: The company of men.* Champaign, IL: Common Ground Publishing.

Green, M.C. & Brock, T.C. (2000). The role of transportation in the persuasiveness of public narratives, *Journal of Personality and Social Psychology*, 79(5), 701–21.

Health Promotion Board (2019). *Many pathways to a healthy nation: Annual report 2018/2019.* Retrieved from: https://www.hpb.gov.sg/docs/default-source/annual-reports/hpb-annual-report-2018_2019.pdf?sfvrsn=df71c372_0

Kaeberlein, M. (2018). How healthy is the healthspan concept? *GeroScience*, 40(4), 361–4.

Khamzina, M., Parab, K.V., An, R., Bullard, T. & Grigsby-Toussaint, D.S. (2019). Impact of Pokémon GO on physical activity: A systematic review and meta-analysis. *American Journal of Preventative Medicine*, 58(2): 270–82.

Lamsal, T. (2014). *Globalizing Literacies and Identities: Translingual and transcultural literacy practices of Bhutanese refugees in the US (Doctoral dissertation).* Louisville, KY: University of Louisville. Retrieved from: https://ir.library.louisville.edu/cgi/viewcontent.cgi?article=1788&context=etd

Lee, I., Shiroma, E.J., Kamada, M., Bassett, D.R., Matthews, C.E. & Buring, J.E. (2019). Association of step volume and intensity with all-cause mortality in older women, *JAMA Internal Medicine*, 179(8), 1105–12.

Ministry of Health Singapore (2020). National Steps Challenge. Retrieved from: https://www.healthhub.sg/programmes/37/nsc

Movember (2015). *The Movember origin story.* Retrieved from: https://au.movember.com/story/11213/

Murray, L., Elmer, S. & Elkhair, J. (2018). Perceived barriers to managing medications and solutions to barriers suggested by Bhutanese former refugees and service providers, *Journal of Transcultural Nursing*, 29(6), 570–7.

New Zealand Government (2020). Family Violence, It's not ok: Faith Communities. Retrieved from: http://www.areyouok.org.nz/i-want-change/faith-communities/

Newton, D., Keogh, L., Temple-Smith, M., Fairley, C.K., Chen, M., Bayly, C., Williams, H., McNamee, K., Henning, D., Hsueh, A., Fisher, J. & Hocking, J. (2013). Key informant perceptions of youth-focussed sexual health promotion programs in Australia, *Sexual Health*, 10(1), 47–56.

O'Brien R., Hunt K. & Hart G. (2005). 'It's caveman stuff, but that is to a certain extent how guys still operate': Men's accounts of masculinity and help seeking, *Social Science and Medicine*, 61(3), 503–16.

Petraglia, J. (2007). Narrative intervention in behavior and public health, *Journal of Health Communication*, 12(5), 493–505.

Phiddian, E., Hoepner, J. & McKinnon, M. (2019). Can interactive science exhibits be used to communicate population health science concepts? *Critical Public Health*, 30(3), 257–69.

Reid, S. (2019). International students: We need to talk about sex, *Navitas Insights*. Retrieved from: https://insights.navitas.com/international-students-we-need-to-talk-about-sex/

Richman, A., Webb, M., Brinkley, J. & Martin, R. (2014). Sexual behaviour and interest in using a sexual health mobile app to help improve and manage college students' sexual health, *Sex Education*, 14(3), 310–22.

Rosenthal, D.A., Russell, J. & Thomson, G. (2008). The health and wellbeing of international students at an Australian university, *Higher Education*, 55(1), 51–67.

Ruiz-Muelle, A. & López-Rodríguez, M.M. (2019). Dance for people with Alzheimer's disease: A systematic review, *Current Alzheimer Research*, 16(10), 919–33.

Simpson, S., Clifford, C., Ross, K., Sefton, N., Owen, L., Blizzard, L. & Turner, R. (2015). Sexual health literacy of the student population of the University of Tasmania: Results of the RUSSL Study, *Sexual Health*, 12(3), 207–16.

Singhal, A. & Rogers, E.M. (1999). *Entertainment-Education: A communication strategy for social change*. New Jersey: Lawrence Erlbaum Associates.

Storey, D. & Sood, S. (2013). Increasing equity, affirming the power of narrative and expanding dialogue: The evolution of entertainment education over two decades, *Critical Arts-South-North Cultural and Media Studies*, 27(1), 9–35.

Tassi, P. (2018, 27 June). 'Pokémon GO' is more popular than it's been at any point since launch in 2016, *Forbes*. Retrieved from: https://www.forbes.com/sites/insertcoin/2018/06/27/pokemon-go-is-more-popular-than-its-been-at-any-point-since-launch-in-2016/#7943fbb1cfd2

Victoria State Government (2019). Footy stars have your back when it comes to racist bullying. Victoria State Government: Education and Training. Retrieved from: https://www.education.vic.gov.au/about/news/Pages/stories/2019/stories-antiracistbullyingAFL.aspx

Waling, A. & Fildes, D. (2017). 'Don't fix what ain't broke': Evaluating the effectiveness of a Men's Shed in inner-regional Australia, *Health and Social Care in the Community*, 25(2), 758–68.

Whitelaw, S., Baxendale, A., Bryce, C., MacHardy, L., Young, I. & Witney, E. (2001). 'Settings' based health promotion: A review, *Health Promotion International*, 16(4), 339–53.

Wilson, N.J., Cordier, R., Doma, K., Misan, G. & Vaz, S. (2015) Men's Sheds function and philosophy: Toward a framework for future research and men's health promotion, *Health Promotion Journal of Australia*, 26(2), 133–41.

Wisconsin Health Literacy (2017). Let's talk about medicines for refugee and immigrant populations. Retrieved from: https://wisconsinliteracy.org/health-literacy/programs/past-programs/for-refugee-and-immigrant-populations.html

Woodall, J. & Freeman, C. (2019). Promoting health and well-being in prisons: An analysis of one year's prison inspection reports, *Critical Public Health*. Retrieved from: doi: 10.1080/09581596.2019.1612516

World Health Organization (WHO) (1978). *Declaration of Alma-Ata*. Geneva: WHO.

———(1986). *The Ottawa Charter for Health Promotion*. Geneva: WHO.

———(2015). The first 20 years of the journey towards the vision of Healthy Islands in the Pacific. Retrieved from: https://iris.wpro.who.int/bitstream/handle/10665.1/10928/9789290617150_eng.pdf

———(2020a). *Nurturing Care Framework: Why nurturing care?* Retrieved from: https://www.who.int/maternal_child_adolescent/child/nurturing-care-framework-rationale/en/

———(2020b). *Baby Friendly Hospital Initiative*. Retrieved from: https://www.who.int/nutrition/topics/bfhi/en/

———(2020c). The Ten steps to Successful Breastfeeding. Retrieved from: https://www.who.int/nutrition/bfhi/bfhi-poster-A2.pdf?ua=1

———(2020d). *Types of Health Settings: Health promoting prisons*. Retrieved from: https://www.who.int/healthy_settings/types/prisons/en/

Zhou, C., Occa, A., Kim, S. & Morgan, S. (2020). A meta-analysis of narrative game-based interventions for promoting healthy behaviors, *Journal of Health Communication*, 25(1), 54–65.

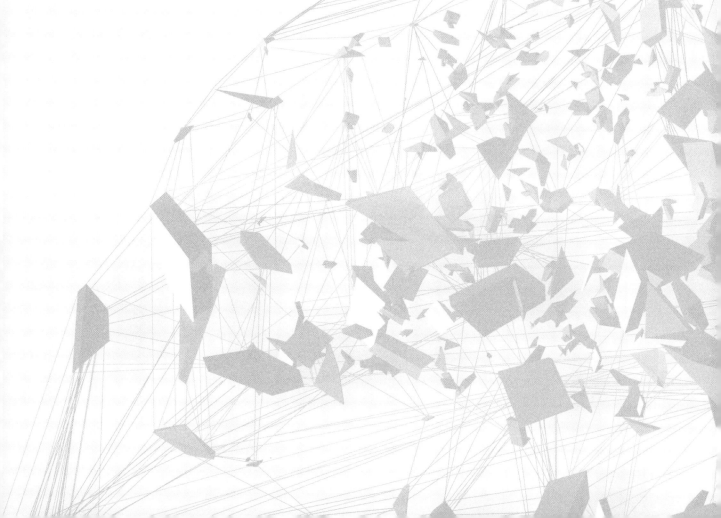

PART 2

Effective communication

Ethics, risk and health promotion

Rod Lamberts

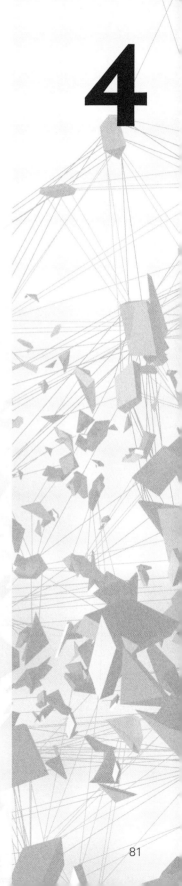

4

LEARNING OBJECTIVES

At the completion of the chapter, you will be able to:

- Apply basic ethical decision-making heuristics to health promotion.
- Understand and appreciate the core principles of risk and how non-specialists might understand risk and make risk-related decisions.
- Articulate and justify critiques of health promotion guidelines informed by ethics and principles for risk perception.
- Adapt perspectives on ethics and risk perception to guide and appraise health promotion endeavours.

Introduction

This chapter introduces basic concepts in ethics, ethical decision-making and risk perception, and examines how they might facilitate the critique of health promotion principles.

The first section outlines what ethics 'are' for the purposes of health promotion and how they relate to morals and laws. It then presents an array of ethical perspectives and decision-making shortcuts that can be applied to health promotion.

The second section provides an overview of some well-known and tested views on risk perception, before considering specific exemplars that offer insights into how we make sense of risk numbers in health and risk-related communication.

Following the overview sections, the chapter closes with examples of codes of ethics from recent health promotion literature and a critique of attempts to create strict ethical and practice criteria for health promotion. It suggests that guidelines for how to think about health promotion need to be flexible, transparent and reflective.

Basic ethical principles

Key concepts: Morals, ethics and the law

A rudimentary discussion of ethics needs a clear delineation between three important terms: morals, ethics and laws.

These concepts all concern judgements of right and wrong, or good and bad, but they locate the basis of these in different places. Teasing apart the differences between them is more than a philosophical exercise: it has practical implications as well, particularly because in practice they can actively clash. While people may argue about the nuances between morals, ethics and the law, there are generally agreed demarcations between these interrelated concepts.

Morals, broadly speaking, tend to concern *personal* values and considerations of rightness, or appropriateness. They are likely to be entwined with an individual's family, community or culture, and may only be tacitly understood by the people who hold them.

'Ethics' refers to considerations of what people should do, usually publicly articulated and often through formal codes and guidelines. The creation of such guidelines involves critical reflection on morals and also laws. Ethical guidelines help professionals choose between options and make decisions that they can justify within their professional community. This is why having a code of ethics is considered to be a necessary characteristic of a professional organisation or society.

In democratic systems, the law ' … tries to create a private space where individuals can live according to their own ethical beliefs or morality [and] … tries to create a basic, enforceable standard of behaviour necessary in order for a community to succeed and in which all people are treated equally' (The Ethics Centre, 2016, para. 9).

To behave ethically is not always to behave morally or legally. For example, a person finds out that a member of their profession, working in a government department, has been incompetent in undertaking their professional duties. This person may feel a moral responsibility to tell the truth regardless of consequences, and so wants to expose the incompetence. Their professional code of ethics could provide contradictory advice: revealing professional incompetence may be required, but in doing so it could bring the profession into disrepute, which is something the code prohibits. On top of this, the law may also have a position, for example, that says the person will be prosecuted for divulging confidential government matters. The 'right' thing to do here is not unambiguous and it depends on perspective. Table 4.1 presents a useful summary of common ethical positions and a selection of **heuristics** for framing ethical choices.

Heuristic – a decision-making rule or process; essentially, a shortcut that enables decisions to be made without having to exhaustively analyse every possible option or perspective

Table 4.1   Common ethical theories and decision-making heuristics

Some common ethical perspectives	
Deontology	Right and wrong are decided against objective moral duties. The right or wrongness of an act is not determined by its consequences, but by the extent to which acts align with duty.
Consequentialism	The only way to make judgements of the right or wrong of an action is on its consequences. This can get trickier when we include foreseen and unforeseen consequences.
Intuitionism	As it sounds, using one's immediate reactions or intuition to judge right or wrong.
Normative	Standards of good and bad, right and wrong for a group. This could be a professional group, a society, a religion or other group. Normative theory describes how people within this group *ought* to think and behave, not necessarily how they actually think and behave. The main aim of this branch of ethics is the consideration, study or formulation of norms about conduct and appraisals of character that can be deemed valid. Pursuits into normative ethics often consider ethics in practical situations.
Utilitarianism	Choices between actions are based on creating the greatest number of positive states for the greatest number of people. It places the needs of the many over the needs of the few. What constitutes a 'positive state' is contestable.
Some heuristics for making (and justifying) ethical choices	
Golden rule	Choosing the action that would result in outcomes that you would be happy to have happen to you. Probably best known as 'do unto others as you would have them do unto you'.
Mentor test	Deciding what to do based on whether you would be happy if your action or decision were judged by an esteemed person in your life such as a parent, teacher or leader.
News (or publicity, or broadcast) test	Imagining how comfortable you would feel if what you were intending to do were broadcast to your community.
Mirror test	Asking yourself if what you were intending to do would cause you shame: could you look at yourself in the mirror without shame if you acted in the manner you are considering?
Role-model test	Considering how you believe a personal role model would act in the situation you find yourself. This is often represented in United States popular culture as 'What would Jesus do?'
'Promise keeping'	Reflecting on your intended action to see if by doing (or not doing) it, you are breaking a promise. A promise does not have to be explicitly made; it can be implicit, like certain behaviours associated with jobs.

Source: Adapted from Lamberts (2012), pp. 132–3.

In the case of health promotion, particularly when the interpretation and communication of risk is critical, a rudimentary appreciation of different ethical positions has direct, practical utility. A health promotion professional will often have to make decisions about what kind information to present to lay people as well as how much to present, what to leave out, when to present it and how. There are ethical implications for all of these choices.

Although the incorporation of ethical principles will not tell us which decision is 'right', it will clarify a variety of perspectives from which to make decisions explicitly and transparently. You can never be absolutely sure you made the right decision, but by formally considering the ethics of the situation, you can at least justify the decisions you have made in ways that can be shared and critiqued.

How risky is risky? Making sense of the numbers

Decisions about our health are among the most important decisions we routinely make. There is more health information around than ever before, and it is more accessible than ever before. But availability of information is not the same as utility of information: having access to health communication does not automatically mean the person is able to understand it – or, better yet, able to choose between competing options.

Critical to making health decisions for ourselves and our loved ones is making determinations about risk. Much like in health promotion, '"risk communication" means communication intended to supply laypeople with the information they need to make informed, independent judgments about risks to health, safety and the environment' (Morgan et al., 2002, p. 5).

In this section, we take a brief look at some risk communication and perception fundamentals that are useful to health promotion. Everyone has biases and can experience difficulties understanding and making risk-related health decisions (Kremer, 2014).

Defining hazard, risk and uncertainty

Hazard, risk and *uncertainty* are three terms that often appear together and are sometimes (incorrectly) used interchangeably.

A 'hazard' is a behaviour, object, attitude or circumstance that has the potential to bring about undesirable consequences. Hazards are *uncertain* if their likelihood and outcomes cannot be quantified and expressed systematically or in terms of their probability. 'Risk' refers to the meaningfully quantified, measured and probabilistically expressed likelihood of a hazard occurring.

Thus, *hazards* are something about which we may wish to make a *risk* calculation. For example, if cigarette smoke is the hazard, the likelihood of getting lung cancer from cigarette smoke can be calculated and expressed as a risk. If we cannot make such a calculation, then the likelihood of a hazard occurring, and the damage it may inflict, is *uncertain*.

Relative versus absolute risks

One other important distinction for health promotion needs to be made here: the difference between *relative* and *absolute* risk (Newson, 2018).

In the context of health, an absolute risk could be the likelihood a group of people will experience a negative health effect under specific conditions, whereas relative risk would be the likelihood one group of people will experience a negative health effect under specific conditions compared to the likelihood that another group under different conditions experiences that same negative health effect. To make this easier to understand, consider the following example, adapted from the European Food Information Council (2017).

Imagine you want to communicate the risks of developing bowel cancer associated with eating bacon over a 10-year period. Two key questions to address and communicate would be:

1. Does eating bacon increase the risk of developing bowel cancer at all?
2. Is the risk greater if you eat no bacon, versus eating a lot of bacon?

In this example, question one concerns *absolute risk*. That is, the likelihood that people who do not eat bacon will have bowel cancer after 10 years. Question two concerns *relative risk*: the likelihood people who eat a lot of bacon will have bowel cancer after 10 years, compared to the likelihood for people who eat no bacon. The example is laid out in Figure 4.1.

No bacon – absolute risk	Lots of bacon – absolute risk
$\frac{6}{100}$ people have bowel cancer after 10 years	$\frac{9}{100}$ people have bowel cancer after 10 years
If you don't eat bacon, you have a 6% chance of developing bowel cancer over 10 years.	If you eat a lot of bacon, you have a 9% chance of developing bowel cancer over 10 years.

No bacon compared to lots of bacon – relative risk
$\frac{9}{100}$ is 50% more than $\frac{6}{100}$
People who eat lots of bacon are 50% more likely to develop bowel cancer than people who eat no bacon over 10 years.

Figure 4.1   An example of absolute versus relative risk: bacon and bowel cancer

You can see how confusing absolute risk with relative risk could give a dramatically different and misleading impression of the likelihood of having bowel cancer after 10 years, based on your consumption of bacon.

Slovic and colleagues (2004) characterise risk in three fundamental ways:

- risk as feelings (fast, instinctive, intuitive reactions to danger)
- risk as analysis (logic, reason, scientific deliberation and management of hazard)
- risk as politics, which arises when the first two clash.

For our purposes, this could be further simplified into a dichotomy in which technical articulations of risk (analysis) contrast with social, cultural or emotional ones (risk as feelings and risk as politics). In essence: risk framed either technically or socially.

This can be articulated as Sandman's now well-known social equation for risk: Risk = hazard + outrage, where outrage is the emotional reaction people may experience should the hazard occur (Sandman, 1988). Outrage may have nothing to do with the technical realities of the risk. In this risk equation, it pays to be at least as focused on discovering and understanding the outrage as the technical or expert assessment of the risk. It is often the case that the thing people are *expressing* outrage about may not be what they are actually upset about.

For example, parents may object to being legally obliged to vaccinate their child before they are allowed to take advantage of public childcare in a number of Australian jurisdictions (National Centre for Immunisation Research and Surveillance, n.d.). Their objection may be expressed as vaccination being something they claim will cause their child harm, but they may be feeling more outrage at having government authorities usurp health decisions they would normally make on behalf of their child.

There are numerous theories and a vast literature considering the plethora of ways we might study and analyse perceptions of risk. There are far too many to cover in this chapter, so a brief overview of some of the more practical ones is provided here before we look at how people make sense of risky numbers in health contexts.

Examining risk perception

Psychological and sociocultural approaches shed some of the most revelatory and pragmatic light on risk perception for the purposes of health promotion. Such approaches focus on how individuals think about risk.

Possibly the most straightforward and immediately applicable psychological theory of risk in communication focuses on what we consider to be 'better' or 'worse' risks. Fischhoff and colleagues (1981) present a series of risk–choice dichotomies which, though simple, provide a useful starting point against which to consider how your intended audiences might be perceiving a health risk. For example, as Table 4.2 shows, we may consider a risk to be more acceptable if we choose to expose ourselves to it rather than having it thrust upon us without consultation. Of course, simple pairs like this will rarely account for the entire complexity of the contexts in which risk perception and communication operate in practice, but they do help inspire us to critically appraise risk perception and communication.

For the purposes of effective communication, the 'mental models' approach (Bostrom et al., 1998) provides a relatively complex, detailed and well-tested mechanism for teasing out how both lay people and experts construct risks in their minds. Mental models provide 'maps' to facilitate comparison between differing perspectives.

Table 4.2   The relative acceptability of a risk: A selection of simple pairs of priorities

Worse risk	Better risk
Imposed	Voluntary
Other control	Own control
Little or no benefit	Clear benefits
Unevenly distributed	Fairly distributed
Human made	Natural
Catastrophic	Statistical
Untrusted source	Trusted source
Exotic	Familiar
Children	Adults

Source: Adapted from Fischhoff et al. (1981).

Information about the mental models people have in their minds about a risk and its context is gathered through a combination of methods – usually surveys, interviews and focus groups. The results are often literally 'mapped out' diagrammatically, using 'mind maps' to show relationships between concepts, issues and stakeholders. The relationships may be overt or explicit, and therefore more amenable to analysis. Lay and expert models can be compared, and the similarities and differences between them used to guide communication interactions and activities.

Sociocultural approaches to risk (Pigeon, 2008) view risk as more than an individual – or psychological – phenomenon. Individual approaches to risks are intrinsically embedded in, and influenced by, broad social mores. Sociocultural perspectives provide pathways for considering how people decide on the acceptability of a risk, based on the organisation of their society, and cultural considerations and values. Such approaches recognise that the perception, experience and relative acceptability of a risk is not based solely on individual assessments and experience. For example, a person's perspective of the acceptability of a risk may vary depending on whether they have been raised in a **hierarchical**, **egalitarian**, **authoritarian** or other culture. Sociocultural theories of risk acceptability enable context-sensitive consideration of the implications of notions of fairness and equity, as well as the pivotal role of politics.

Before looking at some of the ways in which people may struggle to make sense of the statistics when considering risk, we briefly look at a phenomenon that is remarkably simple to understand and is often potent in its effect: framing. In essence, framing refers to the possibility that the same facts can be communicated in different ways – and influence people differently – without misrepresenting or distorting those facts. For example, in what is now a classic study in the communication of medical-related risk, McNeil et al. (1982) asked three different types of people – patients with a variety of chronic medical conditions, graduate students and physicians – to imagine they had lung cancer. They were then asked which of two therapies – radiation or surgery – they would choose to treat the condition.

Hierarchical – a society in which there are clear political ranks, and usually an overt chain of command for making decisions about matters such as policies, laws and how to spend tax dollars

Egalitarian – a society in which people are essentially considered to be equal in terms of making decisions; ideally, a society that uses deliberative and consensus strategies for decision-making regarding its citizens

Authoritarian – a society in which the power and decision-making rests solely, or predominately, in the hands of a ruling class or group, or even a single individual

From the perspective of health promotion, one of the most revealing findings was as follows. In one part of the study, half the participants from the three groups were told the likelihood of being *dead* one year after radiation treatment was 32 per cent. That is, 32 per cent of people receiving it were dead one year after treatment. The other half were told that the likelihood of *surviving* after one year after radiation treatment was 68 per cent. Statistically, this reflects exactly the same situation – the only difference was how it was framed.

Overall, among the group given death statistics, 18 per cent chose radiation over surgery. Among the survival statistics participants, 44 per cent chose radiation over surgery. This pattern of results was present for all three participant types. Framing had a potent effect over and above the communication of a simple statistical fact, even among the physicians.

As Gigerenzer and colleagues (2008) emphasise in their work, which aimed to improve understanding of health statistics, statistical illiteracy among doctors and patients:

a. is common to patients, physicians (and politicians) [parentheses added];
b. is created by non-transparent framing of information in a way that may be unintentional (i.e. a result of lack of understanding) or intentional (i.e. an effort to manipulate or persuade people); and
c. can have serious consequences for health (p. 54).

Risk is usually expressed quantitatively, at least among experts. By using numbers, we strive to explain as objectively as we can the parameters that characterise a risk, and simultaneously try to avoid subjectivity as far as possible. But in health communication contexts, even when using basic numbers, the interpretation of test results can be ambiguous.

In fact, before we even try to ask questions about how we should respond to health-risk information, we need to appreciate that the mere presence of numbers can have an undue influence on our perception of a risk, regardless of how accurate, or even relevant, those numbers are. Case study 4.1 touches on this further as it considers the example of health star ratings for food. The intertwined concepts of **anchoring-and-adjustment** offer one of many common examples of the effects of influence.

Anchoring-and-adjustment – an example of a heuristic (see Table 4.1)

In the following example, people were asked to estimate how many headaches they have in a month, something many people are unlikely to know for certain (West and Meserve, 2012). The answers differed depending on which of these two questions they were asked:

1. How many headaches do you have a month – 0, 1, 2 – how many?
2. How many headaches do you have a month – 5, 10, 15 – how many?

Estimates were systematically higher for responses to the second question. The mere presence of uncontextualised numbers as a suggested baseline influenced people's estimates of their personal experience of headaches. They used the suggested numbers as an anchor and determined their estimates accordingly: higher anchoring numbers led to higher subsequent estimates.

CASE STUDY 4.1 Practical food information, or misleading distraction?

The Health Star Rating (HSR) system is a joint initiative by the Australian federal, state and territory governments, and implemented by public health and consumer groups in 2014. The following extracts provide information about the initiative as well as critiques of the HSR system.

The Australian government's HSR website describes its position on the system (Commonwealth of Australia, 2019):

What is a Health Star Rating?

The Health Star Rating is a front-of-pack labelling system that rates the overall nutritional profile of packaged food and assigns it a rating from ½ a star to 5 stars. It provides a quick, easy, standard way to compare similar packaged foods. The more stars, the healthier the choice.

Why do we need a Health Star Rating?

Most products carry a Nutrition Information Panel which provides important information about the contents of the food. But as shoppers we are busy, so the Health Star Rating provides an easy way to compare similar packaged food and helps you make healthier choices.

Choosing foods that are higher in positive nutrients and lower in risk nutrients that are linked to obesity and diet-related chronic diseases; (saturated fat, sodium (salt), sugars and energy), will help contribute to a balanced diet and lead to better health.

Speaking in 2015 on the first anniversary of HSR implementation, Senator the Hon. Fiona Nash, Assistant Minister for Health noted:

The [HSR promotion] campaign shows how easy the Health Star Rating makes it for shoppers to find the healthiest version of a food on the supermarket shelves (Prime Creative, 2015).

Criticism of the HSR system

A year after implementation, researchers Lawrence and Pollard (2015) stated that:

The system is supposed to help consumers discriminate between similar foods within the same food category that contain different amounts of undesirable ingredients. It should, for instance, help compare two loaves of bread in terms of their salt content.

(cont.)

(cont.)

However, the following issues are notable:

• it is not compulsory, so industry can choose to use it if they wish, therefore
• industry predominately use it on discretionary – or junk – foods (fresh fruit and vegetables are not labelled), and
• the system focuses on nutrients within products, rather than taking a food-based perspective, which is how most consumers think about and purchase their food.

Additionally, research suggests the presence of *any* health information on a label can be enough to make people think the food contained within is 'healthier', regardless of what that food is (Lawrence & Pollard, 2015).

QUESTIONS

1. How could risk perceptions influence the way people interpret HSR?

2. Would it be better if it were compulsory to put these ratings on all food packaging? Why or why not?

3. What is the most defensible position to take as a health promoter (what should a health promoter promote about the HSR system)? How, specifically, would you justify your position (Lawrence & Pollard, 2014; Commonwealth of Australia, 2020)?

ELSEWHERE IN THE WORLD

The Chilean warning label system

In 2016, Chile was the first country worldwide to implement a front-of-package (FoP) warning label to guide consumers' decisions at the point of food purchase (Reyes et al., 2019). Several countries have since followed this model.

Another cognitive bias of particular relevance to making health decisions is called 'base-rate neglect'. This is where we an entire risk scenario is generalised on the basis of just a few, poorly contextualised instances of that scenario. A pertinent example of this in Australia is fatal shark attacks.

From 2001 to 2010, there were 12 fatal shark attacks around Australia (Williamson & Raoult, 2018). From 2011 to early 2014, there had already been seven (Pepin-Neff, 2014) fatal shark attacks. This was interpreted by government and media outlets as an increasing trend in shark attacks. In essence, their reactions were predicated on at least two assumptions about the situation. First, that these events represented a relative increase in shark attacks in circumstances where humans and sharks were coming into contact; and, second, that these events were connected. It led to the

Western Australian government putting drumline traps near popular beaches to catch and kill sharks, to protect people from what they saw as an increased threat.

As Pepin-Neff (2014) reminds us, there is a base-rate neglect problem with this interpretation of the statistics, in context, and it resulted in dramatic culling of endangered shark species. What is critical here is that we do not know how often people and sharks are near each other without anything happening. If there has been a significant increase in human–shark encounters of all kinds, then it is possible that these fatalities, while horrifying, do not represent a disproportionally large increase in attacks.

Does this mean that numbers are useless, even harmful, when striving for clear communication of health information? Actually, no. However, the influences they have may not always be as unambiguous as we might hope.

Technical risk equations may describe a situation accurately and in great detail, and they can certainly help us make better-informed decisions about health. What they can never answer, though, is the question, 'Should I accept this risk?' That still comes down to judgements based on many other factors.

This brief look at risk perception reveals how complicated and context-entwined our relationship with risk concepts and risk-related numbers can be. In the same way that ethics-based assertions make little sense without reference to context and perspective, there is probably no situation in which it makes sense to expect there would be a *context-independent* answer to questions like 'Is this an acceptable risk?'. So how does this apply to health promotion more specifically? To address this question, the next section reviews critiques of attempts to create universal codes and core competencies for health promotion professionals.

Ethical decision-making and obligations in health promotion

There will never be a perfect system in health promotion for deciding exactly what 'the right thing' to do is across all possible contexts and situations: the world is a messy place, as the previous two sections have demonstrated. This means that approaches to making decisions about appropriate health promotion need to be flexible enough to adapt to the contexts in which they are applied. Bull and colleagues (2012) propose that:

> The nature of ... [health promotion] activities involves constant reflection of values across multiple cultures of what is regarded as good and bad health promotion practice. It also involves the consideration of issues related to equity, not only in the distribution of scarce resources in vulnerable communities, but also negotiating distribution of power among various actors and stakeholders. The understanding of what constitutes health and well-being is highly variable, as is the understanding of the good, the fair and the acceptable (p. 9).

In this section we consider a critique of indicative ethical and professional health promotion standards. Doing this underscores the difficulties health promoters face when communicating in situations that are at times ruptured by competing social, cultural, political and technical forces. This complexity is what drives us to look for codes, rules or simple steps to provide simplicity and shows why this striving for simplicity can be so elusive, perhaps even futile.

Health promotion needs to incorporate more than health information that is based on research from the highest levels of the traditional hierarchy of evidence (i.e. randomised control trials and meta-analyses). As Carter and colleagues (2011) note ' … simplistically applying such hierarchies can devalue investigation into both the human subjectivity and the social and cultural complexity that are so important for health promotion' (p. 465). For health promotion, having the best possible technical evidence is only the beginning.

Insights based on ethical principles and information about how people perceive and make choices about risks can provide pragmatic tools for health promotion practitioners to be more effective. By applying such insights, practitioners can avoid the trap of seeking universal principles and methods for health promotion and can encourage them to treat contextual diversity as an inevitable reality to be incorporated, rather than a problem to be fixed or avoided.

There is no single, globally agreed set of ethical guidelines for health promoters, though there have been a number of attempts to articulate one, and they share many characteristics (Bull et al., 2012). In the interests of brevity, we use just one of these to serve as an example of the variety of articulations available.

The International Union for Health Promotion and Education (IUHPE) describes itself as ' … a global professional non-governmental organisation dedicated to health promotion around the world' (IUHPE, n.d.). Among the myriad resources offered by the organisation, the Health Promotion Accreditation System Practitioners Application Form provides a comprehensive list of skills and areas of focus that are critical for anyone interested in becoming formally accredited in health promotion:

1. Enable change. Enable individuals, groups, communities and organisations to build capacity for health-promoting action to improve health and reduce health inequities.
2. Advocate for health. Advocate with, and on behalf of, individuals, communities and organisations to improve health and wellbeing and build capacity for health promotion action.
3. Mediate through partnership. Work collaboratively across disciplines, sectors and partners to enhance the effects and sustainability of health promotion action.
4. Communication. Communicate health promotion actions effectively, using appropriate techniques and technologies for diverse audiences.
5. Leadership. Contribute to the development of a shared vision and strategic direction for health promotion action.
6. Assessment. Conduct assessment of needs and assets, in partnership with stakeholders, in the context of the political, economic, social, cultural, environmental, behavioural and biological determinants that promote or comprise health.
7. Planning. Develop measurable health promotion goals and objectives based on assessment of needs and assets, in partnership with stakeholders.
8. Implementation. Implement effective and efficient, culturally sensitive and ethical health promotion action, in partnership with stakeholders.

9. Evaluation and research. Use appropriate evaluation and research methods, in partnership with stakeholders, to determine the reach, effect and effectiveness of health promotion action.

While not overtly a code of ethics, this accreditation system features nine essential requirements for health promotion professionals, most of which inevitably inspire ethical consideration.

It only takes a cursory scan of the IUHPE criteria to begin to see the potential for ethical dilemmas. For example, the first one, 'Enable change', has as a sub-point the imperative to 'Use health promotion approaches which support empowerment, participation, partnership and equity to create environments and settings which promote health' (IUHPE n.d.). Such sentiments are without question noble, but the realities of implementing communication and action that enable change may have unpredictable and unintended effects that will differ depending on context. The guidance afforded by ethical heuristics and an appreciation of context-specific risk elements would facilitate a practitioner's capacity to adhere to this criterion. Consider Case study 4.2 as an example.

CASE STUDY 4.2 Harm-reduction versus harm-eradication

Pill-testing has been a contested issue in Australia, with state governments taking different positions in response to research and clinical findings. Consider for context the following 2019 headlines from *The Guardian*:

- 'NSW government to ignore most recommendations from inquest into drug deaths at music festivals' (McGowan, 2019)
- 'Australian Capital Territory pushes for national pill-testing after study finds it encouraged people to ditch unsafe drugs' (Karp, 2019)

Two positions are observed in these stories: prohibition, which seeks to eradicate drug use, and harm-minimisation, which seeks to reduce harm. Each of these is discussed.

Prohibition – strive to remove the source of the harm

Core argument

- For people who do not take pills, there are no harms associated with consuming pills. There are, relatively, more harms among people who do take pills, because they take pills.

Proposed solutions?

- Prohibit the availability and consumption of pills.
- Enforce this by punishing suppliers and consumers.

(cont.)

(cont.)

Assumptions

- Prohibition is possible; that is, it will remove the risk of consuming pills because they will ultimately become unavailable.
- Allowing pill-testing will:
  - be seen as condoning illicit drug use (counteracts messages of prohibition) and
  - may encourage some people to start consuming pills, who otherwise would not have.

Pertinent evidence

- Prohibition has failed. People continue to access and consume pills, regardless of their legality.
- Pill-testing does not lead to increased use.

Harm-minimisation: support and facilitate pill-testing

Core argument

- It is sensible to accept that pills will continue to be available and that some people will choose to consume them; therefore, we should make it safer to do so.
- Many people consume pills without experiencing harm.

Proposed solution

- Facilitate pill-testing as a strategy to lower both relative and absolute risk of pill-taking by informing potential consumers about what their pills contain and allowing them to decide what they will do with that information.

Assumptions

- People will keep consuming pills, regardless of their legality (Williams, 2019).
- Pill-testing is sufficiently effective to minimise 'enough' potential harm.
- Consumers are, or can / will be, interested in using pill-testing services.
- Consumers will act 'rationally' according to the information the service provides.

Pertinent evidence

- Prohibition has never succeeded in eliminating illicit drug production, supply and consumption (Morelato et al., 2019).
- Pill-testing is not technically perfect; that is, testing can only identify what is already in existing databases and test for specific and known substances (Haggan, 2019).
- Identifying potentially harmful substances is not a guarantee that the consumer will not still take the pill.

QUESTIONS

1. Pills taken for non-medical/recreational reasons are not always lethal (or even harmful). Should this message be promoted? Why or why not?

2. How do you reconcile that fact that some recreational substances are legal and regulated (though clearly potentially very harmful) while others are not?

3. What is the most defensible position to take as a health promoter (i.e. what should a health promoter promote)? How, specifically, would you justify your position (Thomas, 2018)?

ELSEWHERE IN THE WORLD

An inventory of on-site pill-testing interventions in the European Union

At least seven European Union countries (Austria, Belgium, France, Germany, the Netherlands, Spain and Switzerland) have trialled pill-testing (EMCDDA, 2001). The technical details of pill-testing vary between the countries, as does their legal status.

Empowering one group of people may well mean removing some measure of power and influence from another. This is a situation with myriad ethical implications. As Case study 4.2 (pill-testing) demonstrates, giving consumers of illicit drugs information about the ingredients in their pills is intended to empower them to make informed decisions about whether to ingest these pills. However, if your perspective on illicit drug consumption is that the only way to protect people is to deny access, then the proponents of prohibition and zero-tolerance can be perceived by drug users as threateningly disempowering. Further, the ways in which risks are perceived and communicated in this case vary considerably, with strong appeals to emotion frequently eclipsing empirical evidence.

Criterion 8, 'Implement effective and efficient, culturally sensitive, and ethical Health Promotion action in partnership with stakeholders', provides another example of worthy ideals in theory that could be problematic in practice.

What ethical criteria would you apply in situations in which the medical and epidemiological evidence suggest one course of action, but entrenched habits or traditions dictate a competing one? Even perfunctory examples like this illustrate the need for decision-making advice in health promotion to guide practitioners in thinking about complex situations, rather than striving to create prescriptive lists or codes that inevitably fail to deliver foolproof measures or options.

Bull and colleagues (2012) encapsulate this need in their description of the challenges facing health promotion as a series of tensions:

> Usually the challenges we are confronted with do not present themselves as choices between the obvious good or bad, right or wrong, but rather as choices between degrees

of good and degrees of bad, or good or bad from the perspective of various interests. This constitutes situations of tension, and health promotion literature delineates several such tensions. There is a tension between individual freedom and individual responsibility .... There is also a tension between considerations towards the individual and considerations towards the community .... Distribution of power is another contentious topic within health promotion, with empowerment being a central value of the field. For instance, how does one balance top-down and bottom-up approaches in practical decision-making ...? Other tensions relate to differences in views, values and practices between various groups of professionals, academics, practitioners and communities ... (p. 9)

Such tensions, it seems, could best be tackled through ethical guidelines that help health promotion professionals reflect on possible paths that are also flexible enough to be adapted to the contexts in which they are operating. Bull and colleagues (2012) also note in their survey of health promotions professionals that the vast majority (83% of respondents) saw a ' ... need for a [code of ethics] for health promotion indicat[ing] that health promoters encounter such a wide range of topics and issues that codes from other fields would not suffice' (p. 13). Clearly, this type of response is asking for a code tailored for health promotion specifically. It may be better, however, to offer ethical and risk-based tools to stimulate reflection when making decisions, rather than seeking to create a universal, prescriptive code.

LEARNING ACTIVITY 4.1

Do alcohol warning labels 'work'?

According to research by Coomber and colleagues (2015), the DrinkWise Australia's 'Get the facts' alcohol labelling program failed ' ... to effectively transmit health messages to the general public' (p. 1). Consider this piece of research in the context of the goals, intentions and interest groups associated with DrinkWise Australia (DrinkWise, 2020a) and the 'Get the facts' initiative (DrinkWise, 2020b).

First

Each person should visit and read the three sources mentioned above and take notes in response to the following questions:

1. To what extent would you say 'Get the facts' works?
2. What indicators of success or failure are being used by DrinkWise and the researchers?
3. Did they make these indicators explicit?
4. Did the organisation and the researchers measure success in the same way?
5. Do you agree with their approach to the 'Get the facts' labelling initiative?
6. If you were to ask the organisers of the initiative two questions, what would they be?

Second

Form groups of 3–5 people. In your group, discuss your responses. Ensure everyone provides clear rationales for any conclusions in response to the questions.

Third

As a group, decide how you would approach alcohol labelling.

1. Would you do it at all, or do you not think it is worth it? Why or why not?
2. If you think labelling is not the best approach, propose an alternative.
3. If you *would* do it but in a modified form, would you concentrate on specific people, specific alcohol-related risks or specific geographic locations? Again, justify your decisions.

Your goal as a group is to reach consensus and to justify clearly why you chose your particular approach. The ethical heuristics and risk-perception information in this chapter should help guide you.

In considering the importance of reflection, the inescapable influence of context and the utility of ethics, Carter and colleagues (2011) emphasise that ethical decisions are driven by values, and that this knowledge needs to be incorporated into health promotion thinking and action. They propose a framework of five principles for planning and evaluating health promotion that incorporate this approach.

The first principle emphasises that health promotion thinking must be flexible enough to be able to respond flexibly to the mores of different contexts. The second insists that both evidence-based (i.e. technical evidence) and ethical-based reasoning must be used in concert, and that the values that drive both of them should be made explicit. Related to this, the third principle encourages health promoters to 'Clearly specify the evidential and ethical concepts that are valued or devalued in each situation, and the dimensions along which these vary' (Carter et al., 2011, p. 468). The fourth principle expands on this by advising health promoters to pay attention to the specific ways in which the valued and de-valued concepts interact and are traded off against each other. Finally, the fifth principle highlights a critical value underlying this framework: 'Prioritize procedural transparency: be certain that processes used for reasoning, defining, and trading off can be explained clearly' (Carter et al., 2011, p. 468). For these authors:

> This prioritization of transparency reveals our own values, arising in part from the enlightenment-influenced, democratic society in which we live. Transparency also has pragmatic benefit, as it allows people to make informed judgments by comparing described values with their own, and the steps undertaken with their own procedural standards (Carter et al., 2011, pp. 468–9).

The importance of being transparent about the processes of, and decision-making about, choices seems widely, if often implicitly, shared by many across the health promotion and risk-communication spaces (see, e.g. Kremer, 2014; Lundgren & McMakin, 1998; Gigerenzer et al., 2008; Bull et al., 2012).

It is assumed that providing transparency will facilitate people making their own choices in ways that minimise the effects of biases that communicators bring to their work. This is both a noble and, on the face of it, logical position to take. But it is not without ethical implications itself. For example, providing transparency assumes that people really do want to make their own choices (rather than simply have experts tell them what to do), and that this transparency will provide information that people are actually capable of accessing, understanding and applying. See Case study 4.3 for an example of how complicated this process could be.

Even these few examples form the basis of a persuasive case for the utility of ethics and risk-perception research when making decisions about how to think about, practise and evaluate health promotion efforts in more nuanced ways than simply following a set of rules. There is, of course, much more that could be taken into account than we have considered here. For the purposes of this chapter, though, there are three core themes to remember.

First, the importance of transparency in communicating facts and sources, as well as information about the processes that lead you to the positions you choose to promote. By being transparent about what you included and excluded, what you prioritised (and how), you provide critical information that will help people to interpret and apply the facts and information provided.

Related to transparency is reflectivity. Transparency will be more effective if you openly and iteratively reflect on the information you have, the decisions you make, what you know and do not know, and how you understand all that. Being reflective about your practice, biases and decision-making priorities, for example, facilitates transparency.

Finally, there is flexibility. Simply put, striving for flexibility provides a valuable counterpoint to seeking and applying guidelines, methods and practices as though they are universal, interchangeable and independent of context. Flexibility involves recognising that each health promotion context is unique, and therefore will require active and explicit reflection about what are the best approaches.

CASE STUDY 4.3 They said, they said: Red meat and cancer

The following extracts put forward three positions with respect to recommendations about the consumption of red meat and links between red meat and cancer. Read each extract and then consider the questions that follow.

From the Fox Network:

Public health officials for years have beseeched Americans to limit their consumption of red meat and processed meats, fearing they may be linked to certain diseases. But a new study challenges that very notion.

Published Monday in the *Annals of Internal Medicine*, the study challenges those widespread recommendations to limit the intake of red and processed meats, saying there is no need to cut back.

'The panel suggests adults continue current unprocessed red meat consumption' while also suggesting that adults 'continue current processed meat consumption,' (Johnston et al., 2019) according to the study's guidelines (Genovese, 2019).

From the Harvard T.H. Chan School of Public Health:

A controversial 'dietary guidelines recommendation' published in *Annals of Internal Medicine* suggests that adults can continue to consume red meat and processed meat at current levels of intake.

This recommendation runs contradictory to the large body of evidence indicating higher consumption of red meat—especially processed red meat—is associated with higher risk of type 2 diabetes, cardiovascular disease, certain types of cancers, and premature death (Harvard School of Public Health, 2019).

From the World Health Organization (WHO) Q&A on red meat, processed meat and cancer risk:

Red meat was classified as Group 2A, probably carcinogenic to humans. What does this mean exactly?

In the case of red meat, the classification is based on limited evidence from epidemiological studies showing positive associations between eating red meat and developing colorectal cancer as well as strong mechanistic evidence.

Limited evidence means that a positive association has been observed between exposure to the agent and cancer but that other explanations for the observations (technically termed chance, bias, or confounding) could not be ruled out.

Processed meat was classified as carcinogenic to humans (Group 1). Tobacco smoking and asbestos are also both classified as carcinogenic to humans (Group 1). Does it mean that consumption of processed meat is as carcinogenic as tobacco smoking and asbestos?

No, processed meat has been classified in the same category as causes of cancer such as tobacco smoking and asbestos ([International Agency for Research on Cancer] IARC Group 1, carcinogenic to humans), but this does NOT mean that they are all equally dangerous. The IARC classifications describe the strength of the scientific evidence about an agent being a cause of cancer, rather than assessing the level of risk (WHO, 2015).

QUESTIONS

1. Should you address the differences in interpretation of the article from the *Annals of Internal Medicine* between Harvard and the Fox Network? Why or why not?

2. Would transparency about the processes the two organisations followed in their reporting on the article help people make informed decisions about their consumption of red meat? Why or why not?

(cont.)

(cont.)

3. What is the most defensible position to take as a health promoter (what should a health promoter promote about the dangers or benefits of eating red meat)? How, specifically, would you justify your position (Cancer Council New South Wales, n.d.)?

Ethics, risk and health promotion: Weaving it together

Health promotion is undertaken in complex environments, and often this means that what suits one context may not suit another. Therefore, health promotion practitioners can benefit from flexible, transparent guiding principles so they might adapt their endeavours to the contexts in which they are operating.

But how do we decide what is critical for such principles? This chapter presented a number of ethical theories and decision-making heuristics that could be applied in guiding and critiquing health promotion activities. Adopting an ethics-inspired perspective provides an established language with which to reflect upon, and make explicit, the rationales we use when making decisions about health promotion. This helps make our actions transparent, and the differences in perspectives offered by various ethical heuristics can facilitate flexibility in health promotion planning, delivery and evaluation.

The final section of the chapter presented a brief review of some critiques of health promotion codes of ethics and practitioner guidelines. Although it is understandable that health promoters would want tools to facilitate them doing the best job they can, it is clear that prescriptive criteria will not provide the flexibility required for diverse health promotion contexts. The theme of flexibility emerged as one of three key recommendations to support health promotion efforts adapted to the variety of requirements demanded by diverse contexts.

We also know that health promotion efforts are likely to incorporate risk communication. Like health promotion, risk communication is affected by myriad social, cultural, political and other contextual factors that have little to do with pertinent scientific or expert information.

In another similarity with health promotion, risk communication may need to address public pleas for certainty in situations where scientific and expert consensus does not exist. This, again, is where the need for the flexibility to engage with the specifics of each health promotion context will be critical to success. As Raman and Pearce (2017) succinctly suggest, under such circumstances, rather than seeking absolutes where none exist, 'We are better off trying to facilitate improved ways of appraising and coping with entirely normal uncertainties and reasons for disagreement.' In short, we need strategies for how to think about our tasks, rather than rules for doing them. Fortunately, the abundant literature on risk communication contains invaluable practical advice for health promotion practitioners to do this.

This leads us to what may be the most critical recommendation, that effective health promotion requires transparency: of process, of values and of evidence. Carter and colleagues' (2011) assessment submits that transparency can be enhanced by the application of ethical perspectives and decision-making in health promotion guidelines. Transparency, they argue, should not only further accountability in health promotion, but 'this transparency should increase the effectiveness of risk communication' (Carter et al., 2011, p. 470). Not only can health promotion be improved by the application of sound risk-communication principles; risk communication can be improved by an ethos of transparency in health promotion.

Of course, it is easy to sit back and advocate for greater flexibility and transparency in health promotion, but how do we incorporate these in our planning and activity? It is here that the third theme that emerged from application of risk and ethics to health promotion – reflectivity – comes into play.

Reflectivity is essential to being both transparent and flexible. If active reflection on the processes and decision-making rationales is not applied to health promotion endeavours, they will remain hidden. And if they remain hidden, they will not be amenable to explicit critique and improvement – and your ability to be flexible in the face of changing contexts will be diminished. Ethical decision-making heuristics offer powerful tools for overtly describing and justifying rationales for health promotion decisions. The literature on risk-communication theory and practice includes innumerable avenues for analysing and addressing many of the challenges a health promoter may confront. Regular reflection, both formally and informally, is critical to assessing the extent of your success, and for suggesting ways to improve.

LEARNING ACTIVITY 4.2

Health promotion code of practice and ethics – critical, could be useful, or completely pointless?

This chapter contends that a universal, prescriptive code of practice or ethics for health promotion is likely to be of limited practical use. It suggests that we need guidelines for how to think about health promotion, rather than checklists and codes.

It is easy to offer idealised advice for practitioners that makes theoretical sense, but to what extent do such perspectives reflect reality for health promoters 'on the ground'?

Do you agree? Do you disagree? Maybe you think it's not important, either way?

For this activity, your job is to argue for having very clear codes and guidelines. Think about what cases you can make to support this position and try to pre-empt arguments against them.

You can do this on your own, in pairs or in small groups.

Make sure you clearly justify your arguments. It is not sufficient to simply assert your points without substantiating them with a clear rationale, preferably backed by evidence.

Throughout this activity, make sure you explicitly incorporate the three core themes of transparency, reflectivity and flexibility, both in your process and in your final code or guidelines.

Summary

Health promotion undertakings require a sensitivity to the nuances of the diverse contexts in which they operate. Based on existing critiques of worthy, but rigid, attempts to create and agree upon prescriptive guidelines for health promoters, this chapter proposes that broad guidelines for *ways of thinking* about tasks in context would be more useful than strict codes.

This chapter recommends that efforts to productively enable, even enhance, health communication can benefit from the incorporation of ethical and risk-perception perspectives. It presents examples of common risk and ethics perspectives on decision-making and suggests that applying these will help health promoters effectively to critique and improve their practice by applying three principles: transparency, flexibility and reflectivity.

Ultimately, there is no single, universally applicable approach to health promotion that will work across all possible contexts. By applying guidelines that promote reflection and transparency, health promoters can maximise their ability to flexibly respond to the vagaries of each unique situation they confront and maximise their likelihood of success.

REVISION QUESTIONS

1. How do ethics, morals and laws differ?
2. What is the difference between relative and absolute risk – can you create your own example to explain this difference?
3. Name two ways in which risk perception and ethics can help critique health promotion activities
4. Describe the three principles recommended in this chapter to guide thinking about health promotion.

FURTHER READING

Bernstein, P.L. (1998). *Against the Gods: The remarkable story of risk*. New York: John Wiley & Sons.

Dawson, A. & Grill, K. (2012). Health promotion: Conceptual and ethical issues, *Public Health Ethics*, 5(2), 101–3.

Neher, W.W. & Sandin, P.J. (2017). *Communicating Ethically: Character, duties, consequences and relationships* (2nd ed.). New York: Routledge.

Singer, P. (2011). *Practical Ethics* (3rd ed.). Cambridge: Cambridge University Press.

Slovic, P. (2002). *The Perception of Risk*. London: Earthscan Publications.

REFERENCES

Bostrom, A., Fischhoff, B. & Morgan, M.G. (1998). Characterizing mental models of hazardous processes: A methodology and an application to radon. In R.E. Löfstedt & L. Frewer (eds.), *The Earthscan Reader in Risk and Modern Society* (pp. 225–37). London: Earthscan Publications.

Bull, T., Riggs, E. & Nchogu, S.N. (2012). Does health promotion need a code of ethics? Results from an IUHPE mixed method survey, *Global Health Promotion*, 19(8), doi: 10.1177/1757975912453181

Cancer Council New South Wales (n.d.). Meat and cancer (Website). Retrieved from: https://www.cancercouncil.com.au/21639/cancer-prevention/diet-exercise/nutrition-diet/fruit-vegetables/meat-and-cancer/

Carter, S.M., Rychetnik, L., Lloyd, B., Kerridge, I.H., Baur, L., Bauman, A., Hooker, C. & Zask, A. (2011). Evidence, ethics, and values: A framework for health promotion, *American Journal of Public Health*, 101(3), 465–72.

Commonwealth of Australia (2019). About Health Star Ratings (Website). Retrieved from: http://www.healthstarrating.gov.au/internet/healthstarrating/publishing.nsf/Content/About-health-stars

———(2020). Formal review of the system after five years of implementation (June 2014 to June 2019). Retrieved from: http://www.healthstarrating.gov.au/internet/healthstarrating/publishing.nsf/Content/formal-review-of-the-system-after-five-years

Coomber, K., Martino, F., Barbour, R.I., Mayshak, R. & Miller, P.G. (2015). Do consumers 'Get the facts'? A survey of alcohol warning label recognition in Australia, *BMC Public Health*, 15(816).

DrinkWise (2020a). About (Website). Retrieved from: https://drinkwise.org.au/about-us/about/#

———(2020b). Get the facts: Labelling on alcohol products and packaging (Website). Retrieved from: https://drinkwise.org.au/our-work/get-the-facts-labeling-on-alcohol-products-and-packaging/#

The Ethics Centre (2016, 27 September). Ethics, morality, law – what's the difference? The Ethics Centre (Website). Retrieved from: https://ethics.org.au/ethics-morality-law-whats-the-difference/

European Food Information Council (2017, 1 March). Absolute Risk vs. Relative Risk: What's the difference? EUFIC. Retrieved from: https://www.eufic.org/en/understanding-science/article/absolute-vs.-relative-risk-infographic

European Monitoring Centre for Drugs and Drug Addiction (EMCDDA) (2001). *An inventory of on-site pill-testing interventions in the EU*. Retrieved from: https://www.emcdda.europa.eu/attachements.cfm/att_2879_EN_pill_testing_fact_files.pdf

Fischhoff, B., Lichtenstein, S., Slovic, P. & Keeney, D. (1981). *Acceptable Risk*. Cambridge, MA: Cambridge University Press.

Genovese, D. (2019, 1 October). Why the red meat guidelines you've been following could be wrong, *Fox Business*. Retrieved from: https://www.foxbusiness.com/lifestyle/red-meat-guidelines-health

Gigerenzer, G., Gaissmaier, W., Kurz-Milcke, E., Schwartz, L.M. & Steven Woloshin. (2008). Helping doctors and patients make sense of health statistics, *Psychological Science in the Public Interest*, 8(2), Retrieved from: https://journals.sagepub.com/doi/10.1111/j.1539-6053.2008.00033.x

Haggan, M. (2019). Pill testing: Passing the test, *The Australian Journal of Pharmacy*, 100(1181), 18–20, 22–[23].

Harvard School of Public Health (2019). New 'guidelines' say continue red meat consumption habits, but recommendations contradict evidence, The Nutrition Source (Website). Retrieved from: https://www.hsph.harvard.edu/nutritionsource/2019/09/30/flawed-guidelines-red-processed-meat/

International Union for Health Promotion and Education (IUHPE) (n.d.). *IUHPE Health Promotion Accreditation System Practitioners Application Form.* Retrieved from: https://www.healthpromotion.org.au/images/Sample_Application_Practitioner_LinkK.pdf

Johnston, B.C., Zeraatkar, D., Han, M.A., Vernooij, R.W.M., Valli, C., El Dib, R., Marshall, C., Stover, P.J., Fairweather-Taitt, S., Wójcik, G., Bhatia, F., de Souza, R., Brotons, C., Meerpohl, J.J., Patel, C.J., Djulbegovic, B., Alsonso-Coello, P.A., Bala, M.M. & Guyatt, G.H. (2019). Unprocessed red meat and processed meat consumption: Dietary guideline recommendations from the nutritional recommendations (NutriRECS) Consortium, *Annals of Internal Medicine,* Retrieved from: https://www.acpjournals.org/doi/10.7326/M19-1621

Karp, P. (2019, 10 December). ACT pushes for national pill-testing after study finds it encouraged people to ditch unsafe drugs, *The Guardian.* Retrieved from: https://www.theguardian.com/australia-news/2019/dec/10/act-pushes-for-national-pill-testing-after-study-finds-it-encouraged-people-to-ditch-unsafe-drugs

Kremer, W. (2014, 7 July). Do doctors understand test results? *BBC World Service.* Retrieved from: https://www.bbc.com/news/magazine-28166019

Lamberts, R. (2012). Ethics and accountability in science and technology. In J.K. Gilbert & S.M. Stocklmayer (eds.), *Communication and Engagement with Science and Technology Issues and Dilemmas – A reader in science communication.* New York: Routledge.

Lawrence, M. & Pollard, C. (2014, 26 February). Food labels are about informing choice, not some nanny state, *The Conversation.* Retrieved from: https://theconversation.com/food-labels-are-about-informing-choice-not-some-nanny-state-23320

———(2015, 13 July). A year on, Australia's health star food-rating system is showing cracks, *The Conversation.* Retrieved from: https://theconversation.com/a-year-on-australias-health-star-food-rating-system-is-showing-cracks-42911

Lundgren, R.E. & McMakin, A.H. (eds.) (1998). *Risk Communication: A handbook for communicating environmental, safety, and health risks* (2nd ed.). Colombus: Battelle Press.

McGowan, M. (2019, 11 December). Drug deaths inquest: Gladys Berejiklian says she is 'closing the door' on pill testing, *The Guardian.* Retrieved from: https://www.theguardian.com/australia-news/2019/dec/11/drug-deaths-inquest-gladys-berejiklian-says-she-is-closing-the-door-on-pill-testing

McNeil, B.J., Pauker, S.G., Sox, H.C. & Tversky, A. (1982). On the elicitation of preferences for alternative therapies, *New England Journal of Medicine,* 306(21), 1259–62.

Miles, F. (2019, 14 October). Is red meat safe to eat or not? Food advice is confusing Americans, *Fox News.* Retrieved from: https://www.foxnews.com/health/red-meat-food-advice-confusing-americans

Morelato, M., Fu, S. & Roux, C. (2019, 17 May). Two perspectives on pill testing, UTS (Website). Retrieved from: https://www.uts.edu.au/news/health-science/two-perspectives-pill-testing

Morgan, M.G., Fischhoff, B., Bostrom, A. & Atman, C.J. (2002). *Risk Communication: A mental models approach.* New York: Cambridge University Press.

National Centre for Immunisation Research and Surveillance (n.d.). National and state legislation in relation to immunisation requirements for child care. Retrieved from: http://www.ncirs.org.au/public/no-jab-no-play-no-jab-no-pay

Newson, L. (2018, 31 January). Calculating absolute risk and relative risk, *Patient*. Retrieved from: https://patient.info/news-and-features/calculating-absolute-risk-and-relative-risk

Pepin-Neff, C. (2014, 14 January). Shark bite statistics can lie, and the result is bad policy, *The Conversation*. Retrieved from: https://theconversation.com/shark-bite-statistics-can-lie-and-the-result-is-bad-policy-21789

Pigeon, N. (2008). Risk, uncertainty and social controversy: From risk perception and communication to public engagement. In G. Bammer & M. Smithson (eds.), *Uncertainty and Risk: Multidisciplinary perspectives* (pp. 349–61). New York: Earthscan Routledge.

Prime Creative (2015, 8 July). Health Star Rating awareness campaign enters second stage, *Food and Beverage*. Retrieved from: https://www.foodmag.com.au/health-star-rating-awareness-campaign-enters-second-stage/

Raman, S. & Pearce, W. (2017, 24 August). Why we should expect scientists to disagree about antibiotic resistance – and other controversies, *The Conversation*. Retrieved from: https://theconversation.com/why-we-should-expect-scientists-to-disagree-about-antibiotic-resistance-and-other-controversies-82609

Reyes, M., Garmendia, M.L., Olivares, S., Aqueveque, C., Zacarías. I. & Corvalán, C. (2019). Development of the Chilean front-of-package food warning label, *BMC Public Health*. Retrieved from: https://doi.org/10.1186/s12889-019-7118-1

Sandman, P. (1988). Risk communication: Facing public outrage. *Management Communication Quarterly*, 2(2), 235–8.

Slovic, P., Finucane, M.L., Peters, E. & MacGregor, D.G. (2004). Risk as analysis and risk as feelings: Some thoughts about affect, reason, risk and rationality. *Risk Analysis*, 4(2), 311–32.

Thomas, M. (2018, 2 May). The pros and cons of pill-testing. Parliament of Australia (Website). Retrieved from: https://www.aph.gov.au/About_Parliament/Parliamentary_Departments/Parliamentary_Library/FlagPost/2018/May/The_pros_and_cons_of_pill_testing

West, R.F. & Meserve, R.J. (2012). Cognitive sophistication does not attenuate the bias blind spot, *Journal of Personality & Social Psychology*, 103(3), 506–19.

Williams, E. (2019, 20 November). Greens leader Shane Rattenbury rues 'missed opportunity' with no pill testing planned for spilt milk, *The Canberra Times*. Retrieved from: https://www.canberratimes.com.au/story/6502385/no-spilt-milk-pill-testing-a-missed-opportunity/

Williamson, J. & Raoult, V. (2018, 27 February). FactFile: The facts on shark bites and shark numbers, *The Conversation*. Retrieved from: https://theconversation.com/factfile-the-facts-on-shark-bites-and-shark-numbers-76450

World Health Organization (WHO) (2015, 26 October). Q&A on the carcinogenicity of the consumption of red meat and processed meat (Website). Retrieved from: https://www.who.int/features/qa/cancer-red-meat/en/

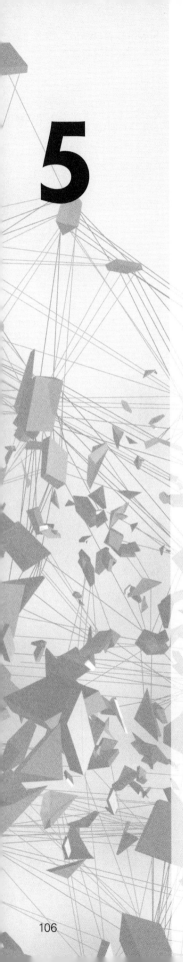

5

Influencing factors and empowering decision-making

Will J. Grant

LEARNING OBJECTIVES

At the completion of the chapter, you will be able to:

- Apply an understanding of audience differences, media framing and psychological biases to assessment of communication challenges.
- Engage with pathways for behavioural and attitudinal change, other than by reciting facts.
- Describe and employ strategies and techniques for overcoming resistance.
- Apply principles of knowledge translation towards putting evidence into action.

Introduction

Imagine you have been tasked with persuading a frightened, confused and injured person to cooperate with a medical professional who is using a complicated piece of new equipment. You see the patient is looking puzzled and is perspiring. From behind you come the ominous-sounding 'pings' of the machine. What do you do?

Whatever you decide, it is likely that you would like to have more information. Why is this person frightened? Why are they confused? Why and how are they injured? What might they be thinking? What might they be feeling?

You are hoping for more information because, in its essence, the scenario described above is inadequate. There could be thousands of reasons the person is frightened, thousands of reasons they are confused and thousands of different things they might be thinking and feeling. If you are to persuade them to follow instructions, you will need to know more. At heart, we all know intuitively that there is no one-size-fits-all message that would persuade everyone who might be frightened, confused and injured to follow medical advice. There is no 'silver bullet' for communication. So what do we do? This chapter seeks to explore this dilemma.

This chapter examines the factors that influence whether people accept or reject health messages, and discusses how to engage and empower people to formulate their decisions based on credible and trustworthy information. The chapter begins with an exploration of perceptions of public health and medical framing, before turning to why facts do not, in and of themselves, convince people to change their behaviour. It then outlines the factors that influence acceptance or rejection of a message or idea, and how we can overcome resistance with empathy and by finding common ground.

The chapter encourages you to think of communication not as an end goal – some state of message clarity we might strive for – but as a continuing, dialogic process through which we can empower those with whom we are working.

Understanding perceptions

This chapter began with a scenario of persuasion: asking you to imagine how you would persuade a frightened, confused and injured person to cooperate with a medical professional. If we are to successfully communicate with an audience – on any topic, with any goal – then it is essential first and foremost that we abandon any idea of a 'one-size-fits-all' or 'silver-bullet' approach to communication. This idea may disappoint. Many coming from a scientific background may hope that logic and facts are universal languages, and that the straightforward facts of the matter will connect with anyone. That is not the case.

This section explores the ways in which people might perceive the work done in public health, and how the media frames various health issues.

Public health – hero, nanny or not thought of at all?

Those working within public health have a storied understanding of their effect on the world. From foundational narratives of John Snow's cholera map (see Rogers, 2013) to lists of the 10 great public health achievements of the 20th century (CDC, 1999), public health scholars, students and their supporters regularly talk of the ways in which vaccines, clean drinking water, safety regulations and other interventions have transformed lives around the world.

These have been, of course, significant interventions and achievements. To reduce them to very simplistic terms, these interventions have been integral in dramatically increasing the duration and quality of human lives around the world (Roser et al., 2019), and this has been – all other things being equal – something humans in general (probably) want.

There is nothing wrong with celebrating these successes. The effects on the world of the ideas and people in public health have been enormous. But self-describing in such a transformative, positive light may cause people working in public health to be blinded to how the rest of the world sees the discipline. For argument's sake, we could narrow it down to three potential ways the rest of the world sees public health. One is positive: like the internal picture, as 'hero'. One is neutral: for many people, the field is probably not thought of at all. But the third view is hostile: the field of public health is considered as the 'pointy, scolding end of the freedom-hating nanny state'.

The Centers for Disease Control and Prevention's (CDC) list of Ten Great Public Health Achievements in the United States makes for fertile ground to tease out these attitudes. The list includes such things as vaccination, motor-vehicle safety, safer workplaces, control of infectious diseases, safer and healthier foods, family planning, water fluoridation and tobacco control (CDC, 1999). Undoubtedly, many of us encounter the results of these interventions in our lives every day – putting on seat belts, vaccinating children or seeing the designated smoking areas around public buildings. Many might consider them as part of a narrative; for example, that 'cars are in general getting safer', or 'families are getting smaller'.

Yet, while significant proportions of society are interested in health (see Lamberts et al., 2010), we would be deluded if we thought such interventions formed an important part of most people's dinner-table conversations. While we do not have data on dinner-party conversations, we can draw a proxy from a social media platform such as Twitter. As Zhao and Jiang (2011) have shown, health is typically the topic of less than 5 per cent of tweets. If health is talked about in households, then individual health issues (shown through the most commonly found words such as ageing, skin, sick, hurts, cough) or global pandemics, when they occur ('flu, swine, #H1N1 and, of course, COVID-19), are far more likely to be discussed (Zhao & Jiang, 2011) than the more incremental public health interventions those in the public health community might hold dear. It is doubtful if sugar taxes, the widths of footpaths and health star ratings ever make it to most people's dinner-party conversations. Perhaps if these issues had more relevance to individuals, this might change (see Case study 5.1).

Meanwhile, a third discourse can be far more hostile. For some, the achievements of public health – such as the CDC's list above – were unwelcome interventions at the time, and only the start of more interventions to come. While those who hold this view may have come to grudgingly accept some of the main interventions, for those who hold these views public health remains the unwelcome front of the **'nanny state'** (Jochelson, 2006). We can see such discourse today in debates over a proposed introduction of a sugar tax; for example, Marar's (2018) assertion that 'a sugar tax is another attack on freedom and personal responsibility'. Yet, these kinds of assertions

Nanny state – a pejorative term for government intervention in typically health-related areas, particularly regarding what people do, eat and drink

have probably emerged alongside nearly every public health intervention. Jochelson (2006), for example, traces similar discourse in the 19th century:

> The first British Public Health Act, passed in 1848, gave local government powers over the water and sewerage systems and was opposed for being 'paternalist' and 'despotic'. For one newspaper 'a little dirt and freedom' was 'more desirable than no dirt at all and slavery' (p. 1150).

At this point it should be recognised that such a line of argument is far from an unbiased assessment of a field of work. Cries of 'Nanny state!' are very often made by or on behalf of those who wish to continue benefiting from the status quo (Monbiot, 2013). So, how should we in health promotion deal with these attitudes?

First, it would be foolish to think we could change these attitudes by asserting that they are incorrect. People have every right to pay attention to – or ignore – whatever issues they want. But more importantly, it would be erroneous to simply assert that the work of public health is not interventionist, as the libertarians decrying the 'nanny state' argue. The label 'nanny state' is clearly pejorative, but the work of public health is, by its very nature, interventionist. We may very much desire to change people's lives for the better, but the fact we want to change people's lives at all will be unwanted by some. Perhaps the wisest course of action is to recognise people's existing attitudes (and the underlying economic environment supporting them) and to build from there. Later sections of this chapter explore what to do.

CASE STUDY 5.1 Wash your hands!

Hand hygiene is simple, but not common

Perhaps ever since public health workers started advocating it, we humans have been poor at washing our hands. As Borchgrevink and colleagues noted in 2013, barely anyone did the recommended 20 seconds of good, hard scrubbing with soap to maintain hand hygiene. Just 5.3 per cent of their sample washed their hands for 15 seconds or longer (Borchgrevink et al., 2013). Even among people you would think would know better – researchers working in laboratories with viruses, hospital staff, for example – perfect handwashing has been hard to enshrine (Hamblin, 2020; Yong, 2020).

But that was 'pre-pandemic'.

Changing behaviour in response to a threat

This chapter is being written during a time of significant reaction to the COVID-19 pandemic. One of the main defences against the spread of the virus has been the practice of good hygiene, in particular covering coughs and sneezes with masks and elbows and washing hands frequently. Governments around the world commenced

(cont.)

(cont.)

significant mass-information campaigns to encouraging the practice, and others on social media dived in to reinforce the messages. Verified peer-reviewed statistics on handwashing may only be available long after the pandemic, and so it is difficult to know what handwashing practices are like at the time you are reading this. But the available anecdotes (Hamblin, 2020; Yong, 2020) already suggest mass movement towards better hand hygiene.

QUESTIONS

1. What do you think has caused people to change their behaviour in this way at the population level?

2. The COVID-19 pandemic brought about a time of great uncertainty, and in eastern Australia came very soon after a prolonged and highly destructive bushfire season. Communications in both of these situations included brief 'dot point' communications and instructions on what people could do to stay safe. Thinking about personal motivations and values, do you think this communication approach is effective, and why or why not? Support your answer with examples.

ELSEWHERE IN THE WORLD

Global Handwashing Partnership

Established in 2001, the Global Handwashing Partnership (https://globalhandwashing .org) works through programs and advocacy initiatives to strengthen handwashing practices locally, nationally and internationally. One such advocacy initiative is the promotion of Global Handwashing Day, which is held on 15 October each year. This is an opportunity for groups around the world to raise awareness of the proper way to wash hands, using soap and water as a way to prevent disease. In Indonesia, for example, school students have given performances about handwashing (including handwashing songs) and have filmed instructional videos on proper handwashing technique, which have been shared on social media.

Framing

The ways people think about the interventions proposed by the public health community (or, indeed, the ways people think about any public topic) depend enormously on the **framing** of the topic in the media they are exposed to. As Chong and Druckman (2007, p. 100) describe it:

> virtually all public debates involve competition between contending parties to establish the meaning and interpretation of issues. When citizens engage an issue – be it social security, foreign aid, a hate-group rally, affirmative action, or the use of public funds for

Framing – a way of presenting an issue so as to promote particular interpretations of the causes of the issue and potential solutions; framing can influence perceptions of who or what is responsible for the issue

art – they must grapple with opposing frames that are intended by opinion leaders to influence public preferences.

George Lakoff (2004), in his classic *Don't Think of an Elephant!* holds that:

> frames are mental structures that shape the way we see the world. As a result they shape the goals we seek, the plans we make, the way we act, and what counts as a good or bad outcome of our actions. In politics our frames shape our social policies and the institutions we form to carry out policies. To change our frames is to change all of this. Reframing is social change (xv).

To draw on the example of a sugar tax, a public health advocate might frame it as a sensible intervention that might save lives and money. We can see, for example, Demaio (2016) describing such policies as 'good', 'sensible' and 'practical'. While readers of this text may well agree with Demaio's conclusions and the evidence he uses to support them, the terms 'good, sensible and practical' are adjectives, not context-free facts. They are ways of framing a reader's thinking so as to associate a sugar tax with values of sensible, practical – good – public policy. However, if we were to turn to a libertarian – or an advocate for the sweetened-beverage industry – we might instead see words that frame sugar taxes as an attack on freedom or personal responsibility. Satyajeet Marar (2018), for example, decries the concept of a sugar tax as an 'immoral', 'experimental', 'nanny state' intervention that will not work ('we know that they have not reduced obesity rates in the four countries that have experimented with them'), and that will have a strong effect on employment:

> But even putting all these points aside, sugar taxes are fundamentally immoral because they punish people for making free and informed choices to indulge themselves using their hard-earned cash. When we use the tax system to single out drinking, eating or other human pleasures rather than immoderate consumption of these products which is the ultimate issue, we send the implicit message that human adults cannot be trusted to exercise these activities responsibly and diminish the role of individual accountability as a result (Marar, 2018).

It should be stressed at this point that both these arguments – that the sugar tax is a good and sensible intervention that will save lives and money, and that it is an immoral intervention in people's freedoms – weave both factual evidence and values. The factual evidence in both arguments is testable (Will it save lives? Is it an intervention in people's lives?), but in this case is probably true. Both also are seeking to associate these facts with value assertions about the role government should play in people's lives. What Marar and Demaio are seeking to do is to frame the policy in light of particular values. It's worth asking: 'Which of these values do we personally hold most dear?'

Importantly, acknowledging the frame used by an opponent – even to negate it – could still work to reinforce the opponent's frame. There are those, for example, who might see the headline of Demaio's article, 'Sugar tax is not nanny state, it's sound public policy', and walk away only with a slight reinforcement of the association between 'sugar tax' and 'nanny state' (see the backfire effect, later in this chapter).

Why facts do not work

Working in the world of scientifically based medicine and health – whether conducting research directly or working to implement the results of that research into policies and behaviours in the wider world – we are trained to orient ourselves towards facts. We are trained to remember a series of facts throughout our education, and trained to think, along lines famously articulated by philosopher of science Karl Popper (2005), that the progress of knowledge hinges on the gradual establishment and refutation of facts. As Popper argued, a theory is falsified 'if we discover a reproducible effect which refutes the theory' (p. 66). Put simply, minds are changed by facts.

But the world – including in fact the scientific world (Kuhn, 1962) – does not work like that. People do not change their minds based on facts.

Personal values and beliefs

Throughout the 2020 COVID-19 pandemic, polling company Civiqs released data on concerns about the coronavirus outbreak in the United States. Separated by political affiliation, the result (shown in Figure 5.1) is stark: Democrats were far more likely to be concerned about the pandemic than Republicans. Though there may be some

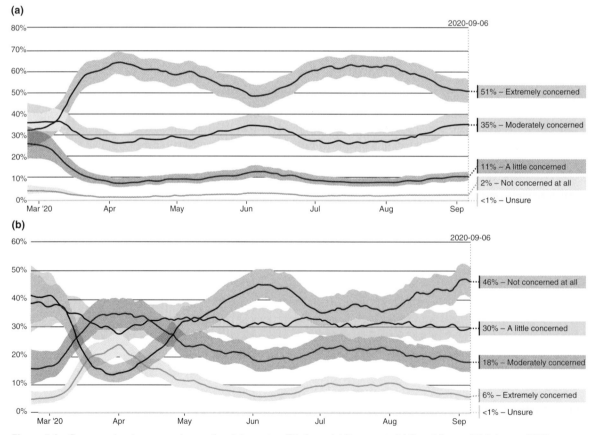

Figure 5.1   Concern about a coronavirus outbreak by party affiliation – (a) Democrat; (b) Republican – 25 February 2020 to 6 September 2020

Source: Civiqs (2020a, 2020b).

demographic differences between the two groups – Democrats were more likely to live in cities, Republicans were more likely to be older – there's no profound difference in their risk profile towards the disease such as would warrant this divide. Instead, to understand the differences displayed in Figure 5.1, we have to recognise that our worldviews and values dramatically influence how we see the world in general, and how we process information.

Demonstrating this, a range of scholars have used objectively neutral mathematics questions – that is, questions where there is a right and wrong answer – to show that our political orientations and worldviews shape how we approach even technically neutral data. The results of these studies demonstrate that politically polarising topics such as gun control (Kahan et al., 2017) and climate change (Nurse & Grant, 2019) dramatically affect our ability to answer these neutral mathematics questions. As Nurse and Grant (2019) note, even those having high mathematical ability use so-called 'system two' or systematic logical thinking 'to rationalize their beliefs in the face of contradictory evidence' (p. 3).

LEARNING ACTIVITY 5.1

Individually or in small groups, run a search online for the phrase 'sugar tax'. Then select three or four articles from the first two pages of results. As most search engines provide slightly tailored results, members of the group may get slightly different results. Taking those articles, search for the phrases or keywords used to support – or argue against – a sugar tax, being careful to highlight concrete, falsifiable evidence (e.g. rates of obesity going up or down; tax collection going up or down) and values assertions (e.g. freedom or greater good).

QUESTION
What value assertions were raised for (in defence of) the policy? What values were raised against the policy?

EXTENSION QUESTION
Which of the lines of concrete evidence and which values were more appealing to you or to other members of your group? Why?

Remember that it is legitimate to use logic to critique your own or another student's (or the writer's) evidence and to use that evidence, but it is not acceptable to critique their values.

Confirmation bias

Building on our worldview-dependent interpretation of neutral information, there is also evidence that our news-seeking behaviours are highly selective. Here, **confirmation bias** means that we all 'notice and give more credence to information that agrees with views we already hold. We are attuned to seeing and accepting things that confirm what we already know, think and believe' (Grant & Lamberts, 2014). This manifests

Confirmation bias – the seeking or interpreting of information and evidence in ways that are partial to existing beliefs, expectations or hypotheses (Nickerson, 1998)

in a range of health scenarios; for example, when exploring vaccination information, 'people select more belief-consistent information compared to belief-inconsistent information' and perceive 'belief-confirming information as being more credible, useful, and convincing' (Meppelink et al., 2019, p. 129).

The backfire effect

So, if we notice the things we like, what does that mean for the things we do not like? Nyhan and Reifler (2010, p. 307) note that 'individuals who receive unwelcome information may not simply resist challenges to their views. Instead, they may come to support their original opinion even more strongly'. This is the **backfire effect**. Importantly, the backfire effect suggests that attempting to correct misinformation by 'putting out the correct information' is likely not only to be ignored but may even further entrench opposed views. Examples can be found in a range of decision-relevant areas, again vaccination (Thornock, 2017), public health decisions in politics (Nyhan & Reifler, 2010) and nutrition (Skurnik et al., 2005).

Backfire effect – the effect whereby individuals who are presented with information that contradicts their prior beliefs come to support their original opinion more stridently (Nyhan & Reifler, 2010)

Overcoming resistance

The goal of this chapter is not to wallow in the fact that people do not listen to facts, but instead to provide pathways through which to engage with audiences and to overcome resistance to the health behaviours we might want to instil. This section focuses on a number of crucial communication tactics you can employ to overcome resistance in your audience.

Using empathy in communication

This chapter began with a scenario – of a frightened, confused and injured person who you were trying to get to cooperate with a medical professional. There was little information in the scenario: nothing about the language spoken, nothing about why the person was confused or about their injury. Information about all of these would be useful to help persuade the person to engage. But perhaps more than anything, beginning from a standpoint of **empathy** might make all the difference.

Empathy – the ability and practice of seeking to understand and share the feelings of another

Learning activity 5.2 explores an activity called 'The Rant'. Participants are asked to 'rant' to a partner on a topic that infuriates them – a clear negative emotion. (This could similarly be done with a range of other negative emotions, such as in the scenario at the beginning of the chapter, fear.) Following the rant, the partner is asked to introduce the person, detailing something that they care deeply about. Here, the concept of infuriation and care are treated as two sides of the same coin, in that someone is only infuriated when something they value is being negated.

So, why does empathy help with communication? At its core, empathy is about understanding both the nature of someone's emotional state and what has brought that state into being. It should be noted that a truly empathetic engagement will mean that you, too, are open to sharing your feelings, and indeed to changing your mind. It may well be that the reasons someone is not following your advice are legitimate and compelling. Is it truly empathetic, for example, to attempt to convince inpatients in mental health facilities not to smoke? (See Connolly et al., 2012.)

If you are able to understand what someone values, then you will be more able to persuade them of what you want. This means more than acknowledging and attempting to salve the negative emotions they may be experiencing and the resistance they may be displaying. Instead, it means attempting to understand what is driving them, and then engaging with that. It provides you with a shared position to start from, rather than a dichotomy of right and wrong.

LEARNING ACTIVITY 5.2

This activity asks you to engage in a small piece of role-play exploring empathy and listening. It takes 10 minutes for a group of 20 participants, longer if there are more. It can be played with any number of participants but is best played with an even number.

First, form a circle, and within that find a partner. In the first part of the exercise, each pair takes two minutes to 'rant' to their partner about a topic that makes them extraordinarily frustrated. The topic can be anything – the failures of your sporting team, poor share-house etiquette, teenagers who don't pick up their washing. While one person is ranting, their partner must listen quietly, without saying anything, nodding, smiling or engaging in any way. When one partner has ranted for two minutes (set a timer – be strict about this), swap so the other partner can rant about their topic, with the same rules.

Q1: Both roles here can be quite difficult. How easy or hard was it for you to rant about something for two minutes? Likewise, how easy or hard was it for you not to react to the person ranting? How did it make you feel to not get any reaction from your audience? For each of these questions, explore why.

Following the rant, everyone then takes a turn to introduce their partner to the group, using this specific format: 'Hi everyone, I'd like to introduce my new friend … they care deeply about … ' Here, the task is to reverse the negative emotion of the rant by looking for the positive values that drive that emotion. For example, is it love for their community, desire to make a difference or perhaps belief in the importance of mutual respect?

Q2: How did being introduced in such a positive way make you feel, and why?

This activity builds deep listening skills and asks us to find ways to empathise even with people we disagree with. We may have different opinions, but we all share some common values and that is a place to start productive communications.

Source: Adapted from a workshop at Alan Alda Center for Communicating Science, Stony Brook University, New York.

EXTENSION QUESTION
Can the values different participants have articulated be ranked? Which are perhaps closest to their deep values of life; which might be trivial manifestations of deeper feelings?

Identifying common ground

How can we engage with someone who has deeply held beliefs that are potentially radically opposed to our own? It is not always possible. Case study 5.2 documents the story of two college students in the United States: one an Orthodox Jew, the other an avowed white nationalist. Rather than ignoring and ostracising each other, Matthew Stevenson (the Orthodox Jew in this story) reached out to the white nationalist (Derek Black) and found a way to include him in college society. Eventually, after many shared dinners and conversations, Derek disavowed his former ideology. Of course, it took bravery on the part of Matthew to make an offer of openness to someone whose ideology considered him to be subhuman; it took bravery to step beyond that ideology and accept Matthew as a person. At the heart of this story of personal transformation is the recognition that no productive conversation can happen without the interlocutors finding **common ground**. To do so, Derek and Matthew had to start with something they did share: dinner, Arabic grammar or marine aquatics. It is unlikely that, had they started with a discussion of the politics of race, any productive or sensible conversation would have been possible. Common ground is an essential beginning for any successful communication.

Common ground – points of shared values or interests between two or more individuals

CASE STUDY 5.2 A narrow slice of common ground

The story of a white supremacist

Derek Black had grown up immersed in racism and hate. His father, Don, had launched the neo-Nazi website Stormfront and his mother, Chloe, had once been married to Ku Klux Klan Grand Wizard David Duke. Derek's childhood had included road trips to help his father organise white supremacist rallies, and at the age of 10 years Derek launched a white nationalist website for children (Saslow, 2016).

When Derek finished high school, he enrolled at the New College in Florida, where he could study medieval European history. But during his time there Derek also began something of a double life. He concealed his political views from his new friends, while continuing to espouse them away from the college. But this double life was not to last. Eventually Derek's fellow students discovered his secret and he was summarily ostracised (Solomon, 2016). Some of Derek's classmates saw an opportunity. 'Ostracizing Derek won't accomplish anything,' one wrote. 'We have a chance to be real activists and actually affect one of the leaders of white supremacy in America … Who's clever enough to think of something we can do to change this guy's mind?' (Saslow, 2016).

Inclusion, not exclusion

Matthew Stevenson was the only Orthodox Jew at New College. Figuring he might be able to change Black's ideology, Matthew reached out: 'What are you doing Friday night?' He decided his 'best chance to affect Derek's thinking was not to ignore him or confront him, but simply to include him' (Saslow, 2016).

Derek accepted. That night, there was not as many people at Matthew's dinner group as usual, but the conversation was polite. Derek returned the next week, and the next. Eventually, attendances increased and the dinners grew back to their former size. On the rare occasions when Derek directed conversation during those dinners, it was about the specifics of Arabic grammar, marine aquatics or the roots of Christianity in medieval times. He presented as smart and curious, and mostly he listened (Saslow, 2016).

Eventually, Derek disavowed his former ideology. 'After a great deal of thought … I have resolved that it is in the best interests of everyone involved to be honest about my slow but steady disaffiliation from white nationalism. I can't support a movement that tells me I can't be a friend to whomever I wish or that other people's races require me to think of them in a certain way or be suspicious at their advancements' (cited in Saslow, 2016).

Thinking fast or slow

Nobel prize winner Daniel Kahneman's *Thinking, Fast and Slow* presents a useful dichotomy between the fast, instinctual and emotional 'system 1' form of thinking, and the slower, more deliberative and more logical 'system 2' form of thinking (Kahneman, 2011). Ostracism would appear to be a natural response; however, it is an example of a system 1 response; a 'knee-jerk' reaction. If we are to affect change – any change – then we have to engage our strategic brains.

QUESTIONS
Reflect on Matthew's actions of inclusion rather than exclusion. Imagine you were in the same situation – do you think you could respond the same way? Why or why not?

EXTENSION QUESTION
Issues in health are sometimes contentious and hotly contested; an example is vaccination. Examine some of the reasons people resist or campaign against vaccination and see if you can identify the underlying values that cause them to do so. Based on your findings and Kahneman's dichotomy, develop a system 2-type response, building upon the common ground (values) you can identify.

The scenario that began this chapter – of a frighted, confused and injured person you are trying to convince to engage with a medical professional – draws significantly from Learning activity 5.3. In this exercise, participants are asked to imagine a significant gulf in communication between people from two radically different time periods. Like Tolstoy's unhappy families, there are myriad ways people can fail at this exercise – cajoling, using jargon familiar only to modern medical professionals, lying, relying on the ethos of medical expertise. But there is a certain unity in those who are successful in this exercise: they recognise intuitively that it is the speaker's job to speak in ways – whether words, tone, metaphors or examples – that resonate with the audience.

This is a fundamental point of communication. As the audience always decides if communication is successful, it is our job as we seek to communicate to work, with respect and empathy, to use their words and metaphors, to echo their tone. Different styles of communication will work with different people; our job must always be to work first to understand what will work with that audience.

LEARNING ACTIVITY 5.3

Engage in some role-play to explore different communication approaches. This activity takes 10 minutes and can be played with any number of participants. There are two rounds.

First, divide the group into pairs and spread out around the room. It works best if everyone is standing up. In each pair, decide who will be person A and who will be person B.

In the first round, each person plays as one of two personas:

Person A: You are from a time 500 years ago, when superstition ruled, outside ideas were treated as the work of the devil and people were treated harshly – sometimes burned at the stake. You've stepped through a wormhole in time and have landed here in the present day.

Person B: You are from the present day. You're waiting around to receive an important phone call, but you've just noticed Person A, who seems agitated and confused. Introduce yourself to Person A and try to make them feel okay with the phone call you are about to receive. Can you convince them that the mobile phone is not the work of the devil?

Person B, has 2 minutes to make Person A okay about the phone.

Once the two minutes is up, discuss as a group. Is anyone getting burned at the stake for this 'magic' talking device? Why? What was said or done that made them feel this way? Was anyone who played Person A happy with the phone? Why? What was said or done that helped them accept this new idea?

Remember, it is the audience who gets to decide whether this moment of communication is successful, not the speaker.

This exercise unearths a range of topics in the communication of complex information. There are the negatives, such as:

- The emptiness of assertions of fact
- The dangers of relying on unfamiliar jargon (e.g. phone, computer, electricity, which should all be familiar to the audience)
- The dangers of attempting to explain how something works, particularly when we are likely to be uncertain ourselves
- The dangers of lying

Then there are the benefits of focusing on the audience and communicating with them by focusing on their needs:

- Using language and metaphors familiar to the audience
- Concentrating on why something is used or is useful – tell them what is in it for them!

In the second round, swap roles. Person B is now from the past, Person A from the present. However, this time in the journey through the wormhole, Person B got their finger caught on the edge of the wormhole and it really hurts – it might be broken. Person A, can you convince them to put their finger into an x-ray machine? Again, you have 2 minutes.

Afterwards, discuss. Was anyone getting burned at the stake for using this machine that could see inside people? Why? Was anyone happy to put their hands in the x-ray machine? Why? Other similar topics can be explored here as the first round, as well as:

- The danger of focusing on the 'shiny science machine'
- The danger of appeals to authority
- The need to focus on the audience; in particular, the values of the audience
- The power of empathy, reflected through tone, words and body language
- The power of 'show, don't tell' – did anyone playing Person A volunteer to put their own hand in the x-ray machine first?

Source: Adapted from a workshop at Alan Alda Center for Communicating Science, Stony Brook University, New York.

QUESTION

How might the principles used in this exercise be applied to health promotion? Answer with respect to these scenarios:

- Talking to new parents about vaccination
- Implementing a water and sanitation hygiene program with communities in a developing country
- Advocating with policy makers for climate-mitigation strategies to address health risks

How and where knowledge can be translated for people to use

How, then, do we use insights from this chapter to translate our knowledge for public benefit? Here, we explore **knowledge translation** (Straus et al., 2009, p. 165) and the levers available to influence behaviour.

Knowledge translation – a dynamic and iterative process of applying research or other forms of knowledge to improve health care

Knowledge translation and its purpose

Our goals in health promotion – or, more broadly in the communication of any science – often revolve around the idea of getting expert knowledge into action among those who can use it. It's worth noting Straus and colleagues' (2009) highlighting of the significant variety in synonyms for knowledge translation, including 'implementation science', 'research utilisation', 'dissemination and diffusion', 'research use' and 'knowledge transfer and uptake' (2009). As the WHO (n.d.) notes, 'knowledge derived from research and experience may be of little value unless it is put into practice'.

The purpose of knowledge translation is simple. As this chapter has stressed, people – even medical practitioners (see Cabana et al., 1999) – do not make health decisions based on direct assessment of scholarly meta-analyses. We make decisions and change behaviours on the basis of a range of values, emotions, opportunities, social network influences, attitudes and knowledge. Only by working with these various factors in mind can we successfully translate knowledge into action.

Where knowledge can be used

If we seek to put knowledge into action, there are a range of levers we might be able to pull, depending on our own particular influence and power as well as knowing what is available. Following traditional political theories, we can place these levers on a spectrum, from carrot (incentive) to stick (deterrent) – or from costs and punishments for negative behaviour to inducements or incentives for positive ones.

Governments have access to a range of options to serve as costs and punishments for negative behaviours. These include fines, increased taxes, regulatory changes and custodial sentences. While custodial sentences are not often talked of directly in health promotion circles, they have been used to stop fraudulent purveyors of dubious cures and in efforts to enforce prohibition of sales of alcoholic beverages in the United States. Like custodial sentences, fines are also less critical to the world of health promotion but have been used in a variety of areas to stop medical fraud.

Taxes, however, offer a far more nuanced tool for the adjustment of societal behaviour. Governments around the world have used taxes in a range of health promotion interventions, raising the price of behaviours that have a negative health effect and typically using the proceeds of the tax to support other health benefits. Perhaps the most recognisable example has been the gradual increase in tobacco taxes around the world, which have done much to reduce smoking rates (Bader et al., 2011) but not necessarily in all communities (see Case study 5.3). Another example can be seen in taxation interventions in alcoholic beverages, such as the Australian government's taxation of 'ready-to-drink', pre-mixed beverages (Gale et al., 2015).

Individuals also have the ability to influence the health environment around them, using negative inducements. Most classically, individuals and societies have regularly used the social pressures of stigma and shame to punish those considered to have committed anti-social behaviours and to deter others from committing such behaviours (Kahan, 1999; Scruton, 2000). Contemporary societies have typically (though not exclusively) moved away from overt use of stigma and shame, but it would be foolhardy to assume that more hidden, quieter shaming does not occur. Have you ever looked askance – or been looked at askance – at publicly unhealthy behaviour?

Flipping that notion around, individuals (and communities) also have significant ability to positively influence norms towards healthy behaviours: role-modelling, setting norms and affirming positive behaviours can all induce positive health behaviours in individuals and communities. Positive health behaviours can also be reinforced in the policy sphere, by providing incentives and rewards for desired behaviours, comparatively reducing the price of healthier food or through the norming of advertising. All of these are areas where effective communication in health promotion can contribute.

CASE STUDY 5.3 A deadly choice is a healthy choice

Disparities in smoking rates

Decades of anti-smoking campaigns in Australia, stretching back to the 1970s (Pierce et al., 1986), appear to have had a significant effect on smoking rates in general. As documented by Greenhalgh, Scollo and Winstanley (2019), 35 per cent of Australian adults smoked in 1980, but by 1998 this had reduced to 26 per cent, and by 2016 to 13 per cent. Among Aboriginal and Torres Strait Islander peoples, despite a decrease in the proportion of people smoking from 54.5 per cent in 1994 to 41 per cent in 2018, the percentage of smokers remained significantly higher in 2018 than for the wider Australian population, at almost 30 per cent higher (Greenhalgh et al., 2019). This is where initiatives such as Deadly Choices come in.

Deadly Choices

Deadly Choices is a health campaign working to:

> empower Aboriginal and Torres Strait Islander peoples to make healthy choices for themselves and their families – to stop smoking, to eat good food and exercise daily … In Aboriginal slang, if something is 'deadly' it is great. As such a Deadly Choice is a good choice, and we encourage community to make such choices each day (Institute for Urban Indigenous Health, 2018a, para. 1).

Deadly Choices seeks to foster this community empowerment by using a range of techniques explored in this chapter: framing messages in ways that resonate with the values of the Aboriginal and Torres Strait Islander communities involved with the campaign; using appropriate and meaningful language and metaphors; and engaging spokespeople from the communities to represent the campaign. For example, Aboriginal and Torres Strait Islander sports stars act as ambassadors talking about their own healthy choices, to encourage people to make healthier choices for themselves. The ambassadors are also included in posters and promotional material for campaigns such as the Deadly, Smoke Free Spaces pledge.

Program and impact

Deadly Choices runs a tobacco education program, which runs for six sessions in schools and community environments. It covers topics such as the history of tobacco use in Aboriginal and Torres Strait Islander peoples, the negative health effects of smoking and passive smoking, addiction, smoke-free spaces and where to get help (Institute for Urban Indigenous Health, 2018b). Data collected between 2016 and 2018 indicated a downward trend in smoking rates (53% to 39%) with 6545 smoke-free pledges made – with potential to directly affect 28 666 people (Duff & Parter, 2019).

(cont.)

(cont.)

QUESTIONS

1. What elements of the Deadly Choices tobacco education program and pledge do you think could influence a person's decision to make a healthier choice?

2. Search for a health promotion initiative happening in an area close to you (in your town or state/territory) that targets a particular cultural group. How is that culture represented and integrated in that initiative? Is it effective? How do you know?

ELSEWHERE IN THE WORLD

Atii! Reduce second-hand smoke

This program produced Inuit-specific materials and resources in multiple languages and dialects to focus on reducing harms associated with second-hand smoke (Pauktuutit Inuit Women of Canada, 2020).

Summary

This chapter has sought to articulate one key argument: that those hoping to promote health must recognise there can never be a 'one-size-fits-all' communication message that can be applied to all audiences. Every group of people, and individual, we deal with comes to us with their own preconceptions, biases, worldviews and beliefs; all happily receive new information that agrees with their prior beliefs; and all will crankily reject information that contradicts them. If we hope to change health attitudes, knowledge and behaviours for the better, we must proceed by working with what is already there. This is not a call to abandon our task. Instead, if we embrace a pathway of health promotion that begins from a stance of empathy, seeks to find common ground and works to incentivise the good in ways that resonate with the worldviews and values of the people we are working with, then success is possible.

REVISION QUESTIONS

1. What are media frames and what do they do?
2. What ideas does the 'nanny state' framing seek to associate with public health interventions?
3. Who is likely to be prone to confirmation bias?
4. What are the key elements of knowledge translation?

FURTHER READING

Grant, W. & Lamberts, R. (n.d.). Life in a Herd (Podcast series). The Wholesome Show. Retrieved from: http://wholesomeshow.com/life-in-a-herd

Kahneman, D. (2011). *Thinking, Fast and Slow*. New York: Farrar, Straus and Giroux.

Saslow, E. (2016, 15 October). The white flight of Derek Black, *The Washington Post*. Retrieved from: https://www.washingtonpost.com/national/the-white-flight-of-derek-black/2016/10/15/ed5f906a-8f3b-11e6-a6a3-d50061aa9fae_story.html

REFERENCES

Bader, P., Boisclair, D. & Ferrence, R. (2011). Effects of tobacco taxation and pricing on smoking behaviour in high risk populations: A knowledge synthesis, *International Journal of Environmental Research and Public Health*, 8(11). Retrieved from: doi:10.3390/ijerph8114118

Borchgrevink, C.P., Cha, J.M. & Kim, S.H. (2013). Hand washing practices in a college town environment, *Journal of Environmental Health*, 75(8).

Cabana, M.D., Rand, C.S., Powe, N.R., Wu, A.W., Wilson, M.H., Abboud, P-A.C. & Rubin, H.R. (1999). Why don't physicians follow clinical practice guidelines? A framework for improvement, *Journal of the American Medical Association*, 282(15), 1458–65. doi:10.1001/jama.282.15.1458

CDC (Centers for Disease Control and Prevention) (1999). Ten great public health achievements – United States, 1900–1999, *Morbidity and Mortality Weekly Report*, 48(12).

Chong, D. & Druckman, J.N. (2007). A theory of framing and opinion formation in competitive elite environments, *Journal of Communication*, 57, 99–118.

Civiqs (2020a). How concerned are you about a coronavirus outbreak in your local area? Democrat Party (Website). Retrieved from: https://civiqs.com/results/coronavirus_concern?uncertainty=true&annotations=false&zoomIn=true&party=Democrat

———(2020b). How concerned are you about a coronavirus outbreak in your local area? Republican Party (Website). Retrieved from: https://civiqs.com/results/coronavirus_concern?uncertainty=true&annotations=false&zoomIn=true&party=Republican

Connolly, M., Floyd, S., Forrest, R. & Marshall, B. (2012). Mental health nurses' beliefs about smoking by mental health facility inpatients, *Journal of Mental Health Nursing*, 22(4).

Demaio, A.R. (2016, 12 October). Sugar tax is not nanny state, it's sound public policy, *The Conversation*. Retrieved from: https://theconversation.com/sugar-tax-is-not-nanny-state-its-sound-public-policy-59059

Duff, D. & Parter, S. (2019, 2–4 April). Deadly Choices effective monitoring and evaluation: Measuring our impact. Presented at *National Tackling Indigenous Smoking Workers Workshop*, Alice Springs, Northern Territory.

Gale, M., Muscatello, D. J., Dinh, M., Byrnes, J., Shakeshaft, A., Hayen, A., MacIntyre, C.R., Haber, P., Cretikos, M. & Morton, P. (2015). Alcopops, taxation and harm: A segmented time series analysis of emergency department presentations. *BMC Public Health*, 15, 468. Retrieved from: https://doi.org/10.1186/s12889-015-1769-3

Grant, W. & Lamberts, R. (2014, 3 October). The 10 stuff-ups we all make when interpreting research, *The Conversation*. Retrieved from: https://theconversation .com/the-10-stuff-ups-we-all-make-when-interpreting-research-30816

Greenhalgh, E., Scollo, M. & Winstanley, M. (2019). *Tobacco in Australia*. The Cancer Council. Retrieved from: https://www.tobaccoinaustralia.org.au/

Hamblin, J. (2020, 6 February). 20 seconds to optimize hand wellness, *The Atlantic*. Retrieved from: https://www.theatlantic.com/health/archive/2020/02/hand-wellness/606181/

Institute for Urban Indigenous Health (2018a). Deadly Choices (Website). Retrieved from: https://deadlychoices.com.au

———(2018b). The Deadly Choices Tobacco Education Program explores the historical journey of tobacco use, its acceptance, and its impacts on community (Website). Retrieved from: https://deadlychoices.com.au/programs/tobacco-education/

Jochelson, K. (2006). Nanny or steward? The role of government in public health, *Public Health*, 120, 1149–55.

Kahan, D.M. (1999). The progressive appropriation of disgust. In S.A. Bandes (ed.), *Critical America: The passions of law* (pp. 63–79). New York: New York University Press.

Kahan, D.M., Peters, E., Dawson, E.C. & Slovic, P. (2017). Motivated numeracy and enlightened self-government, *Behavioural Public Policy*, 1(1).

Kahneman, D. (2011). *Thinking, Fast and Slow*. New York: Farrar, Straus and Giroux.

Kuhn, T. (1962). *The Structure of Scientific Revolution*. Chicago: University of Chicago Press.

Lakoff, G. (2004). *Don't Think of an Elephant! Know your values and frame the debate*. White River Junction, VT: Chelsea Green Publishing.

Lamberts, R., Grant, W.J. & Martin, A. (2010). Public opinion about science, *ANUPoll*. Retrieved from: http://cpas.anu.edu.au/files/ANU%20Poll%202010%20Public%20 Opinion%20About%20Science.pdf

Marar, S. (2018, 1 May). A sugar tax is another attack on freedom and personal responsibility, *Spectator Australia*. Retrieved from: https://www.spectator.com .au/2018/05/a-sugar-tax-is-another-attack-on-freedom-and-personal-responsibility/

Meppelink, C.S., Smit, E.G., Fransen, M.L. & Diviani, N. (2019). 'I was right about vaccination': Confirmation bias and health literacy in online health information seeking, *Journal of Health Communication*, 24(2). doi:https://doi.org/10.1080/1081 0730.2019.1583701

Monbiot, G. (2013, 16 July). Cigarette packaging: The corporate smokescreen, *The Guardian*. Retrieved from: https://www.theguardian.com/commentisfree/2013/ jul/15/cigarette-packaging-corporate-smokescreen-liberty

Nickerson, R.S. (1998). Confirmation bias: A ubiquitous phenomenon in many guises, *Review of General Psychology*, 2(2). doi:https://doi.org/10.1037/1089-2680.2.2.175

Nurse, M.S. & Grant W.J. (2019). I'll see it when I believe it: Motivated numeracy in perceptions of climate change risk, *Environmental Communication*. doi:10.1080/1 7524032.2019.1618364

Nyhan, B. & Reifler, J. (2010). When corrections fail: The persistence of political misperceptions, *Political Behaviour*, 32, 303–30.

Pauktuutit Inuit Women of Canada (2020). *Atii!* Reduce Second-Hand Smoke (Website). Retrieved from: https://www.pauktuutit.ca/health/tobacco-cessation/atii-reduce-second-hand-smoke/

Pierce, J., Dwyer, T., Frape, G., Chapman, S., Chamberlain, A. & Burke, N. (1986). Evaluation of the Sydney 'Quit For Life' anti-smoking campaign. Part 1. Achievement of intermediate goals, *Medical Journal of Australia*, 144(7), 341–4.

Popper, K. (2005). *The Logic of Scientific Discovery*. London: Routledge.

Rogers, S. (2013, 15 March). John Snow's data journalism: The cholera map that changed the world, *The Guardian*. Retrieved from: https://www.theguardian.com/news/datablog/2013/mar/15/john-snow-cholera-map

Roser, M., Ortiz-Ospina, E. & Ritchie, H. (2019). Life Expectancy. OurWorldInData.org (Website). Retrieved from: https://ourworldindata.org/life-expectancy

Saslow, E. (2016, 15 October). The white flight of Derek Black, *The Washington Post Sunday*. Retrieved from: https://www.washingtonpost.com/national/the-white-flight-of-derek-black/2016/10/15/ed5f906a-8f3b-11e6-a6a3-d50061aa9fae_story.html

Scruton, R. (2000). Bring back stigma, *City Journal*, Retrieved from: https://www.city-journal.org/html/bring-back-stigma-11807.html

Skurnik, I., Yoon, C., Park, D.C. & Schwarz, N. (2005). How warnings about false claims become recommendations, *Journal of Consumer Research*, 31(4). doi:https://doi.org/10.1086/426605

Solomon, D.J. (2016, 17 October). Shabbat dinner helped turn around this ex-white supremacist, *Forward*. Retrieved from: https://forward.com/news/352094/shabbat-dinner-helped-turn-around-this-ex-white-supremacist/

Straus, S.E., Tetroe, J. & Graham, I. (2009). Defining knowledge translation, *Canadian Medical Association Journal*, 181(3–4), 165–8. doi:10.1503/cmaj.081229

Thornock, B.S.O. (2017). Heralding the pariahs: What the narratives of vaccine hesitant parents can teach us about the backfire effect and physician-patient relationships, *Annals of Public Health Reports*, 1(1). doi:10.36959/856/485

World Health Organization (WHO) (n.d.). Aging and life-course: Knowledge translation (Website). Retrieved from: https://www.who.int/ageing/projects/knowledge_translation/en/

Yong, E. (2020, 25 March). How the pandemic will end, *The Atlantic*. Retrieved from: https://www.theatlantic.com/health/archive/2020/03/how-will-coronavirus-end/608719/

Zhao, X. & Jiang, J. (2011). An Empirical Comparison of Topics in Twitter and Traditional Media. Singapore Management University School of Information Systems Technical Paper Series. Retrieved from: http://www.mysmu.edu/faculty/jingjiang/papers/TechReport(Zhao2011).pdf

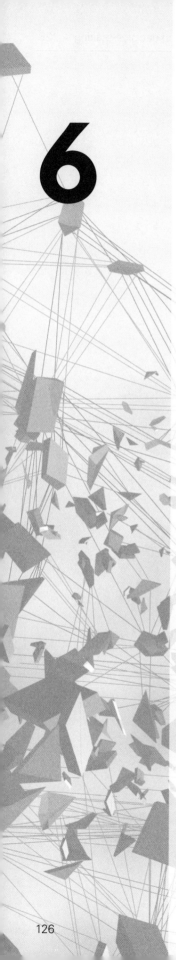

6

Components of effective communication

Lindy A. Orthia

With contributions from Amy R. Dobos

LEARNING OBJECTIVES

At the completion of the chapter, you will be able to:

- Identify communication needs in a health promotion context.
- Think critically and constructively about your audience.
- Tailor communications to people, time and place.
- Develop appropriate communication aims.
- Craft communications that are accessible and clear.

Introduction

It is common for people to believe they can change others' attitudes and behaviours just by making their specialist knowledge publicly available, but that is rarely the case, including in health promotion (see Chapter 5). For any health promotion initiative to be effective, it must employ appropriate communication techniques. This chapter explores some basic steps to maximise the chance your audience will engage with your communication efforts.

There are five primary factors to consider when undertaking any communication act: audience, content, context, aim and medium. Chapter 7 discusses the 'how' of working with different communication mediums. The current chapter raises questions about the other four factors (audience, content, context, aim) and how they intersect.

The following section outlines two big steps you must take when commencing work on a communication strategy: (1) gather information about the problem you are trying to address and (2) plan how best to tackle it. The chapter considers questions of audience and aim, respectively, both of which are important to get right if you wish to avoid wasting your resources on vague or untargeted initiatives. The final section presents two techniques for enhancing your communication's accessibility and clarity.

Identifying a communication need

Health promotion initiatives can be expensive, both in terms of money and the time and other resources needed to implement them. There can also be an **opportunity cost** if an initiative is poorly implemented, and poorly implemented initiatives can undermine future health promotion activities on the same topic. For all of these reasons, planning is critical to getting a health promotion initiative right. You need to plan in advance what you will do, when or where you will do it, and with whom. You also need to know exactly why you are doing it. Specifying the communication need you are trying to address will ensure your efforts are not spent on irrelevant matters and will enable you to evaluate your success (discussed in Chapter 8).

Opportunity cost – inefficiencies that result from squandering an opportunity, or to the opportunities you miss while focusing your efforts elsewhere

Conducting an environmental scan

The first step in any initiative is to conduct an environmental scan. This is a technical term for finding out everything you can about your health topic and what different stakeholders are saying about it, before you commence your own communications on the topic. In other words, an environmental scan ensures your communication will be evidence-based. Most people can communicate – most of us can speak or write or sign – but often our communication efforts go unnoticed or have unexpected effects. Basing communications on evidence rather than assumptions is a critical element of effective health promotion, especially when you're starting out.

Incorporating different kinds of evidence into your planning will increase the likelihood of success. This is because you will better understand the environment in which you are communicating and the people you are communicating with. You will also learn from other health promoters' experiences, as reported in the academic literature, and from the common lessons health promotion researchers have brought together to build theories. Health promotion initiatives based on social and behavioural theories tend to be much more successful than those not using theory (Glanz and Bishop, 2010), because theories are the product of accumulated, systematically evaluated experience. When considering theories, identify the role of communication within them. For example, the Health Belief Model associates individuals' actions with their perceptions of the threat of disease or the benefits of action, which can sometimes be influenced by communication products, including health promotion campaigns (Munro et al., 2007). Social Cognitive Theory requires the audience to pay attention and retain ideas, which can be promoted through entertaining communications such as television and radio drama (Smith et al., 2007).

Your environmental scan can be broad or narrow, but the more comprehensive it is and the more regularly you update it, the better prepared you will be to respond to challenges and capitalise on opportunities. An environmental scan might begin with a comprehensive review of the health, medical and communication research on your topic, as you would do when conducting a literature review for a research project. Health promotion initiatives frequently draw upon **grey literature** as well as peer-reviewed research but, as with all information, always think critically about your sources.

In practice, an environmental scan for health promotion is much broader than a literature review (Charlton et al., 2019; Wilburn et al., 2016). Depending on your topic, the environmental scan might include reviewing:

Grey literature – formally produced works that have not undergone a rigorous peer-review process but are nonetheless considered relatively reliable, such as reports, working papers and program reviews by governments, non-government organisations and international bodies such as the World Health Organization

- examples of health promotion materials, such as factsheets, leaflets and flyers, websites and blogs, videos, podcasts and popular books
- discussions on social media
- coverage by mass media
- data and governance documents from hospitals, clinics and other health providers
- government legislation, policies and budgeting measures
- community sector activities, including patient advocacy, political lobbying, community support and public information
- private-sector activities, e.g. DNA-testing services if your topic is genetics-related
- unpublished interview or survey data from health and medical professionals, patient groups, community organisations, policy makers and other stakeholders
- direct discussion with key collaborators and stakeholders about what they think are the most important contextual factors shaping this topic right now.

When considering what to include in your scan, two acronyms can help you brainstorm. 'STEP' (or 'PEST') is commonly used in the field; it stands for the **s**ociocultural, **t**echnological, **e**conomic and **p**olitical aspects of a topic (Charlton et al., 2019). Our alternative, 'SPICIE', breaks this down further by covering a topic's **s**ocial, **p**olitical, **i**deological, **c**ultural, **i**nstitutional and **e**conomic aspects. Both can help you remember that the health knowledge you possess is only part of the picture. People's ideological beliefs, cultural norms, social limitations and institutional affiliations, as well as broader political and economic factors and technological supports or hindrances, all shape the communication environment in which you are operating. Think about an environmental scan as a rich map of the communication landscape.

To ensure your scan is comprehensive, you may wish to follow a protocol with clear steps, and some are available in the research literature and online. For example, health promoters in charge of a campaign on the human papilloma virus (Wilburn et al., 2016, pp. 2–4) followed a seven-step protocol that included internal steps for managing the environmental scan, including determining their team's capacity, delegating tasks and creating a timeline with incremental goals. These internal factors can be as critical to success as scanning the external factors.

Using information, and gaps, to plan an initiative

Once you have completed your environmental scan, you will be aware of which initiatives are already underway for your topic. You can then see which, if any, are relevant to your region, target audience or other factor of interest. Use the knowledge you have gained to compare *the initiatives that already exist* to *the initiatives that are needed*. Are there gaps? Can you identify unmet needs? Has an important audience been overlooked? A useful medium under-utilised? Is there urgent new information yet to be communicated?

The gaps you identify will often provide the foundation for your initiative, in conjunction with information about what has worked in the past that is worth repeating. Use good practice as a model for the future. But do so critically, taking into account new evidence of what is effective, new knowledge of your topic, the changing circumstances of your audiences and stakeholders, and developments in media usage. The best health promotion initiatives combine existing and new approaches in ways appropriate to context.

Sometimes the gaps you find might actually be big blank spots without any information to guide you! If so, you may have to use your best judgement, combined with trial and error, to find out what will be effective. Not every health promotion topic has been comprehensively researched, so there are times when you will need to pioneer a new approach (see Case study 6.1).

However, even with the best-laid plans, the world continues to turn, and this can present unexpected obstacles and new opportunities. To respond to them, remain flexible. If you are attuned to current events and debates related to your topic, you can capitalise on them to boost your campaign's reach and keep it relevant (see Chapter 7).

CASE STUDY 6.1 Visual communication of Alzheimer's disease research

Amy R. Dobos and Lindy A. Orthia

Alzheimer's disease in Australia

Dementia is the second-leading cause of death of Australians, and almost half a million Australians are living with it (Dementia Australia, 2020). Alzheimer's disease, the most common form of dementia, can cause memory loss, deterioration in social skills and

(cont.)

(cont.)

emotional unpredictability (Dementia Australia, 2020). It is often stigmatised, partly because medical research does not yet fully understand it, and because its biological causes are essentially invisible (Dobos et al., 2015).

Can research on Alzheimer's disease be communicated visually?

In 2012, science communicator Amy Dobos was working for non-profit organisation Alzheimer's Australia, communicating with its subscribers about recent developments in Alzheimer's research. She wanted to enhance subscribers' understandings of this research by using visual images that summarised each development. However, her environmental scan revealed little previous research about creating effective medical images for non-specialist audiences, so Dobos conducted her own research to explore this (Dobos et al., 2015).

Dobos created four images intended to communicate different aspects of Alzheimer's disease research: two depicting social and emotional aspects, and two depicting biological (genetic and biochemical) aspects (Figure 6.1). She then surveyed a subset of the organisation's subscriber list, asking them to interpret each image.

Dobos and her co-researchers discovered that images about the emotional and social aspects of Alzheimer's disease were more likely to be interpreted in the way they intended, while images about the biological aspects were often confusing for subscribers. Subscribers were also more likely to become frustrated with biological images considered ambiguous than social–emotional images that were ambiguous. They also found it easier to interpret images accompanied by words, in an infographic rather than photographic style.

Research directs communication choices

Dobos's research helped her to create communication products in a way that kept her messages clear. Her future designs were informed by knowing the engagement potential of combining written and visual communication forms. Communication is a science in itself and must be based on evidence wherever possible, to enhance its effectiveness. Sometimes the best way to find out if something is effective is to ask the intended audience.

QUESTIONS

1. Why might information about biological aspects of Alzheimer's disease research be harder to communicate visually than information about its social or emotional aspects?

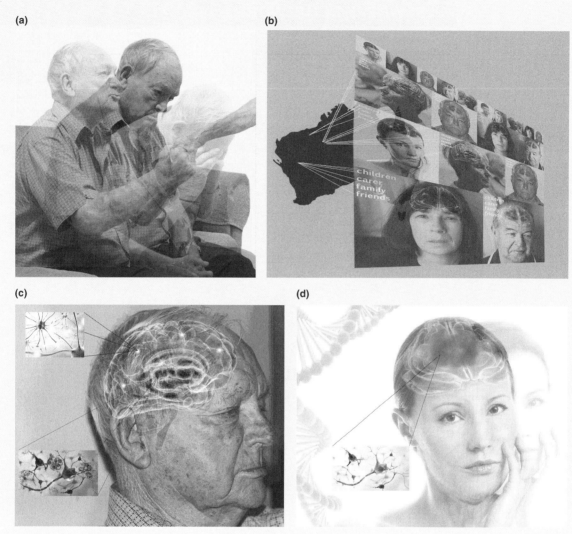

Figure 6.1   The four images tested by Amy Dobos. Images (a) and (b) depict emotional and social aspects of Alzheimer's disease, while (c) and (d) depict some biological characteristics of the disease
Source: Dobos et al. (2015).

2. What do you think the consequences might have been if Dobos had used her images without testing their effectiveness first?

3. Choose another health issue. Based on the findings of this case study, try to develop visual communications about your chosen health issue. Test the clarity of these messages on other people and reflect on what worked and why.

ELSEWHERE IN THE WORLD

World Alzheimer Reports

The annual World Alzheimer Reports (Alzheimer's Disease International, 2020) communicate about state-of-the-art research into Alzheimer's disease. The reports always contain images, but they tend to be generic images, not ones designed to communicate about specific research projects, unless they are infographics that blend words and pictures. Purely visual communication about Alzheimer's research remains a difficult task.

Images from US National Institute on Aging

The US National Institute on Aging has a website (US Department of Health & Human Services, 2020) devoted to highlighting images and videos available in the public domain that can be used to communicate about Alzheimer's disease. Many of the images are quite technical and would likely require interpretive words for them to be well-understood by most people.

Knowing your audience

When asked to consider the audience for your health promotion initiative, whom do you picture? It's very common to conceptualise an audience as 'the general public' and to give it no further thought, especially when working on topics related to general health matters such as diet and exercise, rather than clinical conditions or stigmatised activities. But knowing your audience matters if you are to reach it and communicate with successfully. You may wish to reach millions of people with your health promotion initiative, but even so, each one of the millions is a unique person who is engaging with your messages as an individual. Understanding the diversity within the rich population you are communicating with will help target your efforts.

Moving beyond 'the public' as an audience

Let's break down this idea of 'the public' – it can mean a lot of different things, but when health promoters use the term, we are often talking about people untrained in the Western paradigm of health and medicine. We might think about health promotion as an 'us-and-them' interaction in which health promoters have the knowledge and everyone else needs to know what we know.

Deficit model – a way of thinking about an audience as deficient in knowledge and as empty vessels waiting to be filled with the information they need in order to create a desired response

There are many problems with this **deficit model,** though. Most importantly, it does not reflect reality. People with no formal training in Western health or medicine *do* have knowledge about health. Their knowledge may come from any number of sources, including: other health promotion activities; popular health books, documentaries and websites; past advice from medical and health practitioners; health traditions outside the Western scientific model; and, importantly, their own experiences with illness and wellness. Ignoring this and assuming they know nothing will likely cause offence, thereby inhibiting communication. In addition, if people's existing knowledge clashes with what you want to tell them, ignoring it will make your communication process slower and more complicated. Strategically, it is to your benefit to find out what they already know and work with it. Treat your communication as a conversation, not a homily or lecture.

It may help you to think about your audience as your communication partners. Using this term acknowledges that communication is a two-way conversation, not a monologue, and that you can learn from each other (Kirk, 2009). It will also help you limit your audience to a manageable reach. For example, to really cultivate a relationship with communication partners you may need to focus on a particular region or community. That, in turn, will help you tailor your communication more precisely, so that you adjust the communication according to feedback from your audience; this will increase your effectiveness (see Case study 6.2).

CASE STUDY 6.2 Face-to-face community involvement with alcohol licensing processes

Alcohol licensing in Christchurch

Alcohol consumption contributes adversely to community health in Aotearoa New Zealand, increasing the risk of illness, injury, violence and death. Up to 2015, there was little community involvement in decisions about applications for alcohol licences in the city of Christchurch and surrounds. Then some sectors of the community began to question some decisions involving 'risky' applications – for example, when applications involved premises in locations close to schools, social services or alcohol treatment centres (Canterbury District Health Board, 2019).

Community engagement project

In 2015, the local health board initiated a project to actively involve community members in high-risk alcohol licensing applications. Their objectives were to increase community knowledge of local applications and the processes involved, and to increase community skills in preparing for licensing hearings (Canterbury District Health Board, 2019, p. 6).

The project was geographically localised, enabling face-to-face and interpersonal contact between health promotion professionals, citizens and other stakeholders such as licensing officials and lawyers. Its communication techniques included a letter to key contacts in the community about having a say, workshops to help prepare community members for hearings and the employment of an Alcohol Health Promoter by the government to coordinate all activities and be a central point of contact.

(cont.)

(cont.)

Results and conclusions

The project met its objectives, demonstrating increased community knowledge and involvement in licensing activities. Key stakeholders interviewed in the evaluation process attributed the project's success to a number of factors. These included the existence of the Alcohol Health Promoter to unify the project for all other stakeholders; partnerships between different agencies that made community participation easy; the passion of community members; and allocating extra resources to areas of high socio-economic deprivation. The letter and workshop were also praised for their effectiveness in communicating meaningful information in an accessible way (Canterbury District Health Board, 2019).

The four 'human' factors contributing to the project's success demonstrated the effectiveness of building dialogical, interpersonal relationships between communication partners. This was made possible by focusing on a geographically local community and building on locals' knowledge of their community. Well-crafted communications were also important, but on their own would likely not have had the same effect in this case.

QUESTIONS

1. In what ways did the project designers demonstrate good knowledge of their audience(s)?
2. What strategies might you employ to develop interpersonal relationships in a health promotion initiative for a geographically large region?

ELSEWHERE IN THE WORLD

Community theatre for HIV/AIDS awareness

Community theatre is an inherently interpersonal communication medium. It is used in many countries across the world – including in Botswana (see UNICEF, 2020) – to provoke community discussions about HIV/AIDS. When used this way, community theatre involves community members creating a performance about HIV/AIDS with characters, settings and scenarios relevant to their community. They perform it for other community members then engage in conversation with the audience about issues the performance raised. The process can create community change by bringing taboo topics into the open and enabling dialogue among people who may not otherwise come together to discuss such issues.

Yarning circles and Dadirri for Indigenous health

Yarning circles and Dadirri (Lowitja Institute, 2020) are two methods used by Aboriginal and Torres Strait Islander communities to communicate about health and other matters

(Laycock et al., 2011). A yarning circle is a particular kind of large group conversation that can provide a safe space for people to express themselves because it involves intimate processes of building trust. Dadirri is a philosophy involving non-judgemental, deep listening to help people talk about sensitive topics such as trauma, knowing they will be heard and will not be interrupted. Both are strongly interpersonal, echoing communication conventions used by Aboriginal and Torres Strait Islander peoples to share ideas since time immemorial. In its report, *Researching Indigenous Health: A practical guide for researchers,* the Lowitja Institute, Australia's national institute for Aboriginal and Torres Strait Islander health research, explains how health researchers and promoters can use these methods effectively (Laycock et al., 2011).

There is another major reason to avoid thinking about your audience as 'the public'. We are all embedded in communication networks far more complex than the us-and-them binary described above. Some people outside the health profession have more material influence than others on how our society manages health. For example, you might want to encourage people to give up smoking, but smokers as a group may not be the most strategic audience to target, depending on your aims. Your audience could be the politicians who determine advertising policies, the lawyers who construct cases against tobacco companies, the journalists and celebrities who drive public opinion, or the corporations that profit from tobacco or its alternatives. Your audience could be other health promoters, if you seek to build a coordinated campaign. Or, even if smokers are your primary audience, consider who smokes and why, and if there are different reasons different groups of people smoke.

Regardless of your intended audiences, tailor your communication to be relevant and appropriate for each of them. Treating people as agents with complex lives who have pressing reasons for their decisions can only enhance your chances of success.

Managing audience barriers, motivators and drivers

Just like you, other people are complex, and your audience members' lives are shaped by all kinds of factors including economic means, language skills, **social capital**, obligations, pressures and abilities. All those factors will affect how each person responds to your initiative, and all will sometimes present barriers to quality communication. For example, having a low income will prohibit some people from engaging with initiatives that cost money or require them to forgo paid work. People who lack confidence in reading or speaking the language of your initiative may find it intimidating to engage with. People who have spent their lives feeling unheard and marginalised may be slow to trust a health initiative produced by members of the dominant culture, with good reason. And, in general, many people have competing demands on their time and often higher priorities. It is to your benefit to make engaging with your initiative easy for them.

Some simple approaches can assist:

- *Choose your placement strategically.* Put your initiative where your audience is – do not expect them to come to you. That means you need to know where they go – whether online or in person – and when they go there.

Social capital – how seamlessly a society operates; at the individual level, it means the ability of a person to effectively negotiate social relationships (e.g. to have their needs met, to access resources, to be heard and to have influence). Social capital can be influenced by the extent to which a person feels they have a shared sense of identity, values and norms with others, and especially with the dominant culture

- *Make it quick.* Demand the minimum possible time from your audience. The more efficiently you can deliver, the better your uptake will be.
- *Link engagement to simple outcomes.* Make it clear what people are committing to by becoming engaged with your initiative. What is it you expect them to do, and have you made that clear? Make their first task quick to complete (read this, watch this, consider this). Then communicate further actions you want them to take (with resources to help them), including significant behavioural changes such as practising safe sex or challenging stereotypes about mental illness.
- *Catch their attention with relevance.* People decide within a few seconds whether to read, listen to or attend something new, based on whether it sounds relevant to them. Make it immediately obvious what your topic is and why it matters to them.
- *Make writing digestible.* Written materials can intimidate if they have large blocks of text and the language is hard to understand. Keep it short and simple to help put your readers at ease, while writing at a level of knowledge and jargon appropriate to them.
- *Make visual and aural material inviting.* If your material is visual, make it legible and attractive. If it involves listening, ensure your sound quality and production values are high. Do not force your audience to work too hard to engage with your ideas. They will quickly lose interest.
- *Make events accessible.* If your initiative involves an in-person activity, is the venue cheap to get to for people with limited funds? Is the location accessible by both public transport and private vehicle? Is the building physically accessible for people with limited mobility, including seating and toilets? Is it culturally comfortable for your audience? Do you need to provide childcare, or food and drinks? Do you need an interpreter and, if so, for what language(s)? Can people with limited hearing or vision participate? Can people participate without having to speak in front of others?
- *Ensure your initiative is culturally appropriate.* If addressing a culturally diverse audience, be inclusive and respectful. If addressing an audience who shares a specific cultural identity – be that based on ethnicity, religion, sexuality, geography, work, hobbies or something else – employ representatives of that community as consultants from the beginning to ensure your health promotion initiative is appropriate throughout.

Culturally competent communication

To attract and maintain a diverse audience, your health promotion practice must be culturally competent. While this term can apply to any situation involving cultural diversity, it usually refers to cultures associated with nationality, ethnicity, language and religion. The term's progenitors defined it as follows:

> A culturally competent system of care acknowledges and incorporates – at all levels – the importance of culture, the assessment of cross-cultural relations, vigilance towards the dynamics that result from cultural differences, the expansion of cultural knowledge, and the adaptation of services to meet culturally-unique needs (Cross et al., 1989, p. 13).

Attention to these imperatives is crucial if health promotion initiatives are to reach audiences whose identities are marginalised within the dominant culture. This is where understanding your audience comes to matter greatly: knowing who your audiences are (culturally speaking) will enable you to employ community representatives as collaborators, consultants and intermediaries to plan your health promotion strategy in a culturally appropriate way.

However, elements of the cultural competence ideal can be difficult to achieve in highly diverse countries whose populations are drawn from many hundreds of indigenous and/or immigrant cultures, since by definition each culture has specific norms, needs and values that cannot be addressed with a single approach (Vertovec, 2007). It is simply not possible to gain meaningful cultural knowledge about hundreds of cultures.

This is one reason the concept of cultural competence has come under criticism even by people who recognise the importance of attention to culture (reviewed by Morrison et al., 2019). Another criticism is that the concept is too superficial, because it does not address structural causes of racial inequality (Morrison et al., 2019). Consequently, the concept of cultural humility was proposed to replace it, incorporating three core dimensions that go deeper than learning knowledge about different cultures: (1) accountability, (2) lifelong learning and critical reflection, and (3) actions that mitigate power imbalances (Morrison et al., 2019, p. 54; see also Tervalon and Murray-Garcia, 1998). While cultural humility focuses on how professionals must approach cultural diversity, a third concept, cultural safety, has also become part of the discourse, focusing 'on the *power* of minoritised peoples to determine whether or not the service relationship has met their needs for respect, equity, culturally appropriate engagement and trust' (Morrison et al., 2019, p. 56; see also Gerlach, 2012).

Together, these concepts demand that service providers – including health promoters – respond to the needs of **minoritised people** in reflective ways that involve listening, respect, self-awareness and humility. In practice, that means communication must be two-way (or multi-way) and must take the form of a continuing conversation, if it is to respond adequately to cultural diversity and redress social inequality.

Minoritised people – a reference to people who have less social power than others in their nation or community because those who are more powerful do not value their culture, interests or needs as much as their own. Minoritised people may constitute a small sector of the population or a numerical majority. Racism, homophobia and sexism are examples of minoritising behaviours

Knowing your aim

Being clear about your aim in communication is as crucial as understanding your audience. As described in Chapter 2, aims should always be SMART, so you can track your progress, know when you are finished, and appropriately evaluate your success.

More specifically, health promotion initiatives can have aims beyond the simple desire to 'disseminate information' or 'educate people'. Just as we need to stop using a deficit model of our audience, if we are to be effective health promoters we need to stop employing simplistic, broad aims like these.

What do you want your audience to know/think/do?

The best way to think strategically about your aims is to consider what change you want to see in the given population. What do you want your audience(s) to know or think or feel after interacting with your initiative? More importantly, what do you want them to *do* or *not do*, to *be* or *not be*?

It can help to separate your aims into three categories: the ultimate or ideal *goal*, concrete *objectives* and step-by-step *tasks*.

The goal is the change you want to see in the population that will fuel your passion. 'Fewer people infected with HIV', 'quicker resolution of 'flu epidemics' or 'better quality of life for people with Down's syndrome' are all goals of this type. As an ideal, such goals may not meet the SMART criteria, though the SMARTer it is the closer you will get to achieving it. In general, your initiative will usually have just one goal, but sometimes more.

The objectives are practical aims that move you towards the identified goal, and they *must* meet the SMART criteria. Objectives should be built into your communication plan and they should be measurable so you can evaluate the success of the initiative. The initiative should ideally have between two and 10 objectives. Examples are 'new HIV infections in the region will be reduced by 5% per cent within one year', 'website visitors who can articulate our key message will double' and '90 per cent of injecting drug users in the region will always use sterile equipment by the end of the project'. Objectives must be meaningful, not trivial, yet also genuinely achievable for you and your audience. They must also be measurable within your timeframe and budget, bearing in mind that some things are difficult to measure directly (see Chapter 8).

Your tasks are the smaller steps you must complete to towards achieving your objectives, and are generally things within your control, such as 'create website', 'publicise website through social media' or 'survey key audience segement about the website's content'. Planning these in advance will help you stay on track and within budget, but be sure always to leave some 'wiggle room' for unexpected expenses, obstacles and opportunities.

Developing a key message

While developing your aims, you should also articulate a number of key messages. Again, it is helpful to differentiate between two types of key messages.

The main type should be succinct yet fully articulated key messages that best represent your aims. Always bring your communication activities back to these key messages, to ensure the initiative literally 'stays on message' when communicating about your topic. Encourage other people to use these key messages when communicating about your topic. Repeating messages reinforces them to your audiences, so using this approach enhances your chances of success. In addition, having a number of key messages makes it possible to tailor your communication to different audiences and contexts while retaining overall consistency.

You may wish to craft one or more slogans. Slogans are very short, catchy versions of your key messages, designed to attract attention. They can provide coherence across a large communication campaign; for example, connecting different initiatives across the world. They might incorporate hashtags, logos or images that contribute to brand recognition on social media and visual communication contexts (see Case study 6.3).

Make sure you put processes in place to test the effectiveness of your key messages and slogans, as well as other aspects of your communication products, including understanding your audience, before you produce the final versions of campaign materials. Ideally, engage key audiences and other stakeholders in evaluation of your ideas throughout the development process, to ensure they remain relevant, effective and unambiguous. **Focus groups** are a useful method for this purpose because they emphasise the sharing of personal responses and promote group conversations among stakeholders rather than surveying individuals. In this way they will yield a breadth of information on a topic and can help you understand *why* people respond in the ways they do to your materials, not just what their response is.

Testing your materials with focus groups can ensure an efficient use of resources and a successful end product. For example, the US-based Safe City Study Group developed a four-step collaborative process to produce a video for display in sexual health clinics (Myint-U et al., 2010). In step 1 the researchers identified a theoretical framework, medium and key messages, and in step 2 worked with a film company to draft ideas for an appealing product that integrated these. Both steps were conducted with information from a detailed environmental scan. In step 3, the researchers conducted three rounds of focus groups with diverse groups of people representing the target audiences: one round for development of the video storylines, one at the scriptwriting stage and a final round during post-production editing. After each round the researchers adjusted their product's dialogue, slogans and other characteristics in response to participants' responses in the focus groups, including to make the characters relatable and to ensure key messages were communicated clearly. Step 4 involved pilot-testing of the final video in clinic waiting rooms.

Focus groups – small groups ranging from 4 to 20 people (most often 6–10), brought together to explore different responses to a topic or product. In health promotion settings, project managers often organise several focus groups to discuss proposed campaign materials. The groups are typically comprised of stakeholders relevant to the intervention, and can be mixed (e.g. patients, doctors and government officials in a group together) or separate (a different stakeholder category in each group)

CASE STUDY 6.3 Key message and slogan in campaigns

Binge drinking in Australia

Risky single-occasion drinking (RSOD), commonly known as 'binge drinking', is associated with increased injuries and violence including sexual coercion, and risk-taking behaviours such as unsafe sexual practices and drink driving. RSOD is recognised as a health problem for young people in Australia, with one-quarter to one-third of young Australians reporting binge drinking monthly or more frequently (van Gemert et al., 2011).

'Drinking Nightmare' campaign

In 2008, the Australian government launched an initiative to illustrate the potential consequences of binge drinking to young people. The key message was 'Binge drinking can lead to injuries and regrets', and it featured mass-media advertisements with the slogan 'Don't Turn a Night Out Into a Nightmare'.

(cont.)

(cont.)

Key message not always identifiable from the slogan

A team of researchers surveyed young people at a music festival in 2009 to evaluate whether they could identify the campaign's key message (van Gemert et al., 2011). Those surveyed were asked to choose between four health messages (the correct one, plus three plausible-sounding but incorrect messages) or to provide their own answer. The researchers found that while about three-quarters of those surveyed chose the correct answer, people who engaged in frequent binge drinking – the most important segment of the target audience – were statistically less likely to recognise the key message from the campaign material. This suggests that either they had not been exposed to the campaign, and/or they had not engaged with it, and/or they did not interpret its message in the way intended.

This case shows the importance of ensuring a key message is communicated well and reaches its key audience. 'Catchiness' is not the only criterion for a good slogan.

QUESTIONS

1. How might you explain the mismatch between the campaign's slogan and key message?

2. Can you devise a better slogan to represent the key message in this campaign?

ELSEWHERE IN THE WORLD

World Patient Safety Day 2019

In 2019, the WHO ran a campaign to mark the first-ever World Patient Safety Day (WHO, 2019). WHO provided materials for health promoters around the world to use in the campaign. These included 18 key messages aimed at six different audiences, including patients, health workers, policy makers, researchers, organisations and health advocates. But the campaign as a whole was united by a single logo and slogan: 'Speak up for patient safety'. The campaign's website demonstrates how key messages and slogans can be different and how they relate to other health promotion materials. It also documents how the materials were used across the globe.

Resolution Communications Guide

RHD Action is the name of a global movement to reduce the burden of rheumatic heart disease (RHD), which affects children living in conditions of poverty and overcrowding (RHD Action, 2020). RHD Action produced a communication guide for supporting the WHO's draft resolution on RHD and demanding governments act on it. The guide includes four key messages and two slogans with hashtags. It advises campaigners to stick closely to these while tailoring communication to local contexts.

LEARNING ACTIVITY 6.1

Imagine you are employed by a hospital as a health outreach officer for new parents. Part of your job is to communicate about the effects of breastfeeding versus formula-feeding on infant health. Now, consider three scenarios.

In scenario 1, you are commencing a 10-week series of workshops about parenting, similar to the workshops you have run for new parents for the past 5 years.

In scenario 2, there has been a contamination scare in two popular brands of infant formula. Six babies have died around the country while others are reporting sick, including in your city. The city council is holding an urgent public meeting about it and has invited you to speak.

In scenario 3, a conservative lobby group has launched a campaign against breastfeeding in public places and has gained the support of a local shopping centre. A pro-breastfeeding group has launched a counter campaign and asked you to address a protest.

For each scenario, brainstorm:

1. Sources of information you would seek out in an environmental scan and key stakeholders you would consult.
2. Who your audiences are. What do you know about them? What do you need to know?
3. Your aims, as far as possible, including goals, objectives and tasks.
4. Your key message/s and points for crafting your communication materials, tailored to each audience and to achieve each aim.

Now, reflect on how each scenario changes your approach to communication. What is different between them? Are any elements consistent across all three? Why or why not?

Making your communication clear

With your audience, aims and key messages at the ready, you now need to craft your communication materials. Location and medium-specific techniques are discussed in Chapters 3 and 7, but to use them successfully you need to master some core skills that apply to communicating about any scientific subject, including health and medicine.

Starting where your audiences are

The most important starting point in crafting communications about health, medicine and science is to understand where your audiences 'are' with respect to knowledge, priorities and familiarity with scientific and medical **jargon**. Jargon is useful for people inside the profession because it functions as a shortcut for complex ideas, so it is not inherently bad, but there is a time and a place for its use.

Jargon – specialist terms used by members of a profession and not often by other people

Consider what your audience/s already know, and work with that, as discussed above. Then consider *what you want them to know* in conjunction with *what they want to know*. The latter will depend on their reason for being interested in your health promotion initiative, which relates to their priorities. Have they asked you to speak to a community meeting about a chemical spill that imminently endangers their safety? Or are you being interviewed on an entertaining radio show about healthy living, good food and good sex? Should you strip back your content to the most urgent issues, or cloak your key messages in fun commentary and humour? Think about what your audience wants – ask them, if you can – to ensure you are pitching your content at the right level. By all means incorporate *what you want them to know* into your communications, if it will be relevant to your audience, but be aware you will lose people if you persist in telling them things that are not of interest to them or important within the context.

Communicating with people in language they can understand is also critical. Using medical jargon that most of your audience is not familiar with defeats the purpose of communication. If they cannot understand what you have said, you have failed. In addition, jargon can alienate people, creating distance between you that can be difficult to reverse. Using jargon they do not understand can cause an audience to feel stupid or that you think they are stupid. If you can, avoid jargon. If there is a technical term that is central to your key message and too useful to leave out, introduce it to the audience, explaining it with everyday language the first time you use it.

Note that not all jargon sounds technical. Sometimes ordinary words are used in a special way in scientific contexts, turning them into jargon. Common examples from public health studies are 'significant at the point-oh-five level', 'sample size' or 'recruitment strategy'; each word on its own is ordinary and familiar to most English speakers, but in these contexts they only make sense to people familiar with quantitative research involving humans. Such uses should be avoided or explained, just like other forms of jargon. It is often simply a matter of taking a few more words to explain a process. Instead of 'significant at the point-oh-five level', you might say 'the chance of this happening by accident is less than one in 20'. Instead of 'sample size', say 'the number of people we tested'. Instead of 'recruitment strategy', use 'the way we found people to take part in the study'. You are saying the same thing in an accessible way and bringing your audience in, rather than excluding them. That is the essence of good communication.

Simplifying complex ideas through metaphor and analogy

Occasionally you will have to communicate a concept that is quite complex, and simply re-expressing it in everyday language is not adequate for explaining it succinctly. The biological and psychological systems we talk about in health promotion frequently have many components, all of which are usually referred to by scientific jargon names, and whose functions are also usually explained in jargon terms.

In such situations, **metaphors** and **analogies** can help you. The advantage of these linguistic tools is they compare something unfamiliar to something familiar, thus aiding clear communication. For example, if you were to compare the structure of a liver cell to a peach, where the peach seed is the cell's nucleus because it is a distinct component in the centre of the cell, you would be employing an analogy. If your audience is familiar with peaches, they would instantly know what you mean.

Metaphor – an object or action using a word or phrase that is not literally applicable; metaphors often take the form 'something is something else' – for example, 'the mitochondria is the battery of a cell'

Analogy – to compare an idea or object with something more familiar; for example, 'the heart functions like a pump'

However, be careful when choosing your metaphor or analogy. First, note any important limitations of your comparison. Using the above example, there are ways a peach is nothing like a cell – for example, in its size. The tiny size of a liver cell may be obvious to you but it will not necessarily be obvious to your audience. There are, of course, other differences between peaches and cells too, so do not let your audience run away with the metaphor.

Second, you must ensure that *what you think is* common ground *is genuinely* common ground. Common ground is influenced by age, culture, language, gender and more. If your audience is not familiar with peaches, the peach analogy would not work. This point applies to both comparative objects and figures of speech. For example, if you use the phrase 'silver bullet' about a new drug, an audience unfamiliar with the phrase would not understand you if they were also unfamiliar with the cultural frame of reference from which the term originates. Not everyone knows that silver bullets are instantly lethal to werewolves.

LEARNING ACTIVITY 6.2

Work in pairs. Each person in the pair is to draw a simple image, using only basic shapes. The image should not be too big or elaborate, about six two-dimensional shapes are enough. They can be touching, inside each other, whatever you like. Keep your image hidden from your partner. When you both have an image ready, sit back to back – no peeking! One of you goes first as the 'sender'. Your job is to describe your image to your partner (the receiver) in enough detail that they are able to draw a copy.

Rules: Only the sender is allowed to speak. The receiver is not allowed to talk, ask questions or communicate in any way with the sender. Senders are not allowed to look at what the receiver is doing.

Once the sender has finished describing the image and is satisfied that the job is done, then compare images. How did you go? Suggested things to discuss:

- What worked well?
- Where did problems occur and why?
- How could they be avoided?
- What was it like working without any feedback?

Things to think about in discussion with your partner include:

- Context – did you know what to expect? Why or why not?
- Pace – was the information provided too quickly or too slowly?
- Repetition – if the receiver missed a step, did they get a chance to find out the information again?

Now swap roles and use the other image. You might want to make it a bit harder by removing the 'jargon' – you can't use shape names. How else can you describe the shapes in your image?

Once you are finished, compare and discuss the process again. Go through the same questions as before and, if you did not use shape names this time, discuss how

(cont.)

(cont.)

you managed to talk about the shapes – what strategies did you use? Did they work? Why or why not?

Now, answer the following questions.

1. How does this exercise relate to communication in a:
   a. brochure
   b. workshop or presentation
   c. grant application?
2. Based on your identification of the strategies that worked, how might you employ these strategies in other communication activities?

Summary

This chapter reviewed some communication principles considered fundamental to good health promotion. Environmental scans can help you to identify what others have done to communicate your topic and to which audience, and can provide information about what worked, what did not and what is left to do. Understanding your audience in as much detail as possible will help you to develop an effective communication strategy. To maximise the effectiveness, wherever possible engage your audience in the development of your strategy or initiative. Set clear targets for what you want to achieve, both large-scale aspirational goals and the steps to get there. Make sure all of them are SMART, so you can measure your progress along the way.

Finally, clear communication is not simply about saying all the words you want to say. It is ensuring that what you want to say is relevant and understandable to your audience. It is not the job of the audience to 'learn' the information; rather, it is the responsibility of the communicator to ensure that the audience understands. Start where your audience is and then take them with you on the journey.

REVISION QUESTIONS

1. Why is it important to start with an environmental scan before designing your health promotion initiative?
2. What kinds of factors enable audiences to engage with a health promotion initiative? What factors promote disengagement?
3. What is the difference between cultural competence, cultural humility and cultural safety?
4. How do goals, objectives, tasks, key messages and slogans relate to each other in a communication strategy?
5. What are some linguistic techniques for communicating about specialised medical and health concepts?

FURTHER READING

Rimmer, A. (2014). Doctors must avoid jargon when talking to patients, royal college says, *British Medical Journal*, 348, g4131.

Talley, J. (2016). Moving from the margins: The role of narrative and metaphor in health literacy, *Journal of Communication in Healthcare*, 9(2): 109–19.

Tervalon, M. & Murray-Garcia, J. (1998). Cultural humility versus cultural competence: A critical distinction in defining physician training outcomes in multicultural education, *Journal of Health Care for the Poor and Underserved*, 9(2): 117–25.

Wilburn, A., Vanderpool, R.C. & Knight, J.R. (2016). Environmental scanning as a public health tool: Kentucky's human papillomavirus vaccination project, *Preventing Chronic Disease*, 13, 160165.

REFERENCES

Alzheimer's Disease International (2020). World Alzheimer Reports (Website). Retrieved from: alz.co.uk/research/world-report

Canterbury District Health Board (2019). *Evaluation of the Community Engagement with Alcohol Licensing Project*. New Zealand: Canterbury District Health Board.

Charlton, P., Doucet, S., Azar, R., Nagel, D.A., Boulos, L., Luke, A., Mears, K., Jelly, K.J. & Montelpare, W.J. (2019). The use of the environmental scan in health services delivery research: A scoping review protocol, *British Medical Journal Open*, 9, e029805.

Cross, T.L., Bazron, B.J., Dennis, K.W. & Isaacs, M.R. (1989). *Towards a Culturally Competent System of Care: A monograph on effective services for minority children who are severely emotionally disturbed*. Washington: Georgetown University Child Development Center.

Dementia Australia (2020). Dementia statistics: Key facts and statistics (Website). Retrieved from: https://www.dementia.org.au/statistics

Dobos, A.R., Orthia, L.A. & Lamberts, R. (2015). Does a picture tell a thousand words? The uses of digitally produced, multimodal pictures for communicating information about Alzheimer's disease, *Public Understanding of Science*, 24(6), 712–30.

Gerlach, A.J. (2012). A critical reflection on the concept of cultural safety, *Canadian Journal of Occupational Therapy*, 79(3), 151–8.

Glanz, K. & Bishop, D.B. (2010). The role of behavioral science theory in development and implementation of public health interventions, *Annual Review of Public Health*, 31, 399–418.

Kirk, L. (2009). Taking a more strategic approach to science communication. In *11th Pacific Science Inter-Congress*, Tahiti, 2–6 March.

Laycock, A., Walker, D., Harrison, N. & Brands, J. (2011). *Researching Indigenous Health: A practical guide for researchers*. Carlton: The Lowitja Institute.

Lowitja Institute (2020). *Researching Indigenous Health: A practical guide for researchers*. Retrieved from: https://www.lowitja.org.au/page/services/resources/health-services-and-workforce/workforce/Researching-Indigenous-Health-Guide

Morrison, A., Rigney, L.-I., Hattam, R. & Diplock, A. (2019). *Toward an Australian Culturally Responsive Pedagogy: A narrative review of the literature*. Adelaide: University of South Australia.

Munro, S., Lewin, S., Swart, T. & Volmink, J. (2007). A review of health behaviour theories: How useful are these for developing interventions to promote long-term medication adherence for TB and HIV/AIDS? *BMC Public Health*, 7, 104.

Myint-U, A., Bull, S., Greenwood, G.L., Patterson, J., Rietmeijer, C.A., Vrungos, S., Warner, L., Moss, J. & O'Donnell, L.N. (2010). Safe in the city: Developing an effective video-based intervention for STD clinic waiting rooms, *Health Promotion Practice*, 11(3), 408–17.

RHD Action (2020). Global Resolution (Website). Retrieved from: https://rhdaction.org/rhdresolution

Smith, R.A., Downs, E. & Witte, K. (2007). Drama theory and entertainment education: Exploring the effects of a radio drama on behavioral intentions to limit HIV transmission in Ethiopia, *Communication Monographs*, 74(2), 133–53.

Tervalon, M. & Murray-Garcia, J. (1998). Cultural humility versus cultural competence: A critical distinction in defining physician training outcomes in multicultural education, *Journal of Health Care for the Poor and Underserved*, 9(2), 117–25.

UNICEF (2020). UNICEF in Botswana (Website). Retrieved from: https://www.unicef.org/botswana/

US Department of Health & Human Services (2020). *Alzheimer's Scientific Images and Video*. National Institute on Aging. Retrieved from https://www.nia.nih.gov/alzheimers/alzheimers-scientific-images-and-video

van Gemert, C., Pietze, P., Gold, J., Sacks-Davis, R., Stoové, M., Vally, H. & Hellard, M. (2011). The Australian national binge drinking campaign: Campaign recognition among young people at a music festival who report risky drinking, *BMC Public Health*, 11, 482.

Vertovec, S. (2007). Super-diversity and its implications, *Ethnic and Racial Studies*, 30(6), 1024–54.

Wilburn, A., Vanderpool, R.C. & Knight, J.R. (2016). Environmental scanning as a public health tool: Kentucky's human papillomavirus vaccination project, *Preventing Chronic Disease*, 13, 160165.

World Health Organization (WHO) (2019). World Patient Safety Day 2019 (Website). Retrieved from: https://www.who.int/campaigns/world-patient-safety-day/2019/campaign-essentials

Understanding and using media in health promotion

7

Merryn McKinnon

With contributions from Mitsuru Kudo and Shino Ouchi

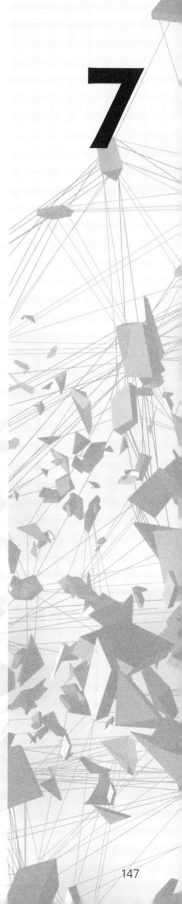

LEARNING OBJECTIVES

At the completion of the chapter, you will be able to:

- Describe the role of media in health promotion and public perception of health issues, using appropriate examples.
- Develop a communication strategy for a health promotion campaign.
- Compare and contrast the strengths and weaknesses of different communication channels.
- Identify and describe news values.

Introduction

The media is a vital tool for health promotion and can be used on a local, national or global scale to share information. By understanding the fundamentals of news and its production, the aim of this chapter is to assist you to produce information and material for the media in a way that will facilitate your story getting coverage. However, as you will no doubt have come to realise after reading the earlier chapters of this text, the media outlet you use is only one small part of your approach to health promotion. In media communications, through whichever channel/s you may choose, the beliefs and values of your audience will always influence how they perceive the topic. How the media presents the topic also plays a key role.

The first section of this chapter looks at general techniques and considerations in the presentation of news by the media, the evaluation of that news by the public and the influence of both of these factors on public perception of health issues. The second section outlines what makes news – the news values that journalists use to evaluate whether they will cover a story – and the strengths and weaknesses of various media channels as tools for communicating health information for different purposes. The final section puts it all together by providing instructions of how to develop a communication plan to strategically ensure your information reaches your intended audiences.

The relationship between media and public perceptions of health

What do we mean when we talk about 'media'?

People can get information from a range of media types. Global communications firm Edelman proposed a 'Media Cloverleaf' in 2011, which outlines the four different spheres of media that can be used to support public engagement. This cloverleaf sits at the centre of all four spheres:

- Traditional media – the typical large media conglomerates that provide news through print, television and radio channels.
- Tradigital media – online-only outlets that tend to be focused on very specific topics (but are optimised for easy discovery by search engines); these tend to be readily shared and often include blogsites.
- Social media platforms – such as Facebook, Twitter, Reddit and Instagram, also used by traditional media to drive further engagement.
- Owned media – content produced by an organisation – for example, stories written and shared by a university or health agency.

When thinking about how to engage your intended audience, you may wish to use all of these spheres, or maybe one or two of them. But this must be determined by knowing where your audience does, or is most likely to, get their information and, of these, which sources they trust.

Information sources and credibility

Trusted sources

What we see in the media is created and influenced by a variety of factors. The type of media used, the outlet and the spokesperson may all influence public perceptions of a topic. Even the topic itself will be interpreted and responded to according to the values and beliefs of the audience, as we have discussed in previous chapters. The Trust Barometer is an annual, global survey asking thousands of respondents from 28 different markets about trust, including their trusted sources such as organisations, sectors or people. The 2020 survey found that online search engines and traditional media are the most trusted sources for information, with owned media third and social media the least trusted source (Edelman, 2020). This is similar to a study conducted in Australia in 2019 by Roy Morgan. The company surveyed about 1000 people for its Media Net Trust Survey, to calculate the Net Trust Score (NTS) for the different forms of Australian media. It found that the Australian Broadcasting Corporation (ABC) was the most trusted media outlet, distrusted by only 7 per cent of respondents, in comparison to the 44 per cent of respondents who distrusted social media (Roy Morgan, 2019). This does not necessarily mean, however, that social media is never trusted as a source. The person or organisation sharing the information on social media will be a mitigating factor.

When it comes to trusted people, the top three most-trusted professions are consistently company technical experts, academic experts and 'someone like me' (Edelman, 2020) – the latter reinforcing the importance of family members and peers, as outlined in the various theories and models discussed in Chapter 2. Interestingly, the second-least trusted persons are journalists (Edelman, 2020). While a particular media source may be trusted, the individual journalist may not be. This means that who the journalist quotes in their stories may be potentially an important contributor to how public audiences respond to and/or perceive a health issue reported in the news. Trust is very important when considering the communication of health issues, as trust influences someone's intention to act on the basis of information received (Sillence et al., 2019). Given that much of health promotion aims to facilitate behavioural change, understanding how people evaluate trust is crucial.

Previous studies have explored how people determine what is 'trustworthy' and credible when they look for health information, and while predominantly looking at online sources, the criteria for 'trustworthy' could arguably be extended offline as well. A systematic review by Sun and colleagues (2019) found 25 criteria used by consumers to evaluate the quality of information; however, of these criteria three could be considered core: trustworthiness, expertise and objectivity. Whether a source is considered trustworthy depends heavily on how the information is presented. Information is considered trustworthy if it is good-quality and relevant, well-designed and presented, and impartial (Sillence et al., 2019). Impartiality and objectivity are largely referring to the same thing: is the information presented in the best interest of the consumer or patient, or that of the information provider? This is analogous to a media article being considered 'balanced', or not. Does it provide all perspectives to an issue or is it giving more credence to one? A note of caution: sometimes, in an attempt to provide all perspectives, media providers can create a 'false balance' – the perception that the debate is equally weighted when in fact it is not. This has been starkly demonstrated by media coverage of measles, mumps, rubella (MMR) vaccination (Jackson, 2011). The overwhelming scientific evidence disproving claims about the vaccine's negative side-effects was often given the same weight as the unsubstantiated views of anti-vaccination groups, creating the public perception that scientists themselves were disagreeing and helping to 'fuel a public health disaster' (Jackson, 2011, p. 1).

Evaluating information

One way people can evaluate the quality or 'trustworthiness' of the information they find is by looking at its source. Is it provided by a reputable source using the best available, peer-reviewed scientific evidence, such as from randomised control trials, or is it from an advocacy group that might have an **agenda** (hidden or explicit) influencing the information they present or the *way* in which they present the information? The latter is called 'agenda setting', whereby the manner in which information is presented is not explicitly telling the reader or viewer what to think so much as what to think about. A study of the results returned by searching 'vaccination' and 'immunisation' on the Google search engine found all of the top-10 results were anti-vaccination sites (Davies et al., 2002). Audiences who have strong information literacy may be able to better evaluate the information presented than those who have limited or weak information literacy.

There are several forms of literacy that someone searching for information needs to have; a lack of even one of these can create barriers to finding or receiving appropriate information. First of all, the audience needs to know how to find information. They then need to be able to understand the information presented. This understanding can be influenced by their reading ability, language comprehension and whether the material is presented in their first language or their second or even third language. The nature of the information provided is also important, as the previous chapters and prior research have discussed (Sillence et al., 2019; Sun et al., 2019). Is it clear, relevant and easy to understand? Finally, information seekers need to have **information literacy** to help them evaluate the quality of the information they find, as it is likely to be inconsistent. A study by Oncel and Alvur (2013) found that parents who used the Google search engine to help them evaluate whether to vaccinate their child against influenza were likely to receive almost an equal number of correct and incorrect information sources in the first page of results, in both English and Turkish languages. Knowing how to distinguish between correct and incorrect sources is important to facilitate informed decision-making.

The influence of framing

Another tool used by the media, and arguably organisations as well, is framing, which was introduced in Chapter 5. Framing features heavily in health stories, particularly in the headlines. Have a look at these example headlines:

Agenda – an aim or reason for doing something. A hidden agenda may be a secret reason for doing something – for example, causing people to doubt the safety or effectiveness of one product so they buy another instead

Information literacy – the ability to recognise the need to seek information, and knowing how to find, evaluate and effectively use the information found

- Doctors battle outbreak
- Researchers declare war on brain cancer
- SARS: A deadly killer
- Latest weapon in battle against HIV/AIDS
- Live bacteria spray is showing promise
- Could Australia have the answer to a COVID vaccine?
- Malaria vaccine research breakthrough
- A clue to stopping deadly virus.

What do you notice? The first four headlines are presenting stories with health as a 'battlefield' and a 'war' to be won against enemies. The next four headlines are more positively framed around hope and insight, leading to success. One word that gets used in relation to health far too often is 'breakthrough' (and you can see it in one of the headlines above). There is nothing wrong with using the word breakthrough, but it needs to be describing a genuine breakthrough. These are examples of real headlines from over the past 10 years. Do we have a commercially available, effective malaria vaccine yet? No. Therefore, was it really a breakthrough? Most 'breakthroughs' are more like the HIV/AIDS vaccine headline – there are promising results and avenues for future exploration, but we really will not know if it is a breakthrough for another 5–20 years. Not quite as catchy as a headline, but accuracy should never be sacrificed for **hype**. Even when you keep your message as accurate as possible, the possibility of unintended interpretations and consequences still exists, as Case study 7.1 shows.

Hype – extravagant, often overstated, claims about a person, place, product or result

CASE STUDY 7.1 What do Japanese public health experts think about health or medical information provided by the mass media?

Shino Ouchi and Mitsuru Kudo

Mass-media coverage of health and medicine – popular but problematic?

While many people in Japan rely heavily on the mass media (e.g. television, newspapers and magazines) for health and medical information, we often hear that health and medical professionals criticise the mass media for its lack of accuracy in reporting on health or medical matters (Hashimoto, 2016; Matsunaga & Tsubono, 2008a; Matsunaga & Tsubono, 2008b; Takahashi, 2008). To explore this issue we interviewed 10 Japanese experts in public health, epidemiology and health communication (Ouchi, 2018). In the interviews, we focused on their views about mass-media reporting on the prevention of non-communicable diseases.

(cont.)

(cont.)

What do public health experts say about mass-media reporting?

Most of the public health experts interviewed recognised the importance and necessity for health or medical researchers to communicate their research findings through the mass media. While maintaining a degree of concern about the potential inaccuracy of media reporting, they acknowledged that the breadth of topics the mass media can communicate to the general, non-expert audience was indispensable in our society today. Some of the interviewees also mentioned that health or medical professionals and journalists should collaborate more, since they both share a primary interest in raising public awareness of health and motivating the public to improve their health behaviours.

Unintended consequences

Health and medical reporting can trigger behavioural change in possibly unexpected, and even unhealthy, ways. One interviewee, a public health nurse, told a story about media reporting on the potentially positive health effects of consuming cocoa. Some people responded to these news stories by consuming too much cocoa, shown by an abnormally high level of glucose in their blood. Other interviewees also told us that people with health problems were prone to turn to 'healthy food' and 'healthy behaviours' featured in mass media reporting as an easy, convenient cure for their health problems, instead of seeking professional medical advice and/or treatment. This suggests that people with lower awareness of how to get and maintain good health would be susceptible to an (occasionally overly) positive, optimistic tone of health and medical reporting, and would not be able to judge the scientific rigour or actual effectiveness in health and medical terms.

What should we be careful about when speaking to the mass media?

The findings of these interviews reiterate the importance of paying careful, detailed attention to our audience. Often, as health promotion professionals we focus on ensuring that the message we communicate through the mass media is accurate, which is understandable since scientific accuracy of media content is vital to health and medical communication. Yet, what is equally – or possibly even more – important is to think very carefully about how the message will be interpreted by the diverse members of the public, how this will influence their behaviours and what health consequences they may possibly experience as a result.

QUESTIONS

1. What media sources would you turn to when seeking health or medical information? Why?

2. Your friend asks you, 'How much can we trust health information in the mass media?' How would you respond?

3. What do you think are the characteristics of mass-media coverage of health or medical issues that attract the attention of an audience? Do you think this is a positive or negative way to attract attention? Explain your answer.

ELSEWHERE IN THE WORLD

Science Media Centre

Science Media Centres (SMCs) (https://www.sciencemediacentre.org/) provide journalists, scientists and press officers with support and resources to ensure the provision of accurate and evidence-based information about scientific topics to publics and policy makers. There are SMCs in the United Kingdom, Australia, Canada, Germany and Aotearoa New Zealand.

The other way framing can be used is to direct the audience's attention to a particular aspect or element of the story. In a study exploring media framing of obesity prevention policy, researchers found that people were more likely to support policies if the media story featured an individual obese child, rather than a story covering the causes and statistics in general terms (Barry et al., 2013). This is similar to what is advocated in fundraising and philanthropic circles. By telling the story of one individual, people can focus their attention, and it makes the issue seem manageable: one person can be helped, whereas trying to 'fix' a problem for 1 million people can seem impossible (Chilcott, 2014). It can also influence perceptions of the 'cause' of a problem. In a study of media coverage of obesity, Kim & Willis (2007) found that while practices in the food industry were identified as a contributing cause to rising obesity rates, the industry was rarely named as a potential solution. The same study also found that television media outlets were more likely to focus on individual, personal causes and solutions to obesity rather than broader, societal ones. The focus of frames can be influenced by cultural background. The Kim and Willis (2007) study explored media from the United States – a highly individualistic culture. Other studies on the framing of health issues in highly collectivist cultures, such as China, found a greater focus on the broader picture, with emphasis on what is best for the society as opposed to the individual (Zhang et al., 2015). The individual versus society focus of a frame can sometimes play out in unexpected ways, especially during times of crisis. This was clearly demonstrated during the COVID-19 pandemic in 2020, where the ways in which these messages were communicated were seen to influence public responses (see Case study 7.2). Regardless of whether you are seeking an investment of time or money, or if you want people to adopt certain behaviours, careful planning of your communication is key. The next section outlines how to develop a communication plan and the different ways it can be used to achieve your desired objective.

CASE STUDY 7.2 Trust and framing in a pandemic

The emergence of COVID-19

The coronavirus pandemic – COVID-19 – was first identified in Wuhan, the capital of Hubei province in China, in December 2019. By February 2020, rates of infection in China had dropped but cases were rapidly appearing in Italy, Iran and South Korea. The WHO declared COVID-19 a pandemic in March 2020. Around the world, countries grappled with how to prevent or slow the spread of the virus and many enacted widespread control measures, many of which had not been seen since the influenza pandemic of 1918. Internationally, health agencies and governments moved to stop the known methods of transmission of the virus, namely close contact between humans and aerosol infection, whereby the coughs and sneezes of infected people produce respiratory droplets containing the virus and infect others. This led to the roll-out of increasingly strict measures to limit contact between people through the cancellation of large events, closure of businesses and educational institutions, restriction of travel within and between countries, and requiring people to remain in their homes.

The initial response from the international community was mixed, with China moving quickly to quarantine citizens, in an attempt to slow the spread of transmission of the disease, primarily through a public health campaign described as a '"people's war" of epidemic prevention and control' (Xinhua, 2020, para 1). This occurred at the same time as reports emerged of doctors being reprimanded for 'spreading rumours' about the virus and leading to concerns that China may have downplayed the severity of the initial outbreak in its communications with the global community (Kuo, 2020). China's rigorous surveillance, immediate isolation of patients and restrictions on public movement were seen as key factors influencing the country's apparent success in controlling the virus (Kuo, 2020), and countries around the world began to implement similar measures, with varying degrees of success and public acceptance.

The role of media in communication about COVID-19

During a pandemic, the media's role in delivering health messages is critical. Media was a key mechanism for public health and other government officials to communicate with national and international populations. Unfortunately, the media can also propagate confusion and misinformation by simply providing that public mechanism to health officials, without appropriate planning and targeting. Repeated news coverage of excessive purchasing of goods, such as toilet paper and pasta, fed panic buying amid unfounded fears by the public of future food scarcity. This caused usually readily available essential resources to be difficult to procure (Carter, et al., 2020), which in turn increased the negative effects on vulnerable populations who may have already struggled to gain access to necessities, due to cost or inability to get to shops.

In Australia, messaging from the federal government was criticised as confusing and rambling; this was not helped by the fact that information often was conveyed to the public through press conferences, where viewing and listening audiences typically cannot hear questions asked by journalists (McInerney, 2020). At first, some Australians did not appear to take the threat of coronavirus seriously, ignoring the health messages that were designed to prevent the spread of the virus (Murphy, 2020a). A survey by media outlet *The Guardian* (Murphy, 2020b) found that this could partially be attributed to a lack of trust in the media; of the survey's 1034 respondents only 35 per cent trusted the media to give them reliable, honest information about the pandemic. Just over half of the sample trusted government. In practice, what this means is that getting people to act on health messages is very difficult when they do not trust the official channels and sources used to communicate them (Murphy, 2020b).

'Us' versus 'them'

A dominant frame used in health messaging from Australian sources was individualistic, telling people that the 'risk to you is low but we need to do what we can to protect the vulnerable and save lives' (Carter et al., 2020). This set up an 'us and them' mentality, whereby the audience perceives that 'we' personally (us) are at low risk, and 'the vulnerable' (them) are not directly spoken to as an audience (Carter et al., 2020). This also ignores the inherent connected nature of communities, and in a pandemic situation this can exacerbate problems. The panic buying and hoarding of toilet paper and other essentials, for example, reflects people prioritising their own perceived needs, which are founded on their fears and anxieties, *above* what is best for society as a whole. Shared vulnerability, the message that 'we are all in this together' is a more effective frame to motivate action than 'us versus them' (Carter et al., 2020). These frames could be seen illustrated in public communication in Australia and Aotearoa New Zealand. The key message used by the Australian government to communicate its COVID-19 response was 'Help stop the spread and stay healthy' (see Figure 7.1). in contrast, the Aotearoa New Zealand government's key message was 'Unite against COVID-19: Together we can slow the spread'.

QUESTIONS

1. Compare the key messages of the Australian and Aotearoa New Zealand governments. Which of these do you think would be more likely to:
   a. Be understood by the community
   b. Motivate community action – and why?
2. If communities do not trust the media or government to provide honest and reliable information in health messaging during a pandemic, how do you think these messages could be communicated in a way that builds trust? Think about the people, information and sources that could be included.

(cont.)

(cont.)

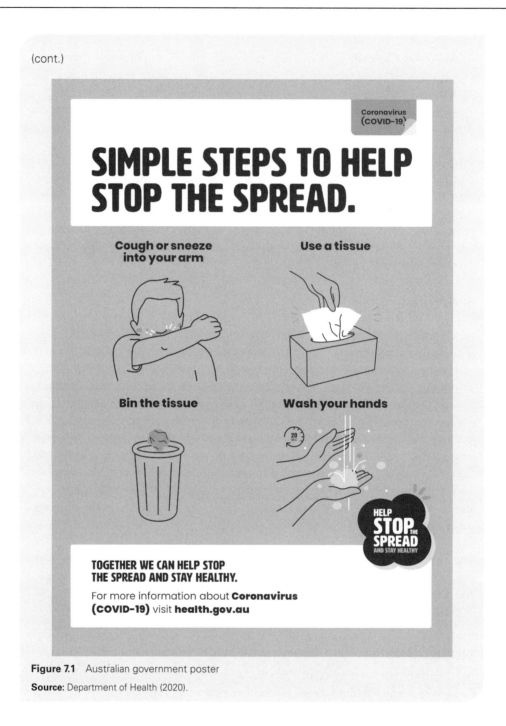

Figure 7.1   Australian government poster
Source: Department of Health (2020).

Communication strategies and plans

There are two main types of communication plans: strategic and tactical. A strategic communication plan is a 'big-picture' plan, usually developed at an organisational level. As an example, the WHO has a strategic communications framework that encompasses all the communication activities it undertakes, across all health issues (WHO, n.d.). The WHO's framework outlines six key principles for effective communication, which are that communications are:

- Accessible – can target audiences receive the information?
- Actionable – are audiences encouraged to take action?
- Credible – WHO is trusted as a source of credible, expert information
- Relevant – the audience sees the information as applicable to them
- Timely – information is provided when audiences need it to make decisions
- Understandable – can audiences understand the information in order to appropriately act?

The WHO's framework suggests different tactics that can be used to apply these principles to its activities, with the aim of improving communication at all levels of the organisation (WHO, n.d.).

The other kind of communication plan is a tactical plan. Tactical communication plans tend to be short-term in nature and focused on achieving a particular outcome. We focus on tactical communication plans in this chapter. These are the kinds of communication plans suitable for use in increasing communication activities to achieve a specific goal or to raise awareness of an issue or event. They can be used to plan and manage communication activities, both within an organisation and from an organisation to an external audience. Both strategic and tactical communication plans usually have the same kinds of information within them – it is really the scale and scope of the two that are different.

Purposes of communication strategies

Regardless of the type of communication activity you are organising, or for which audience, there are lots of different aspects to consider, and a communications plan is one way to make sure you do the job properly. Putting together a communication plan will force you to identify your target audience and the message you want to communicate. It will then help you to identify the channels you will use to get your key message to your intended audience and, most importantly, it can help you plan how to measure your success; more on that in the next section. First, let's look at the different ways communication plans can be applied.

Health promotion practitioners do a lot of communication in almost every aspect of their work. Communication obviously occurs with individuals and groups of all sizes to raise awareness of health issues, but they also to help empower people to make informed decisions about their health. In Chapter 1 we discussed the environmental, economic, political and social influences on health. Health promotion can therefore be a tool for advocacy, to create awareness of issues such as inequality or unmet needs, to influence decisions and lobby for change. It can also be used in capacity building, which incorporates both advocacy and partnerships between people and organisations. This can be done in a variety of ways, with a variety of audiences.

Advocacy

Doctors for the Environment Australia (DEA) is an organisation comprised of health professionals who promote good health through care of the environment. Its 'No Time for Games' campaign began in 2015 and aimed to highlight the effects of climate change on children's health (DEA, 2015). In addition to producing factsheets and reports, the campaign asked medical professionals to sign a pledge declaring a health emergency and supporting four key policy recommendations that aimed to address the negative health consequences created by climate change (DEA, 2018). The list of over 2500 signatories to this pledge was submitted to the federal Health Minister and to leaders of all the major political parties in the lead up to the 2019 federal election. In September 2019, a parliamentary motion to declare human-induced climate change as a most urgent health threat to children was passed, which also called for the decarbonisation of Australia by 2050 (DEA, 2020). Advocacy can be a useful means of creating awareness, momentum and, ultimately, desired change.

Partnerships and networks

Partnerships can be formed between organisations, not-for-profit organisations, government agencies and academic sectors, and are critical to the promotion of health (Estacio et al., 2017). Partnerships and networks can also be a way to extend the reach and influence of your campaign or activities by having more people and organisations involved in delivering activities or communicating your message. For example, World Cancer Day occurs each year on 4 February. In 2017, the National Cancer Control Committee (NCCC) of the Ministry of Health in Indonesia coordinated a national health promotion campaign, coinciding with World Cancer Day and aiming to raise awareness of cancer, including cancer detection and treatment (Giselvania et al., 2018). The NCCC provided national coordination for commemoration of the day and sent out the initial information and proposals to health centres across Indonesia. The centres developed their own activities, which included seminars, media campaigns, celebrity performances and mobile testing for certain cancers. Of the 34 provinces across Indonesia, events were held in 25, involving non-government organisations, professional societies, hospitals, provincial public health services, companies and cancer survivors. The importance of partnerships was seen in 2018, when the NCCC did not provide any coordination, yet events and activities were organised across the country (Giselvania et al., 2018).

Capacity building

Capacity building is a term used in many different fields so there is no unified definition. In terms of health promotion, capacity building has been described as the 'invisible work' (Hawe et al., 1998) that health promotion professionals do to ensure that effective changes are sustained. Capacity building incorporates advocacy and relies heavily on partnerships that work across sectors to produce effective and sustainable strategies (VicHealth, 2012). Capacity building, and the partnerships within them, can operate at four different levels: individual, community, organisational (top down or bottom up, cf Crisp et al., 2000) and system (VicHealth, 2012):

- Individual – building knowledge and skills to influence the individual, with potential for this individual to influence other community members
- Community – influencing change through collaboration, with groups formed by geography, demographic, workplace, shared interests and/or goals
- Organisations – building capacity internally through staff training, restructuring processes and/or allocation and location of resources

- System – capacity building at this level is more complex in scope and may involve multiple partners conducting activities such as advocacy and policy development (VicHealth, 2012).

Health promotion projects may involve multiple levels of capacity building, or only one. Irrespective of the scope of your project, a communication plan can help keep you on track towards achieving your objective.

Core parts of communication plans

At this stage you should have completed your needs assessment, identified your target audience and developed your program, based on the identified needs. Your needs assessment should have identified potential barriers to your intended audience participating in your activity or program or otherwise receiving your message. Perhaps your needs assessment also identified successful communication activities you could emulate? This communication plan is now where the 'rubber hits the road' and you set out how you will get your message to your intended audience.

Objective

What is it that you want to achieve? Your objective needs to be SMART (see Chapters 2 and 6) as this is also what you will be using to inform your evaluation. An objective like: 'To reduce smoking by 100 per cent in New South Wales' is far too unrealistic and not specific enough. What this objective is trying to achieve is huge, but it also does not specify a time frame. If you are trying to evaluate your success against such a goal, then you are setting yourself up to fail. A better, more achievable objective would be 'to reduce smoking in people aged 18–25 by 15 per cent on the Central Coast of New South Wales by 30 September 2021'. It identifies a specific audience and location, a more realistic reduction target and a specific time frame.

Target audience

Whom do you want to communicate with? There may be more than one target audience for your program, but be specific about how you define each audience.

Key message

If people only remember one thing from your communication activities, what would you want that to be? This is likely your key message. Depending on what you are trying to achieve, your key message might be strongly tied to your campaign, like the examples given in Case study 7.2, or if you are running an event your key message might contain the information people need to remember the event, find the details and attend. If you have different target audiences, you may also have different key messages. All key messages should support the objective. If you are stuck for what good key messages are, have a look at advertisements. If someone says to you 'Just do it', 'Because you're worth it' or 'Have a break, have a … ' do you know what brands they are talking about? (Nike, L'Oreal and KitKat.) These are effective key messages and advertisers execute them well.

Communication activities

This is where you set out what you will do. List each activity separately, including its channels, time frame and resources, including human resources. Make sure you also link the activities to your target audience/s and include measures for evaluation so you can know if the activity was successful in helping to achieve the objective. It is very important to remember that every activity you do must reinforce the key message/s of your campaign. This might mean saying the same thing in different ways, but the key message must appear with all communications.

Communication channels

Where will you execute your communication activities? This is another section of the plan where you need to be very specific. It is tempting to say 'newspapers, social media', but which newspapers, specifically? Which social media platforms? This is the section where the adage 'know your audience' is really important. It is also important that you use your resources – including your time – wisely. Invest your energy and efforts in using communication channels (see Chapter 2) where you know your target audience/s are. If you still are not sure, look at the websites of different media outlets to find out their key demographics (sometimes the 'advertise with us' sections contain this information), or search for audience numbers and ratings. When it comes to social media, think about who you could partner with or what other pages or groups share common interests or audiences, and who may be happy to share or promote your content. Tagging other people and organisations in your posts can be a way to boost content. Make sure that you are tagging those who are either involved in your initiative or have a shared interest in it. Tagging lots of different groups and people randomly may actually work against the objective; practise good social media etiquette! Do not forget channels such as community noticeboards (physical and virtual), libraries, sports clubs – list all the places where your audience would likely see the message, to ensure you maximise your chances that they will.

Resources

What do you need to enable these activities to occur and to access these channels? It might be people, money, transport or special skill sets. Planning what you need in advance will help get you organised and may also help you justify what you are asking of those who can supply the resources you need.

Timeline

When will you undertake each activity and how often will you do it? This can be separated into planning, delivery and evaluation phases or you might use time frames (days, weeks, months), or a combination of the two.

Owner

Who is responsible for completing the activity or securing the resources? If you are working with a group and it is a team responsibility, it is still a good idea to have someone designated to take ownership of that particular task or activity.

Indicators

What does success look like? This is where you work out how to evaluate the effectiveness of your program and/or your communication plan in helping you achieve your objective. Choose indicators that are meaningful and can be demonstrated through evidence. Typically, this relies on people doing something – be it turning up to an event, using a new product or service, or changing behaviours. Whatever you choose to measure, it must be related to your objective. Basing measures of success on the creation of a website or giving out leaflets is not meaningful. You may have created a wonderful website, but if no-one is using it, then it is not helping to achieve your objective. Likewise, you could have given out 200 or 2000 leaflets, but if people did not read them then this, too, is not contributing to the achievement of your objective. You may also wish to consider undertaking a **formative evaluation** near the start or part-way through the execution of your communication plan. Such an evaluation can be useful in tracking how you are progressing towards your objective and will give you the opportunity to make any adjustments as needed to keep you on track. There is more on indicators and evaluation in the next chapter.

Formative evaluation – evaluation undertaken in the early stages of planning or implementation of programs and/ or activities, to ensure planned actions are appropriate and will be effective in achieving the desired outcome

Strengths and weaknesses of different media

Once you have begun to think about who your target audience is and what you want to say to them, you can start to plan which communication channels are most appropriate. First, think about your audience: where do they usually go to get information? Where else might you find them? Always use what you know about the information-seeking habits of your audience, to guide your decisions about which media channel/s to use. Each has its own strengths and weaknesses.

Mainstream media

The **mainstream media** is an effective means of getting information quickly to a wide range of audiences. The mainstream media comprises mass outlets such as newspapers, radio and television, and has been fundamental to communication strategies, and many people's lives, for almost a century. Mass media is critical to health promotion; however, each type and outlet has a different level of usefulness and appropriateness for different audiences. It is important to remember that there are highly influential and well-known figures who are prominent on all these platforms. Some well-known figures (including the owners of the media outlet) may use these platform/s to promote their personal opinions and ideologies as part of their coverage of news, and that these may be in contrast or in opposition to advice provided by governments, health agencies and scientists. Coverage of climate change and COVID-19 are recent examples. This can create confusion and contribute to scepticism and distrust, as discussed earlier in this chapter, but this approach is not universal; most journalists and outlets simply want to share accurate, factual and interesting stories with their audiences. Choose your outlets wisely and communicate your message clearly, in a way that does not

Mainstream media – the traditional, established and conventional forms of publishing and broadcast media, such as newspapers, television and radio, which are capable of reaching and thereby influencing large numbers of people. Online media outlets typically are excluded from definitions of 'mainstream media'

facilitate confusion; the mainstream media is extraordinarily effective at getting messages to mass populations.

Television

Strengths Television is an effective means of combining images, people and words to tell a story. One story has potential to reach an audience of millions very quickly. It can be used to create awareness of an issue, using compelling visuals; however, the consequences may not always be as intended (see Case study 7.3). Some television journalists, programs and broadcasters are trusted sources of information and thus are highly influential. Television programs can also be useful in starting conversations on key topics, which in turn can lead to behavioural change.

Weaknesses With the rise of streaming services such as AppleTV, Netflix, Stan and Amazon Prime, free-to-air television channels are increasingly struggling to retain their audiences. In some developing countries, where extremely vulnerable populations may not have access to television at all, the medium is inappropriate for use in health promotion.

CASE STUDY 7.3 The original fear campaign?

The human immunodeficiency virus (HIV) was first transmitted to humans in the 1920s, but it was not until the 1980s that it was recognised as a health condition (Avert, 2019). While HIV was initially associated with men who had sex with men, in 1982 the disease was also found in people with haemophilia and injecting drug users, leading to the use of the name acquired immune deficiency syndrome (AIDS) and the acronym HIV/AIDS (Avert, 2019). In the face of rising infection rates, throughout the 1980s and 1990s, most countries conducted some form of mass-media campaign to prevent the spread of HIV/AIDS, leading to mass media becoming the main source of HIV/AIDS prevention messages (Myhre & Flora, 2000). However, some of these campaigns had unintended consequences.

The Grim Reaper

In April 1987, Australian television showed an advertisement about HIV/AIDS, featuring the mythological persona of Death as 'the Grim Reaper', playing ten pin bowling with men, women and children as the 'pins'. The advertisement was designed to provide people with reliable information on how to prevent HIV and AIDS. It was one of the most effective campaigns ever launched in Australia, with its effects heralded as providing a 'wake-up call', especially bringing HIV/AIDS to the attention of heterosexual audiences (CDC, 2002).

The Grim Reaper ad was extremely memorable – even decades later! And because broadcast media was the sole means of communicating information to mass audiences at that time, this ad 'attained nearly universal exposure' in Australia (Myhre & Flora,

2000, p. 40). It captured the fear and uncertainty of the time, when little was known about how to prevent and treat HIV/AIDS (Power, 2012). However, the ad also had the flow-on effect of creating fear and anxiety in the general Australian population – which was considered a low-risk group overall – without actually changing public knowledge about the disease (Bray & Chapman, 1991). It also created controversy and inspired discrimination as people began to associate the Grim Reaper with people living with HIV/AIDS, especially same-sex attracted men (CDC, 2002).

What worked in the 1980s is not going to work now

In 2012, in response to rising rates of HIV diagnosis in Australia, the Queensland government reprised the Grim Reaper ad – although in a 'softer' form, by showing an actor made up as the Grim Reaper with the catch phrase, 'we shouldn't be making this ad'. The use of a single television commercial was criticised by many HIV/AIDS awareness and prevention organisations, as it was not part of a full campaign to encourage people to seek testing and treatment, or to remind people of best practice in preventing transmission. It was also considered an inappropriate approach to HIV/AIDS prevention and awareness for the 21st century (OIP, 2012).

QUESTIONS

1. In addition to a television ad, what else would you do to develop a campaign for HIV/AIDS prevention and awareness that is better suited to the 21st century? Justify your choices.
2. Reflect on how fear can create stigma and discrimination. What examples of this have you seen locally, nationally and globally?

Radio

Strengths Similar to television, radio can reach large audiences very quickly and easily. As an audio-only medium, radio relies on compelling story telling to remain interesting and engaging. There is a much wider range of radio stations than television, spanning commercial stations, public broadcasting and community run stations that serve particular niche audiences. The latter can be as specific as a university campus radio program or an arts program for a certain geographic audience. Radio personalities and programs are usually trusted sources of information. Radio stations tend to serve particular demographic groups, allowing for easy targeting of an intended audience. Radio is also more easily accessible to remote communities and communities in developing countries that do not have access to television or other mass-media resources. One example is *Bienvenida Salud* (Welcome Health), a radio program run by Minga Peru, a community based organisation in the Peruvian Amazon. The program's content is based on letters sent in by listeners, asking questions about topics such as domestic/family violence, HIV/AIDS, gender equality, human rights and bio-cultural preservation. Bienvenida Salud has been on air for over 20 years and reaches more than 120 000 listeners each episode; program listeners live in one of the most inaccessible regions of Peru (Minga Peru, n.d.).

Weaknesses Radio tends to be relegated to 'background noise', commonly listened to by people at work or while driving or travelling on public transport. This means that people usually are not as focused on the message as they might be when they are watching television, for example. Once something has been said on live radio, it usually disappears, so if a listener misses what has been said, it can be very difficult for them to find that information again without a concerted effort.

Newspapers

Strengths Newspapers can range from local community publications through to nationwide syndicates. Now often available in both print and online editions, newspapers have a longstanding history as a key source of news. Even with the arrival of the first European settlers in Australia in the late 1700s and early 1800s, newspapers were used as a means of communicating health messages – at that time the importance of vaccinating against smallpox (McKinnon & Orthia, 2017). Online versions of newspapers often bring together other supporting materials, such as extended articles and essays, social media content, video and audio clips. Print media provides a source of information to refer back to, and so remains available to its audience for much longer than radio and television.

Weaknesses Access to content is the biggest weakness of newspapers. With the rise of social media and the internet, advertising revenues – which traditional newspapers have relied upon – have reduced dramatically and have caused many newspapers to change their operating models by requiring subscriptions to access their content. People in rural and remote areas do not have the same frequency of access to print newspapers as metropolitan audiences. For some, accessing newspapers may be completely reliant upon having a reliable internet connection. Being able to access information in newspapers requires people to be functionally literate – they must be able to read. This extends to people with visual impairments and conditions such as dyslexia, people unable to access education and immigrant populations for whom English is a second, third or fourth language.

Magazines

Strengths Magazines share many of the same strengths as newspapers. They tend to be broader-ranging in content, with publications tailored to very specific interests, including health. Magazines tend to have a more relaxed writing format than newspapers and journals, which means they can cover issues in greater depth and use images to bring stories to life.

Weaknesses Magazines tend to be published weekly, fortnightly, monthly or even quarterly, which can make them difficult to use if you want to promote something quickly. Other than that, the same limitations as newspapers also apply.

Social media

The internet has made more information available to more people than ever before. But it is important to recognise that some populations do not have ready access to this information because they do not have access to a device and/or the internet. Others may simply not feel comfortable accessing information online. Social media is comparatively new, and for anyone born before the year 2000, even the internet was not commonplace. Not understanding how social media works or how to access different platforms can be a barrier to people accessing information through these channels. Social media should only be used to supplement, never wholly replace, face-to-face communication.

Strengths Social media platforms have developed into a core method of sharing information in societies such as Australia and Aotearoa New Zealand. A wide range of different social media applications (apps) tend to be used by different demographic groups, including cultural groups. For example, Chinese communities in Australia tend to use social media platforms such as TikTok, Weibo, WeChat and RenRen, in addition to Facebook and other mainstream apps. Social media platforms have enabled easy sharing of content, with the emphasis on succinct information, engaging visuals and dissemination of information through 'liking', sharing and/or commenting functions. It provides an excellent way to extend the reach of communication activities by encouraging users to share links to webpages, reports, posters, event links, television, video or radio clips. Using social media with partner organisations to leverage their audiences can help to increase exposure to a message beyond your own social media followers. Beyond disseminating information and encouraging dialogues between users, social media can also be used to create support networks. Studies have found that online social networks can provide social support, which in turn can reduce depression, anxiety and related thoughts and feelings, especially for people who do not have strong in-person social networks (Cole et al., 2017). Curated social media accounts and online events can also be useful tools for advocacy, empowerment and dialogue. For example, Indigenous Health MayDay – #IHMayDay – was 'a day long Twitter festival about Aboriginal and Torres Strait Islander health' (Sweet et al., 2015, p. 673), promoted as a day for 'Aboriginal and Torres Strait Islanders to speak, and for non-Indigenous Australians to participate by listening or re-tweeting' (Sweet et al., 2015, p. 638). Twitter was found to be a useful tool in enhancing connections to culture and community, which in turn supported the social and emotional wellbeing of Aboriginal and Torres Strait Islander people (Geia et al., 2017). #IHMayDay ran annually between 2014 and 2018, with 2018 seeing over 70 million Twitter impressions (the number of times a hashtag turns up in a timeline or search results) of #IHMayDay between 12 May and 11 June 2018 (IHMayDay18Team, 2018).

Weaknesses One of the greatest weaknesses of social media is also its greatest strength – the ease of sharing information. Incorrect information is just as likely, sometimes more likely, to be shared among online networks. The other weaknesses are those outlined at the beginning of this section – social media will help you reach a lot of people, but you do need to be mindful of the barriers.

Other, non-media communication channels

There are so many other ways to get attention to your message, and these can be used to supplement, or be supplemented by, whatever you do in the media campaign. These include:

- newsletters and campaigns delivered by email through apps such as MailChimp, Iterable and EmailOctopus
- posters, brochures, T-shirts, coasters and coffee mugs
- lighting up landmark buildings in your city or town
- wearing a particular colour for a World Awareness Day (e.g. pink for breast cancer or teal for food allergies)
- public transport offers a wide range of opportunities to get your message in front of a captive audience, at stops and stations, on the outside or inside of buses, trams and trains
- roadside signs, flagpoles on major roads or on the front of buildings
- stencils on footpaths, postcards, magnets and art.

The only limit is your budget and your creativity! Whatever you choose to do, make sure it is all part of a comprehensive plan with all the parts working together towards a clearly defined objective.

LEARNING ACTIVITY 7.1

Imagine you are responsible for developing a communication plan to support a health promotion activity or campaign. If you are stuck for ideas, think about causes such as drink driving, mental health awareness or cancer screening. Or use an idea that you might have started developing in the learning activities in earlier chapters.

Develop a communication plan for your activity, making sure that you include all of the elements of the communication plan. Be very specific about your objective, target audience and communication channels.

Once you have a communication plan, develop two different types of materials specified in your communication plan. This can include posts for different social media platforms, brochures, posters, postcards, roadside signs – anything!

EXTENSION ACTIVITY

Find a health promotion campaign or activity, happening near you or online. Have a look at their communication and promotional materials, including media coverage and press releases. Using the materials you find, evaluate:

1. How clearly you can identify the intended target audience/s and key message/s.
2. How well the materials reinforce the key message/s.

What makes news?

Now that you have your communication plan, and you know what media outlets you want to use, how might you ensure that your story gets coverage? Every journalist makes decisions about what stories to cover, based on what they know would be most interesting, relevant and newsworthy to their audience. The easiest way to get your message or material out in the media is by understanding what makes something 'newsworthy'. Newsworthiness is determined by the presence or absence of news values. The following list of news values is indicative. There are other lists – some with more values, some using different words – but the general premise is the same. One key point here is that evaluations of 'newsworthiness' are not simply about news items. Every time someone decides to read an article, a social media post, even an email, they are assessing whether it is 'newsworthy' for them and thus worth their time. Understanding how people evaluate what is interesting and relevant to them, using guiding principles such as news values, can help you in all of your communication activities, not just those directed at the media.

News values

Impact

Is it a big deal? Is it a big thing that will affect a small number of people, or a little thing that will affect a large number of people? Examples could include a global pandemic, the legalisation of voluntary euthanasia or interest rates being raised, which potentially places many people under increased economic pressure.

Timeliness

If it is not 'new', it is not news. Unless it is a new development on an old story. For example, when a new disease such as SARS or COVID-19 is found to be infecting people, stories about them will continue to be run as the situation develops.

Currency

Is it related to current news and events? If your health promotion program is aiming to increase physical activity, for example, and it happens to be running at the same time as the Olympic Games or some other sporting event (on any scale, from local to international), then you can use the focus of the big event to help get more focus on your program.

Proximity

Is it happening close enough for people to be interested or find it relevant to them? This can be something happening in a small community, or about someone from your country taking part in a major international event. A 'local' angle can help to drive relevance and interest.

Novelty

Novelty refers to something that is unusual or surprising. This news value can work well to disseminate to a large audience as people are more likely to share novel or surprising content. But some research suggests that people may choose 'known' or certain health messages instead of novel ones that may challenge their behaviours (Kim, 2015). Choose carefully and attempt to find a balance.

Prominence

Well-known personalities, political figures and organisations can be newsworthy in their own right. Adding any or all of these to a health promotion campaign can increase the appeal to both journalists and publics alike.

Human interest

This is probably the easiest news value to incorporate in health communications. It encompasses ordinary people doing extraordinary things; everyday people, situations and problems. Everyone needs health, so it is easy to use this news value to ensure audience relevance.

Conflict

There's an old journalistic maxim: 'if it bleeds, it leads'. This news value is about wars, fights and disagreements. A note of caution – conflict or disagreement can be hinted at, or worse, made up, so make sure that your intention and meaning is very clearly articulated so that it cannot be misinterpreted.

The more of these news values you can incorporate into your communications with the media, or with audiences generally, the more likely it is that your message will be picked up and shared. Ideally, you will be able to demonstrate some of these news values in your key message.

Writing for the media

The mass media operates on a 24-hour news cycle, meaning that media outlets are constantly looking for material to provide to their audiences. There are certain things you can do to make the journalist's or editor's decision about whether to include your story very easy.

Get to the point

Time is a precious commodity. Editors and journalists – and people scanning news feeds or print publications – often decide within the first sentence or two whether they want to read further. Put your key message and information up the front, in the first sentence, in a way that is engaging and makes it compelling. One way to do this is to follow the conventions of writing a news article: writing in what is called the 'inverted pyramid' (Figure 7.2). This is the format typically used by journalists, whereby the

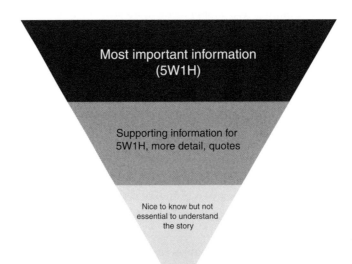

Figure 7.2   The inverted pyramid

most important information is given right at the beginning and the information is presented in a descending order of importance; from most important down to least important.

The most important information is the 5W1H. These are questions that you have likely been asking since you could first talk: who, what, where, when, why and how? They are the key elements of the news story and are linked to news values. Answer as many of these as you possibly can in the first one to three sentences. This is done so that even if someone only reads the first few sentences of a news story, they have the key information and details. Complete Learning activity 7.2 to see how this works in practice.

LEARNING ACTIVITY 7.2

Go to your usual news source – in print, radio, television or online. Have a look for health-related stories. Look at the headlines and read the first few paragraphs of each story.

1. Identify the 5W1H in your health stories.
    a. Sometimes not all of the 5W1H will be present – which ones are most often missing in the articles you are reading?
    b. Why do you think that might be?
2. What news values do you think apply to each story?
3. Can you identify a relationship between the 5W1H and the news values you identified? Describe it, using examples.
4. What is the 'so what' of this article?

Now, combine your headlines and news values with those uncovered by others in your group or class.

Which topics and news values are most commonly used? Are they the same as the ones you identified in your sample?

EXTENSION

Reflect on the dominant news values and topics you and/or your class identified. How might these influence public perceptions of the topics, or of health more broadly?

A note on the how and why – sometimes these are very difficult to explain or articulate in a short news article. This is why sometimes they may not be answered in full, or at all. (Did you find examples of this when you did Learning activity 7.2?)

Make every word count

The way you write your information is important. First, you must write in the tone and style of your intended publication. If it is for a specific news outlet you wish to target, read, watch or listen to how they present stories, and emulate their style. As a general rule, when you are writing for mass media (e.g. in a press release) it is typical to write in paragraphs that are one sentence long. Each sentence should be on average about 18 words. Some can be longer, some shorter. As a guide, if you reach the fourth line of text and you have not yet used any punctuation – stop!

To write concisely and well, every word in a sentence must be contributing something. Use one word if one will do. The same goes for any quotes you include from people. Quotes are useful to add a sense of life and immediacy to a story and help to add the human interest. However, this only works if the quotes are relevant and interesting. Make sure the person you are interviewing and quoting is using language that is free of jargon and easy to understand by a non-specialist audience. Ask them to explain things in a different way if you are not sure what they mean, so the intended audience will also be able to understand.

So what?

The 'so what' of your story (news) is likely your key message. What is the one thing you want people to remember, think or do once they hear your news story? Make it relevant, engaging and short. Earlier chapters have already talked about how to tailor your message to suit your target audience and how to communicate that message clearly. The challenge here is to still do all of that but in a way that can appeal to the news values. Think about your target audience and what you want them to think or do once they receive your information. How can you relate that to what makes news? If you want people to do something then you need to tell them what is in it for them. This also applies to 'calls to action' in social media posts. Imagine someone saying to you 'I need you to give me $500'. You probably would not just hand over the money without knowing why! If you want someone to attend an event, buy a product or change their behaviour, you will first need to tell them what is in it for them – make them want the outcome before you ask them to do something that will create that outcome. A note of caution: you may be 'selling' an idea or an event, or even research results, but it needs to be done in a way that makes it news and not just advertising. Do this by linking it back to the news values and focusing on what makes it relevant and useful for the audience.

Writing a press release

The inverted pyramid is also the best way to structure a press release. This ensures that you get the relevant information to the journalist or editor as quickly as possible, to allow them to judge whether your news is relevant to their audience. Keep it short and snappy – no more than one page is ideal. All of the other writing rules apply. A well-written press release makes the journalist's job easier, which in turn could help you get your message to your audience.

All press releases need to be dated so journalists know which are most recent. You must also tell the journalist when they can use or publish the information. This is done by stating 'for immediate release' on the top of the press release if the information can be used immediately. If you want the journalist to wait to release the information, such as after a press conference or the announcement of competition winners, for example, then you use what is called an 'embargo'. This means that the journalist is free to talk to the contact person, do some research and start preparing the story, but they are not allowed to go public with it until the date and time you specify.

A crucial part of a press release is the inclusion of a contact phone number for the journalist to contact someone if they need more information. Put these details at the bottom of the press release, after text/content and, crucially, after you have put something like ### or <Ends>, where your press release content finishes, otherwise you may find your details published. See Figure 7.3 for a simple example of a press-release structure.

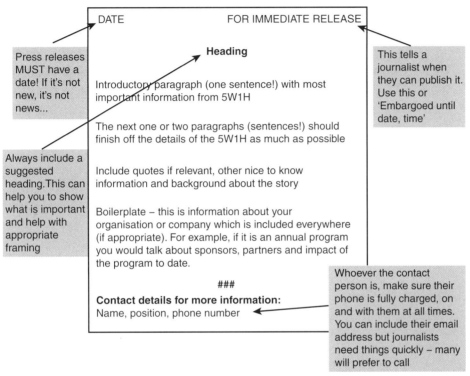

DATE   FOR IMMEDIATE RELEASE

Heading

Introductory paragraph (one sentence!) with most important information from 5W1H

The next one or two paragraphs (sentences!) should finish off the details of the 5W1H as much as possible

Include quotes if relevant, other nice to know information and background about the story

Boilerplate – this is information about your organisation or company which is included everywhere (if appropriate). For example, if it is an annual program you would talk about sponsors, partners and impact of the program to date.

###

Contact details for more information:
Name, position, phone number

Press releases MUST have a date! If it's not new, it's not news...

Always include a suggested heading. This can help you to show what is important and help with appropriate framing

This tells a journalist when they can publish it. Use this or 'Embargoed until date, time'

Whoever the contact person is, make sure their phone is fully charged, on and with them at all times. You can include their email address but journalists need things quickly – many will prefer to call

Figure 7.3   Template for a press release

When you do start to engage with various media outlets and platforms, it is not enough to send a press release or post one tweet. This means that you are expecting your audience to be sitting in front of the exact communication channel you have chosen at the precise time the information is provided, and that they are paying close attention. In reality you need to have a consistent presence on a range of different channels to ensure you capture the audience's attention, and then remind them regularly and often. How effective you are at reaching your audience depends on how well you know your audience, and what media they engage with.

Summary

The media plays an important role in communicating health information to audiences. However, where the news is presented, the people involved and the way the information is communicated in the news can all influence how publics interpret and respond to information. Health promotion professionals undertake a huge range of communication activities, and understanding what makes information 'newsworthy' – interesting, relevant and worth engaging with – is useful in all communication activities. Using a communication plan enables you to ensure that all of your activities, and by extension any activity partners you may have, are working towards a clearly articulated, common objective. This is particularly useful when your goals are related to advocacy or capacity building, which have the potential to change things for populations, not just individuals.

REVISION QUESTIONS

1. Describe the main factors that influence how publics perceive health issues in the news.
2. What are the core parts of a communication strategy?
3. Compare and contrast the strengths and weaknesses of different types of media platforms and outlets.
4. What are news values? Describe them, using examples.
5. Describe the format and give general writing tips for preparing a press release.

FURTHER READING

Cribb, J. & Tjempaka, S. (2010). *Open Science: Sharing knowledge in the global century*. CSIRO Publishing: ePub.
Edelman (2020). *Edelman Trust Barometer 2020: Global Report*. Retrieved from: https://www.edelman.com/trust/2020-trust-barometer
Geia, L., Pearson, L. & Sweet, M. (2017). Narratives of Twitter as a platform for professional development, innovation, and advocacy, *Australian Psychologist*, 52(4), 280–7.

REFERENCES

Avert (2019). *Origin of HIV & AIDS*. Retrieved from: avert.org/professionals/history-hiv-aids/origin
Barry, C.L., Brescoll, V.L. & Gollust, S.E. (2013). Framing childhood obesity prevention policies. How individualizing the problem affects public support for prevention, *Political Psychology*, 34(3), 327–49.
Bray, F. & Chapman, S. (1991). Community knowledge, attitudes and media recall about AIDS, Sydney 1988 and 1989, *Australian Journal of Public Health*, 15(2), 107–13.
Carter, S., Braunack-Mayer, A. & Degeling, C. (2020, 23 March). We need to change our thinking and communication, urgently, to beat COVID-19, *croakey.org*.
CDC (2002, 3 October). AIDS pioneer regrets 'Grim Reaper' demonization of gay men, *The Body*, CDC National Prevention Information Network.
Chilcott, M. (2014, 15 April). Six ways to tell it's a good story, *Fundraising & Philanthropy*.
Cole, D.A., Nick, E.A., Zelkowitz, R.L., Roeder, K.M. & Spinelli, T. (2017). Online social support for young people: Does it recapitulate in-person social support: Can it help? *Computers in Human Behavior*, 68, 456–64.
Crisp, B.R., Swerissen, H. & Duckett, S.J. (2000). Four approaches to capacity building in health: Consequences for measurement and accountability, *Health Promotion International*, 15(2), 99–107.

Davies, P., Chapman, S. & Leask, J. (2002). Antivaccination activists on the world wide web, *Archives of Disease in Childhood*, 87, 22–5.

Department of Health (2020, 15 March). Coronavirus (COVID-19) – Print ads – Simple steps to stop the spread. Retrieved from: https://www.health.gov.au/resources/publications/coronavirus-covid-19-print-ads-simple-steps-to-stop-the-spread

Doctors for the Environment Australia Inc (DEA) (2015). No Time For Games. Retrieved from: https://www.dea.org.au/dea-report-no-time-for-games-childrens-health-and-climatechange-healthy-planet-healthy-people-dea/

———(2018). No Time for Games: Summary Report Update 2018. Retrieved from: https://www.dea.org.au/wp-content/uploads/2018/11/NTFG-Summary-and-Update-2018–11-18-Final.pdf

———(2020, 19 February). #Notimeforgames: A national children's health campaign. Retrieved from: https://www.dea.org.au/notimeforgames-a-national-children-health-campaignnbsp/

Edelman (2020). *Edelman Trust Barometer 2020: Global Report*. Retrieved from: https://www.edelman.com/trust/2020-trust-barometer

Estacio, E.V., Oliver, M., Downing, B., Kurth, J. & Protheroe, J. (2017). Effective partnership in community-based health promotion: Lessons from the Health Literacy Partnership, *International Journal of Environmental Research and Public Health*, 14(12), 1550.

Geia, L., Pearson, L. & Sweet, M. (2017). Narratives of Twitter as a platform for professional development, innovation and advocacy, *Australian Psychologist*, 52(4), 280–7.

Giselvania, A., Jayalie, V.F. & Gondhowiardjo, S. (2018). The role of multisectoral collaboration in Indonesia for successful health promotion, *Journal of Global Oncology*, 4(sup 2), 134s.

Hashimoto, Y. (ed.) (2016). *Nihonjin no Johokodo 2015 (Information Behavior 2015 in Japan)*. Tokyo: University of Tokyo Press.

Hawe, P., King, L., Noort, M., Gifford, S. & Lloyd, B. (1998). Working invisibly: Health workers talk about capacity-building in health promotion, *Health Promotion International*, 13(4), 285–95.

IHMayDay18Team (2018, 11 June). A great big wrap of the news tweeted from the fifth annual IHMayDay, *croakey.org*.

Jackson, T. (2011). When balance is bias, *British Medical Journal*, 343, d8006.

Kim, H.S. (2015). Attracting views and going viral: How message features and news-sharing channels affect health news diffusion, *The Journal of Communication*, 65(3), 512–34.

Kim, S. & Willis, L.A. (2007). Talking about obesity: News framing of who is responsible for causing and fixing the problem, *Journal of Health Communication*, 12(4), 359–76.

Kuo, L. (2020, 10 March). How did China get to grips with its coronavirus outbreak? *The Guardian*.

Matsunaga, W. & Tsubono, Y. (2008a). *Kenkojoho to Media Jyo* (Health information and the media 1), *The Journal of Public Health Practice*, 72(10), 802–6.

———(2008b). *Kenkojoho to Media Ge* (Health information and the media 2), *The Journal of Public Health Practice*, 72(11), 887–91.

McInerney, M. (2020, 26 March). Wrapping the latest COVID-19 news, amid growing push for transparency, action and equity, *croakey.org*.

McKinnon, M. & Orthia, L. (2017). Vaccination communication strategies: What have we learned, and lost, in 200 years? *Journal of Science Communication*, 16(3), A08.

Minga Peru (n.d.). *Our Story*. Retrieved from: https://mingaperu.org/en/our-story/

Murphy, K. (2020a, 22 March). As Australia goes off the coronavirus cliff, the question is how hard will it land? *The Guardian.*

———(2020b, 24 March). Guardian essential poll: One-third say there has been an overreaction to coronavirus, *The Guardian.*

Myhre, S.L. & Flora, J.A. (2000). HIV/AIDS communication campaigns: Progress and prospects, *Journal of Health Communication*, 5(sup1), 29–45.

OIP (2012, 29 August). New Grim Reaper campaign criticised, *Out In Perth.*

Oncel, S. & Alvur, M. (2013). How reliable is the Internet for caregivers on their decision to vaccinate their child against influenza? Results from googling in two languages, *European Journal of Pediatrics*, 172(3), 401–4.

Ouchi, S. (2018). *Masumedia niyoru Kenkoiryokodo ni taisuru Koshueiseisennmonka no Ninshiki* (Public health experts' views of health information provided by the mass media). Unpublished research report. Osaka, Japan: Program for Education and Research on Science and Technology in Public Sphere, Osaka University.

Power, J. (2012, 30 August). The Grim Reaper died in the 80s – time for a new approach to HIV prevention, *The Conversation.*

Roy Morgan (2019, 22 July). ABC still most trusted, Facebook improves, Roy Morgan Finding No. 8064.

Science Media Centre (2012). Science Media Centre: Where science meets the headlines (Website). Retrieved from: https://www.sciencemediacentre.org/

Sillence, E., Blythe, J.M., Briggs, P. & Moss, M. (2019). A revised model of trust in Internet-based health information and advice: Cross-sectional questionnaire study, *Journal of Medical Internet Research*, 21(11), e11125.

Sun, Y., Zhang, Y., Gwizdka, J. & Trace, C.B. (2019). Consumer evaluation of the quality of online health information: Systematic literature review of relevant criteria and indicators, *Journal of Medical Internet Research*, 21(5), e12522.

Sweet, M., Geia, L., Dudgeon, P. & McCallum, K. (2015). #IHMayDay: Tweeting for empowerment and social and emotional wellbeing, *Australasian Psychiatry*, 23(6), 636–40.

Takahashi, K. (2008). *Fu-do fadizumu to kenkou kyouiku* (Food faddism and health education), *Japanese Journal of Health Education and Promotion*, 16(3), 125–30.

VicHealth (2012). *Capacity building for health promotion (Information Sheet). Publication number C-072-CB.* Melbourne: Victorian Health Promotion Foundation.

World Health Organization (WHO) (n.d.). WHO Strategic Communications Framework for effective communications. Retrieved from: https://www.who.int/about/communications

Xinhua (2020, 10 February). Xi stresses winning people's war against novel coronavirus, *XinhuaNet.*

Zhang, Y., Jin, Y. & Tang, Y. (2015). Framing depression: Cultural and organizational influences on coverage of a public health threat and attribution of responsibilities in Chinese news media, 2000–2012, *Journalism & Mass Communication Quarterly*, 92(1), 99–120.

Evaluation – how to measure what works

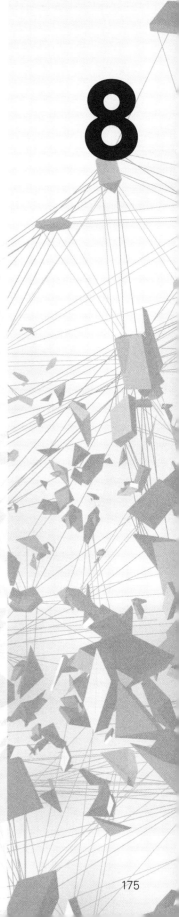

8

Merryn McKinnon

With contributions from Jasvir Kaur, Manmeet Kaur and Rajesh Kumar

LEARNING OBJECTIVES

At the completion of the chapter, you will be able to:

- Describe the role of evaluation in health promotion and program development.
- Define different types of evaluation and describe the role of indicators.
- Identify and describe qualitative and quantitative data-collection methods and critically discuss their strengths and weaknesses.
- Understand the relationship between communication and evaluation.

Introduction

Many of the earlier chapters in this book have mentioned the importance of evaluation at all stages of the planning process. Knowing what works, and why, is just as valuable as knowing what does not work; both contribute to informing and improving your professional practice. There are many different ways of getting information, so how do you know which one is the best for what you are trying to do? How do you know if you are evaluating the right thing in the first place?

This chapter is intended as an introduction to the basic methods you can use in any evaluation. It will also show you how you can use these methods to evaluate the effectiveness of your communication activities, as well as your health promotion activities. Many books and references are available to provide very detailed guidance in evaluation, including the theories and perspectives that underpin them; you may find these useful if you want more information about the foundations of evaluation (see Further Reading at the end of this chapter).

The chapter begins by outlining the relevance of evaluation for health promotion and outlines the key considerations when planning evaluation activities. This includes ethical considerations about what information should be provided to prospective participants. Different types of evaluation and the use of indicators are also discussed, along with the different stages when evaluation can be used to assess an activity. The second half of this chapter provides an overview of the different methods used to collect data in an evaluation, including the strengths and weaknesses of each. The different communication requirements and considerations of each method are also discussed, including how methods can be used to evaluate the communication activities supporting the health promotion initiative, as well as the initiative itself.

Evaluation and health promotion

Competencies – the minimum set of abilities needed to apply knowledge, skills, attitudes and values to differing contexts and at a required standard of performance; core competencies are a common baseline for all roles

Evaluation is an important part of working in health promotion. The Australian Health Promotion Association lists evaluation and research in its Core Competencies for Health Promotion Practitioners (AHPA, 2009; see box below). These **competencies** are informed by Australian state and federal competency documents as well as core competencies from Aotearoa New Zealand and Canadian standards, and so reflect competencies that are core to health promotion nationally and, arguably, internationally. Despite the importance of evaluation being widely recognised, there is evidence that it is rarely done comprehensively in Australia (Lobo et al., 2014) and may be limited – or even discouraged – by political (Huckel Schneider et al., 2016) or funding agency agendas and restrictions (Francis & Smith, 2015). Even if evaluation is done, it might be added as an afterthought or done only because funders require it. The completion of an evaluation does not necessarily mean that the information and insights it provides will be used (Wolfenden, et al., 2016). There are many reasons for this. Lobo and colleagues (2014) identified three main factors that limit program evaluation in health:

1. Organisational factors – evaluation is seen as something done for compliance rather than improvement, or funding agencies have unrealistic expectations of what can be evaluated (in the allocated time, and with the funds available).

2. Capacity factors – practitioners lack the knowledge and skills to design and implement an appropriate evaluation framework.

3. Translational factors – there are difficulties in using the knowledge gained from evaluation in future practice, or in getting target groups involved in programs limited by short-term funding.

They also note that 'supporting health promotion practitioners to conduct evaluations that are more meaningful ... is a shared responsibility ... including health promotion practitioners, educators, policy makers and funders, organisational leadership and researchers' (Lobo et al., 2014, p. 4). Partnerships and collaborations, as this text has already discussed, are invaluable in program design, delivery, communication *and* evaluation. Working together over the life of a project will allow all of the knowledge and insights gained, from both the program and its evaluation, to be shared and used to inform future activities, thereby potentially saving time, effort and resources.

Evaluation and research competencies from the Australian Core Competencies for Health Promotion Practitioners

1.4 Evaluation and research competencies

An entry level health promotion practitioner is able to:

1.4.1 incorporate evaluation into the planning of health promotion programs;

1.4.2 identify appropriate evaluation designs;

1.4.3 design evaluation plans that incorporate process, impact, and outcome measures;

1.4.4 identify evaluation methods applicable to health promotion;

1.4.5 select evaluation instruments;

1.4.6 interpret evaluation findings;

1.4.7 monitor programs and adjust objectives and strategies based on the analysis of evaluation data;

1.4.8 apply and interpret descriptive statistical methods and analyses;

1.4.9 critically analyse quantitative and qualitative data to report on program effectiveness;

1.4.10 communicate evaluation findings;

1.4.11 prepare evaluation research proposals for funding; and

1.4.12 prepare ethics approvals.

Source: AHPA (2009).

Gathering evidence

Much of the rhetoric surrounding health initiatives and policy responses uses the phrase 'evidence-based'. Even the core competencies refer to health promotion practitioners needing 'competencies for planning evidence-based strategies' (AHPA, 2009, p. 3). **Research** and **evaluation** differ, but both are important means of collecting this evidence. If you do not use good evidence, then the quality of the

Research – systematic investigation of materials, methods and sources to develop new insights, understanding and facts

Evaluation – an assessment of the quality, quantity, performance or worth of something

resulting strategies will also suffer; putting garbage into a system will usually lead to garbage coming out! There are also real-world implications of using poor evidence or failing to implement interventions that have been rigorously evaluated and found to be effective. Several studies from around the world, including from low-income countries, have shown failure to use evidence-based guidelines and interventions can lead to increased risk of harm or even avoidable deaths (Haines et al., 2004). Effective communication is also needed to ensure that the stakeholders who are best able to support the implementation of effective programs, such as researchers, practitioners and policy makers, are aware of the evidence and are able to act on it accordingly.

Throughout this book we have talked about the importance of having SMART objectives. These are specific, measurable, achievable, realistic and time specific. This chapter is where we focus on the M – the measurable part of the objective. In the previous chapter we talked about which realistic objectives and measures of these objectives could be included in communication plans. The same principles can be applied to health promotion activities.

Different types of evaluation

Many – if not all – health promotion activities aim to improve health and wellbeing of people and populations by influencing all of the determinants of health. It is also common for one health promotion activity to be part of a larger program of activities, all working to collectively address an identified issue. For example, trying to reduce under-age binge drinking may involve an advertising campaign in the media, educational programs in schools and an increase in the price of pre-mixed alcoholic drinks ('alcopops') through taxes. As an evaluator, you would need to understand which – if any – of these inputs (media, education or tax) was most influential, or if it was a particular combination of some or all of them that is most effective. You also need to be careful that what you are choosing as evidence of success is appropriate and realistic.

As a first step, what are you wanting to evaluate? Are you trying to find out whether a program was run in the way it was intended, or whether it changed something or made a difference to a population more broadly? Each of these questions uses a different type of evaluation; you may use one or more depending upon the aim of your program.

In Chapter 7 we talked about *formative evaluation*. This is used before a program is fully implemented, to ensure it is working in the way intended, and it enables problems to be identified and changes to be made if required.

A *process evaluation* aims to determine whether what you planned to do was implemented as intended, and if this process is working in the way you expected. It does not assess actual outcomes, but it does allow for exploration of how the program functions and its potential effect. Process evaluations are useful sources of information for those wishing to replicate a program, and for explaining to potential funders how a program works.

An *outcome evaluation* is exactly as the name implies – what were the outcomes of this program or activity? Did it achieve what it set out to do? Outcomes can be measured by looking at the target audience of your initiative – what has changed? For example, if you were running a drink-driving campaign with the objective of reducing the frequency of drink-driving in drivers aged 25 years and under, an outcome evaluation would look for changes in the number of drink-driving fines police issued to young drivers or the number of car crashes and hospitalisations involving drink drivers in that age group while the program was active.

Outcome evaluations are a form of **summative evaluation**.

An *impact evaluation* can be done at intervals during and at the end of a program; it aims to show how well a program achieved its intended goal. An 'impact' is measured over a longer term than an 'outcome', and will likely go beyond the original target audience. Building on the drink-driving example given above, an impact would be assessed as whether there was any decrease in drink-driving related offences and whether any injuries were sustained over time for drivers of all ages. An impact evaluation can yield the kinds of results that make compelling evidence for funders and policy makers. Each type of evaluation should use **indicators**, which are an important part of evaluation (see Case study 8.1). They are clear markers that provide 'information to monitor performance, measure achievement and determine accountability' (UNAIDS, 2010., p. 14). Indicators are not the same as objectives; rather, indicators are used to help measure progress against objectives. The way you write an indicator needs to be clear and precise. Because they are measuring progress, indicators also tend to not use directional language (e.g. increase/decrease), and as much as possible it is a good idea to make your indicators SMART (CDC, 2016), just like your objectives.

There are also different types of indicators. The Centers for Disease Control and Prevention (CDC) in the United States describes different types of indicators as:

- *Input indicators* – these measure what kinds of inputs (like resources e.g. staff, money, partnerships) are necessary for a program to be successfully implemented
- *Process indicators* – measure the program's activities and outputs. These can be used to answer who, what, when and where questions
- *Outcome indicators* – is the project achieving what it intended in the short, medium and long term? The long-term outcomes of a project can also be called *impact indicators*, and these tend to be seen in the broader population, not just those targeted by the project. (CDC, 2016)

These input, process, outcome and impact indicators are what UNAIDS (2010) describes as role and/or effect indicators. UNAIDS also describes thematic indicators, which are:

- *Behavioural outcome* – indicators of the effectiveness of initiatives that are designed to influence behaviours
- *Disease impact* – indicators that monitor the disease as well as social and economic consequences of the disease and its broader effects at the individual through to societal and government levels
- *Infrastructure* – indicators that monitor how institutions, services and partnerships (for example) contribute to support an effective program
- *Policy* – indicators of the existence and/or effectiveness of government policies on the health issue of focus

Summative evaluation – an evaluation conducted at the conclusion of a program; used to determine the extent to which desired outcomes were achieved

Indicators – measurable pieces of information that can be used to show progress towards a desired outcome; they are specific, observable, precise and unambiguous

- *Program/service delivery* – these indicators monitor whether programs exist and are effective. Indicators can include services, education, training and measures of attitudes and intentions of the target audience (UNAIDS, 2010, pp. 28–9).

When undertaking an evaluation you may choose to use thematic or process indicators, and it is advisable to use more than one. For example, if you intend to use outcome indicators it is probably a good idea to use some process indicators along the way as well, so you can make changes if needed. Some indicators are likely to be more difficult or expensive to measure than others; you will need to consider this when you are planning your evaluation.

CASE STUDY 8.1 Key performance indicators in evaluation

Girls Make Your Move

The 'Girls Make Your Move' campaign aimed to increase the physical activity of young women in Australia, in response to evidence showing they were less likely to be physically active than young men, often due to issues related to confidence, cultural and social pressures and a lack of time and/or money (Department of Health, 2018).

Girls Make Your Move focuses on girls aged 12–19 years, encouraging them to increase their physical activity, with materials particularly targeting girls aged 15–18 years (Department of Health, 2018). Secondary audiences are parents of girls and women aged 12–19 years and women aged 19–21. The campaign had four key objectives, namely to:

1. Raise *awareness* of the campaign, the benefits of physical activity, how easy it is to be active and the range of different activities on offer
2. Influence *attitudes* about perceived barriers to participation in physical activity and to increase confidence in participation
3. Create and reinforce *intentions* to participate, get more information and use the campaign's resources
4. Change *behaviours* through increasing participation in physical activity and increasing engagement on the campaign's social media platforms and associated offers such as special events and activities (Orima Research, 2019).

The initiative provides information about different types of physical activity through its website, on the Instagram and Facebook platforms and through the use of role models. Sporty Sistas were young women who featured in short videos about activities they loved. The campaign was advertised over three annual phases, in 2016, 2017 and 2018. Communication channels included regional, metropolitan and national television; online video; digital advertising, including display advertisements on search engines, mobile apps and social media; and advertising in regional and metropolitan cinemas.

Orima Research (2019) conducted an evaluation of the Girls Make Your Move initiative after the program had been running for three years. Their evaluation sought to measure the success of the campaign in terms of meeting the aims of the program, as well as the effectiveness of the communication about the program.

Three-phase evaluation and key performance indicators

The evaluation included a key performance indicator (KPI) framework, which mapped against the four campaign objectives. Each KPI was calculated on a scale of 0–100 index points, where 0 showed no indication of the KPI being met and 100 indicated the KPI had been met in full. (This is a highly simplified summary – see Orima Research, 2019 for a full description.)

KPI 1: Awareness

1a) Awareness of the benefits
1b) Awareness of the range of activities and sports available
1c) Awareness of the ease of access to activities and sports

KPI 2: Call to action

2a) Actions taken as a result of campaign exposure
2b) Engagement with campaign website/social media

KPI 3: Intentions

3a) Intentions to participate in physical activity and sport
3b) Intentions to seek information about types of physical activity available

KPI 4: Attitudes

4a) Attitudes to participating in physical activity and sport
4b) Barriers to participation
4c) Confidence in participating (trying something new)
4d) Ability to participate

KPI 5: Behaviours

5) Participation in physical activity and sport (Orima Research, 2019, pp 18–19).

KPI results

The evaluation found that awareness of the campaign was good but had declined over time (83 to 76 points); however, key message recall was very good across the three phases (Orima Research, 2019). Knowledge about where to find information was the poorest performing metric in the first two phases. Changes to the communication materials and approaches in phase 3 resulted in improvements in the awareness KPI.

Results for the intentions and behaviours KPIs were consistent with phase 2, with those exposed to the campaign being more likely to seek information about the campaign or to increase their physical activity than those not exposed (Orima

(cont.)

(cont.)

Research, 2019), although this KPI had declined between phases. The call-to-action KPI, in particular, showed that 56 per cent of respondents aged 12–21 years who had seen the campaign indicated that they had taken one positive action as a result of the campaign. The scores for KPI 2 were high enough to indicate that respondents likely took more than one action, if they did act (Orima Research, 2019).

The attitudes KPI did not show a change in attitudes towards participating in physical activity and sport, which was consistent with phase 2. There were some improvements in the score seen in this KPI, which suggested a decline in the perceived barriers to physical activity among the target audience. However, the difference between those exposed to the campaign and those who were not was not statistically significant, indicating that perceptions were likely influenced by factors external to the campaign (Orima Research, 2019). The results also indicated that the responses from girls aged 12–14 years were significantly different when compared to responses from the same age cohort in previous phases (Orima Research, 2019).

QUESTIONS

1. How could these indicators be used to make changes to the program over consecutive years?
2. Based on the different results seen in the 12–14-year age group in the phase 3 evaluation, what kind of research would you undertake to identify the changes needed to make this campaign relevant in future?

ELSEWHERE IN THE WORLD

This Girl Can

This Girl Can (https://www.thisgirlcan.co.uk/), a program in the United Kingdom, was the inspiration for the Girls Make Your Move campaign in Australia. This Girl Can aimed to inspire and empower young girls and women, of all shapes, sizes, abilities and backgrounds to get active, doing whatever form of exercise they choose and understanding there's no 'right' way to get active.

Us Girls

Us Girls (https://network.streetgames.org/our-work/us-girls) is a program running in England, Wales and continental Europe, designed to increase the participation of girls and young women in physical activity, with a focus on those from disadvantaged locations.

Context matters

Evaluation does not happen in a vacuum. The 'thing' you are trying to measure exists within a broader context, in which individual values and beliefs interact with cultural and societal norms, and are influenced by environmental, structural and economic determinants. Just as the program you develop needs to be appropriate for your audience, so too does the evaluation of that program. This may mean that you need to consider what 'impact' or 'success' looks like for the particular program you are evaluating and the most appropriate way to measure that within the program setting. Imagine you are running a program that is trying to influence the purchasing behaviours of consumers of sugar-sweetened beverages in your local shops. If you tried to evaluate this program by having someone stand right next to the drinks cabinets, asking direct questions of customers and taking notes about what they select for purchase, it would be very difficult to identify whether it was the program or the evaluator who was influencing consumers' behaviours.

There are choices to be made in every aspect of the evaluation planning, which may help to influence the success and usefulness of the evaluation as a whole. For example, what is the best way to collect the data – maybe choosing between a questionnaire or interview? Or maybe it is a choice about who should collect the data. Would using an individual or organisation sharing the same cultural characteristics and understandings of the participant group yield more robust information? Perhaps a more insightful evaluation can be achieved by looking at what people do as a result of participating in the program.

When to evaluate

Don Nutbeam and colleagues (1990) outlined six different stages of research and evaluation for health promotion. Although this framework has been around for several decades now, the stages are still relevant today and are likely to remain relevant into the future.

Stages of research and evaluation

The six stages are as follows:

1. Defining the problem – use existing data (e.g. epidemiological) and needs assessments
2. Creating potential solution/s – draw on behaviour-change theories and models, and what others have done
3. Testing the potential solution/s – identify outcomes and learn how the solution works in practice
4. Implementing the solution/s again – can the solution be repeated or refined using what was learned in stage 3?
5. Reproducing the solution/s – can the solution yield the same results in different locations or contexts?
6. Monitoring performance – analyse costs and benefits; is the program sustainable?

Stages 1 and 2 refer to the needs assessment discussed in the earlier chapters of this book. This is where we attempt to understand as much as we can about the problem, who is most affected (and thus who our target audience is) and what our target audience most wants and needs. From there we can develop a plan of action. Once we begin to implement programs or initiatives in stage 3, through formative evaluation we can look at whether they are working in the way we intended. This then enables us to use preliminary results and feedback to understand how the program is working and whether it is likely to achieve the desired outcome. If it seems to be going wrong, changes can be made to get it back on track. Stage 4 is where we can test any changes or work on refining the solution so that it is as effective as it can be. Once we know a program is working well in one context – for example, in a particular setting or with a certain audience – then in stage 5 we can test whether the same results are seen in the same setting or with the same audience in a larger geographical area. For example, a school-based initiative may be working well in a few schools in a certain regional area. Stage 5 enables you to test whether it works as well across more schools and a wider area, or even several regional areas. Finally, once you have a solution that appears to be working, stage 6, summative evaluation, is where you track how well the program is performing. This stage explores whether the program is consistently achieving good results or its effectiveness is declining over time. Are the benefits of running the solution outweighing its costs? If the solution was supported by a grant or other short-term source of finance, what will happen once that funding runs out?

Where formative and summative evaluations occur in these stages depends on the size and scope of the program. A small program intended for one specific audience or event, for example, could use summative evaluation in stage 3, especially if it is a one-off event. The findings could be used to inform future programs on similar topics, settings or events – even small projects and programs should be evaluated. Each of these stages of research and evaluation will use different activities and different communication strategies within those activities, as shown in Table 8.1. Both the activity and the communication can be evaluated. The next section explores how.

Table 8.1 Stages of research and evaluation, aligned with examples of program and communication activities

Stage	Program activity	Communication activities
1	Needs assessment	Public engagement by recruiting participants to provide feedback/insights; stakeholder engagement; advocacy with potential funders
2	Program design	Pilot testing with members of target audience; briefings/training sessions with stakeholders and partners
3	Program implementation	Development and distribution of promotional materials; media coverage
4	Program refinement	Stakeholder engagement, including target audience
5	Program replication	Promotion through traditional and social media channels; distribution of promotional materials to relevant organisations/audience groups
6	Program monitoring	Reporting to stakeholders, including funders; advocacy with funders and policy makers

Informed consent

Before going too much further into the nuts and bolts of evaluation, a note on the rights of participants and your responsibility as a researcher. If you are going to undertake any research or evaluation involving people, you must ensure that you adhere to the appropriate rules, guidelines and laws of your organisation and country. In Australia, the National Health and Medical Research Council provides guidance in the *National Statement on Ethical Conduct in Human Research* (NHMRC & ARC, 2018), which outlines the legal definitions and requirements for human research. Even though you might only be asking people what they think about a topic or event, there are still certain requirements that you must adhere to. One of the most important of these is informed consent. This means that you have clearly explained to potential participants what you want to find out, what they have to do, the total time required to participate and what you intend to do with the results. Participants also need to know if they may change their mind about participation and, if so, what will happen to their information as well as whether there are any potential negative consequences for them if they withdraw. In short, people need to be given enough information to enable them to make a decision about whether participating in your evaluation is appropriate for, and acceptable to, them.

Do consider how you provide potential participants with information to support their informed consent. Is the information provided in a format and a language they can readily understand? This refers to the actual language being used as well as the 'level' and register (e.g. formal or informal; plain English or technical). Is the participant information sheet filled with complex technical words and jargon? Does understanding it require someone to have a high level of literacy or education? Are your participants legally able to make this decision for themselves (e.g. are they old enough or do they have the appropriate mental capacity)? Again, know your audience and anticipate their needs. Provide translated materials if that is helpful, offer additional information for parents and/or carers where applicable and be available to answer any questions that may arise.

There are different ways of showing that someone has provided consent to participate in research. This includes providing verbal consent to the researcher (which may be recorded in audio or video format), signing a consent form or submitting an online questionnaire. Make sure you are explicit in how participants may provide their consent for your study. It is also advisable to provide a copy of the participant information sheet in plain English, so that participants can refer to it at any time. This information sheet should summarise the main points of the study and provide information about whom to contact if they change their mind or would like to make a complaint about the study and the way it is being conducted.

Considering your participants' needs

As well as ensuring that information is provided to your participants in ways that they can understand, you should also be mindful of creating an inclusive environment. This should occur in your health promotion initiative, anyway, but it is also relevant to any research you conduct with human participants. For example, what language is used in the information sheet, consent form or survey questions? Are you excluding certain groups (e.g. someone with a non-binary gender identity; people from non-English speaking backgrounds)? Can people living with mobility, visual, hearing or other impairments contribute their ideas and perspectives through the data-collection methods you plan to use? Do all potential participants have equal access and opportunity to participate (e.g. can people in rural and remote areas easily participate or is data collection more favourable to those in urban and metropolitan areas)? Is the data collection appropriate to, and respectful of, cultural needs (e.g. the ways in which data is collected, and by whom)?

One final note on your participants. Consider whether you need to contact them separately to collect the data. Is there a way you can embed evaluation activities into the program or event itself? Perhaps this can be done through data collection methods such as live polls, using buttons or tokens to vote or through social media engagement. Some groups in society, often vulnerable groups, are often the target for many programs, initiatives and research and as a result the demands on their time are disproportionate to others'. Consider the potential burden on your participants and explore alternative methods of getting the information you need as best you possibly can, without adding to the demands on their time.

Choosing an evaluation method

Just as there is no one-size-fits-all approach to communication, no single method of evaluation fits all programs and what you might want to find out. There are many different techniques you can use to collect the type of data you want, and you can use these same techniques and data to evaluate your communications. The first step in your evaluation process is to look at the objective of your program or initiative: what is it that you were trying to achieve? If it is an increase or decrease in something, then you will likely need to use numbers – **quantitative** methods – to measure your success or progress. If you are trying to create a change in attitudes, then you will need to hear what people think and believe – you will likely need to employ **qualitative** methods. In some instances, a mix of both, which is called mixed methods (see later in this chapter) is appropriate.

Quantitative methods

A common example of quantitative data is that collected by epidemiologists. By collecting rates of infection or death, for example, they can use these numbers to determine patterns in populations or to predict outcomes. Where are most outbreaks of a disease occurring? Which population groups are at highest risk? Quantitative research methods can also enable relationships between **variables** to be identified using statistical analysis (Choy, 2017).

This section outlines how quantitative data can be used to inform health promotion, some common ways of collecting quantitative data and how it can provide useful information in a communications context.

Counts

This is a simple way to determine how many people need, know about or are affected by something. In health promotion you can use counts, perhaps based on epidemiological data, of the rate of incidence of a disease in a particular area. This could be a useful part of your needs assessment. You can use counts of people over time to determine the influence of an intervention. For example, the number of road fatalities in Australia peaked in the 1970s, with an annual average of 3613 deaths

Quantitative – a deductive process using numerical data to measure the quantity of something; quantitative data is analysed and reported through numerical comparison and statistical analyses

Qualitative – an inductive process using non-numerical data, like words, sounds and pictures, to describe and characterise (but not measure) something; attitudes and objects can be categorised through the development of themes and subthemes

Variable – a factor or part of something that is able to change; it may also be influenced by other factors or variables

(BITRE, 2010). The government implemented a number of initiatives to increase road safety by improving roads and cars; through legislation (e.g. making seatbelt use compulsory for everyone in a vehicle) and enforcement by police and technological means (e.g. speed cameras); and through intensive public education (BITRE, 2010). This led to a drop in average fatalities over time; in 2018 road fatalities had dropped to 1145 in Australia (DITCRD, 2019). These counts tell us some or all of these initiatives have worked, and they may also highlight where more needs to be done (see Learning activity 8.1).

LEARNING ACTIVITY 8.1

The rate of road fatalities in Australia has greatly decreased since the 1970s thanks to the implementation of many different measures, including policy, education and infrastructure. Research has shown that while the current rate of road fatalities has decreased for younger drivers (aged 17–25 years), they are still more likely to be involved in road fatalities than other road users. There has also been an increase in the number of deaths of older road users, particularly those aged 65 to 74 years and older males (DITCRD, 2019). The number of injuries on roads has also increased, at a rate of almost 4 per cent per year since 2013 (DITCRD, 2019).

Imagine you work for a state or territory road safety authority and are responsible for the implementation and promotion of the road-safety strategy and its associated education program.

1. What kinds of resources could you use to identify the rates of road fatalities and injuries in your state or territory – where would you look? Compile a list and choose a resource to use in the next question.
2. Using the resource you identified in 1, identify which two groups are at highest risk in your state or territory. Identify which is the greatest risk for both groups: fatalities or injuries? Justify your assessment.

Keep this information handy and use it again in Learning activity 8.2.

Counts can also be used to measure the outcome of a health promotion initiative. For example, if you were running a program that aimed to change some kind of behaviour, you could compare how many people did that thing (e.g. bought a particular product) before the program with those who did it afterwards, and whether that change is maintained over time. Counts are also useful in evaluating the success of a communication strategy. For example, how many people attended an event or participated in a social media-based competition? Social media and other means of online engagement are increasingly relevant and important tools in engaging audiences, and these can also be used in the evaluation process. Websites can have built-in analytics tools to track how long users stay on a page, what they are reading and the search terms they use. Other counts can be very simple – for example, the number of followers a Facebook page or Twitter or Instagram account gains after a program is launched. While the number of followers tells you something about how visible your program is, it does not necessarily tell you much about those followers, or what they are doing with your program. You can use other metrics, such as 'likes', 'shares' or comments, as indicators of a deeper level of engagement and interest, but this is limited. More can be done, which is discussed in the qualitative methods section.

Questionnaires

A quick note here on the use of the term 'questionnaire' instead of 'survey'. A questionnaire is the set of questions used to gather data for a survey. A survey is the set of questions, as well as the process of collecting and analysing the data.

Questionnaires can provide greater nuance than simple counts alone, as they can be used to get an understanding of perceptions, agreement and disagreement. Questions can be closed or open-ended. Closed questions are those that are essentially 'tick and flick' responses, such as multiple-choice, dropdown items and scales for levels of agreement, such as 'strongly disagree' to 'strongly agree'. Open-ended questions can assist in gathering qualitative data, as these ask for people's opinions and ideas, and respondents are not constrained by pre-set categories.

Questionnaires can provide insights into the effectiveness of communication strategies. For example, questions could be used to identify the most effective communication channel by asking people how they heard about the program or event. Questionnaires can also be useful in evaluating how effective messaging was within a program. For example, are more people aware of an issue or a resource now than they were before they accessed the program? One way to measure change using questionnaires is by giving them to participants at different stages, such as before an event or program starts and again afterwards. Depending upon the program's duration, it may be possible to ask questions in the middle as well, and to track changes over time. Studies that collect data on the same variables over a period of time are called 'longitudinal' studies. Some longitudinal studies run for decades, such as the Household, Income and Labour Dynamics in Australia (HILDA) Survey, which began in 2001 and continues to track over 17 000 people (Melbourne Institute, n.d.).

When using questionnaires, the big challenge is to make sure the questions are fit for purpose. For example, is the question asking about one thing or many? The more 'sub-questions' that are asked within a question, the more likely it is that respondents will not complete the question or the questionnaire. This, in turn, limits the usefulness of the data collected. For example, look at this question:

How often and what kinds of exercise do you do and what are your reasons for this choice?

The question is obviously asking about multiple things – exercise frequency, exercise type and reasons. But the final part of this question is unclear: is the choice referring to the frequency of exercise, the type of exercise, or both? It would be far better to separate it into shorter, discrete questions. All could be answered using closed or open-ended questions, or a mix of both. It depends upon what you want to know. If you already have a scale of exercise frequency (e.g. hours per week) then this will be easy to incorporate as a closed question. Likewise with exercise type, which could be a list of sports or activities where the respondent could tick all that apply. It would also be advisable to include an 'other' response, which enables the respondent to provide details about an exercise that may not be included on the list, to ensure that the data collected is as complete as possible. The 'reasons' part of the question needs to be clarified; either asking for an explanation for each element (time and type) or being more explicit (What are the main reasons you do the exercise/s noted in the previous question?).

If you are using closed questions and scales, then it is important that the scales are appropriate. An organisation that wants to measure visitor satisfaction could ask the question, 'Overall, how satisfied were you by your experience here today?' This is a good question because it is asking the respondent about one thing, their satisfaction with the experience. But if the only possible responses are defined and limited – not at all satisfied, satisfied, quite satisfied, very satisfied – then the data will be strongly skewed towards positive responses. If visitors are not completely dissatisfied but also are not very happy with their experience, the only option they could tick is satisfied. For the organisation, this is still a 'satisfied' result, and therefore they are doing their job properly. But are they?

One other thing to consider is having an internal consistency check in your questionnaire to ensure that respondents are paying attention to the questions and not just choosing any box to tick. Online survey tools often give the option of randomising the order in which possible responses are given. This will help you to identify whether someone is just ticking the first option for every single question, for example. Another way to check is by asking the same kind of question in different ways to see whether the respondent answers in a way that is consistent. Say a visitor notes that they are 'very satisfied' with their overall experience. If the questionnaire also includes the question, 'how likely are you to recommend this experience to others?', you would expect someone who was very satisfied to indicate that they are likely or very likely to recommend the experience to others. If someone notes that they are dissatisfied with their experience, but also likely to recommend it to others, that is a sign that perhaps the responses in that questionnaire are not as valid as you would like.

Golden rules for quantitative methods

This may all seem a bit confusing and overwhelming. There is much to think about to ensure that you get the information you want. Luckily, there are also a great many resources you can use, including online survey tools with suggestions and tips, as well as many reference texts. Here are some golden rules to help make your questionnaire as useful and effective as possible:

- *Keep it short* – as a guide, the questionnaire should not take more than 20 minutes to complete.
- *Be explicit* – ensure your questions are crystal clear and only ask about one 'thing' at a time.
- *Test it* – do the survey yourself, share it with a small group to confirm how long it takes, whether the questions make sense and if the questionnaire is doing what you intend it to (especially if it is all being done online).
- *Respect your respondent* – ask questions that are directly relevant to your objective. Remember that participants are volunteering their time to help you, so keep the questionnaire short and always thank respondents for their time.
- *Keep one question open-ended* – sometimes a respondent may have something to say that could be incredibly helpful or insightful but if your questionnaire does not include a space where they can provide it, that insight might be lost. Always leave space for one question that asks something along the lines of 'Is there anything else you would like to tell us that you have not already shared in your answers?'

Strengths and weaknesses of quantitative methods

A great strength of quantitative methods is that they enable you to get information quickly from a lot of people. Because they are so simple and relatively inexpensive to implement, surveys tend to be used frequently. This also means that people tend to have 'survey fatigue' – they have completed too many of them and do not wish to do any more, which can make getting responses difficult. The use of numerical data allows comparisons and statistical analyses within and between groups. The ability to reduce variables to numbers is a strength and a weakness of quantitative data. To get useful data from quantitative research, you typically need a large sample size, which can be costly and time-consuming or, in resource-poor contexts, simply may not be possible. Reducing variables to numbers may provide you with results; however, you do not gain any insight into *why* these results occur. Quantitative data may help you identify where an issue requiring attention may exist, but it is through the use of qualitative data that a better understanding of the issue and the variables influencing it can be reached. See Case study 8.2 for an example.

CASE STUDY 8.2 Unhealthy diets and chronic disease in Chandigarh, India

Jasvir Kaur, Manmeet Kaur and Rajesh Kumar

Diets high in fat, sugar and salt, and low in fruits and vegetables, represent a major risk factor for chronic diseases such as cardiovascular diseases, diabetes and certain cancers. The prevalence of chronic diseases is quite high in Chandigarh, a city in the north of India. Most of these diseases can be prevented through dietary behaviour modifications. The use of theoretical models in planning health promotion interventions increases the likelihood for an intervention to be effective. This project used an intervention, titled SMART (Small, Measurable and Achievable dietary changes by Reducing fat, sugar and salt consumption and Trying different fruits and vegetables) Eating, to improve dietary behaviour among urban adults in Chandigarh. (For further information on this study see Kaur et al. (2020).)

Using models to assist in planning and implementing an evaluation

The PRECEDE-PROCEED model (Green & Kreuter, 2005) was used to inform the development, implementation and evaluation of the SMART Eating intervention. Each phase of the model was used to systematically develop the initiative.

Phase 1 – Social diagnosis Formative research was used, including a cross-sectional survey and focus group discussions among urban Indian adults from diverse socio-economic backgrounds (i.e. low-income, middle-income and high-income groups). Availability, use and preferences for information technology were assessed during the survey. Guided by the social ecological model, focus groups explored people's dietary behaviours as situated within their sociocultural and interpersonal contexts. In addition, participants' intervention preferences regarding the methods and channels of communication, including language preferences, frequency of messages, duration of the intervention and target audience for intervention implementation, were explored. Focus group participants were recruited with the help of influential people in the local community.

Phase 2 – Epidemiological, behavioural and environmental diagnosis The epidemiological assessment focused on specific health issues such as chronic diseases and their risk factors, and nutritional deficiencies. Focus groups and a cross-sectional survey were used to assess the behavioural (unhealthy diet) and environmental factors (accessibility and affordability of healthy foods) and how these related to prioritised health needs of the community.

Phase 3 – Educational and ecological diagnosis Data collected in phases 1 and 2 was analysed and the results used to select factors that, if modified, would most likely result in sustained behavioural change. Use of the social ecological model helped in identifying multi-level factors that were influencing dietary behaviours.

Phase 4 – Intervention alignment Based on findings from the formative evaluation, the behaviour-change matrix was developed to guide the selection of intervention components. Taking into account the available literature on nutrition education interventions, the national dietary guidelines and focus group participants' preferences for implementation of the intervention, the curriculum of the nutrition education program was prepared. A SMART Eating flip book was developed to guide the families on the use of different components of the intervention:

1. Interpersonal component – a SMART Eating kit including a kitchen calendar, dining table mat (see Figure 8.1), and measuring spoons
2. Information technology (IT) component – including SMS, email, social networking app (WhatsApp) and the SMART Eating website.

Phase 5 – Implementation of the intervention The intervention was implemented at family level over a period of six months, using intervention and comparison groups. One individual was randomly selected from each family for the purpose of measurements. The intervention group received an IT-enabled intervention using a multi-channel communication approach, including the interpersonal and IT components described in Phase 4. The comparison group received a pamphlet on nutrition education.

Phase 6 – Process, impact and outcome evaluation Process evaluation was initiated at the time of the implementation of the intervention. This evaluation was used to assess whether the intervention had been implemented according to the plan, to analyse the factors facilitating and hindering the use of the IT-enabled intervention program and to identify points for improvement. Data included log records of the content delivery, website login/visitor count and use of the social networking app; a home visit following one month of the intervention to assess the use of the SMART Eating kit and whether there were any barriers to using the

(cont.)

(cont.)

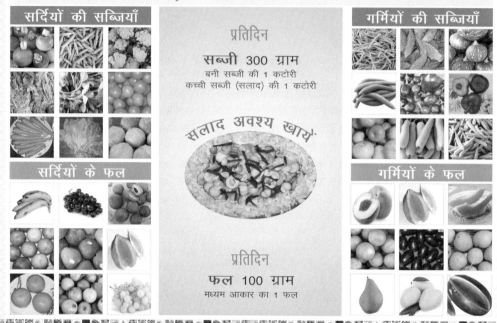

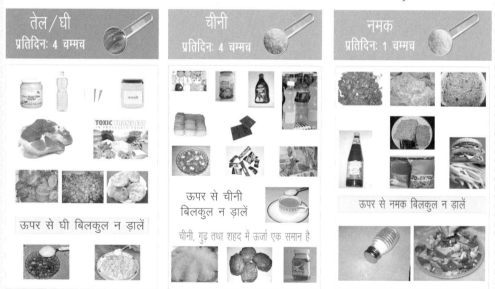

Figure 8.1   Front and back of SMART Eating dining table mat

intervention through different components. Post-intervention feedback was obtained from participants regarding their perception of the effect and their satisfaction with the intervention. The outcome evaluation was done at six months to examine the effect of the health promotion intervention on dietary intakes of fat, sugar, salt, fruit and vegetables, using mixed-effects linear regression models by estimating net mean changes.

Evaluation and conclusion

Overall, the intervention group had significant net mean changes (p<0.001) in their intake of fat, sugar, salt, fruit and vegetables, relative to the comparison group. However, significant net change was not observed for salt intake in the high-income subgroup. Although significant, the magnitude of change for fruit and vegetable consumption was lower in the lower-income groups compared to the medium-income and high-income groups. The post-intervention process evaluation indicated that high costs of fruits and vegetables were the major barrier to healthy eating among the low-income group.

The IT-enabled SMART Eating intervention was found to be effective in reducing fat, sugar and salt intake, and in increasing fruit and vegetable consumption among adults from diverse socio-economic backgrounds. The results show that socio-economic background influences the outcomes. The costs associated with consumption of fruit and vegetables is a major concern for the lower-income group, and increasing prices means that other specific measures should be used to improve access to healthy food for this group. Participants in higher-income groups did not show any reduction in salt intake, which needs further exploration. Reducing fat, sugar and salt intake is not associated with additional household expense; thus it is feasible to implement these interventions even among low-income groups. Future interventions should recruit people from all socio-economic strata to enable deeper understanding of the barriers for different groups and help ensure equity in access to healthy foods.

QUESTIONS

1. Qualitative and quantitative data informed the development, implementation and overall evaluation of the initiative. Is there any other potential data source that could be used to inform or evaluate this initiative? What is it and how could it be used?
2. This case study showed two key results for two different groups:
   - Low-income groups faced barriers to healthy eating due to the prohibitive costs of fruit and vegetables.
   - High-income groups continued to consume too much salt.

   Imagine you are required to design the next health promotion initiative to help address these barriers. For each group answer these questions:

   a. What would you do, and why?
   b. How would you evaluate your success?

(cont.)

(cont.)

EXTENSION QUESTION

This case study shows how socio-economic factors can influence the outcomes of health promotion initiatives. Identify another health issue in which health outcomes are likely affected by socio-economic determinants. What kinds of data-gathering methods would you use to understand these affects, and with whom? Justify your answer.

Qualitative methods

An analysis of numbers alone does not automatically make an evaluation 'good'. Qualitative data enables analysis of written and spoken words, images and observations of people (for example) to explore the questions you are asking in greater depth than is possible with quantitative methods. The previous section introduced one means of collecting qualitative data: through the use of open-ended questions in surveys. Such questions can be included in questionnaires and are also useful in data-collection methods such as interviews and focus groups, using video or audio recordings, or text-based diaries, in print, online and using electronic devices such as smartphones and tablets. Some of the methods described here require the researchers to have specific communication skills and abilities.

Interviews

Interviews enable participants to provide detailed responses about their thoughts, feelings and experiences. Interviews can be more time-consuming to undertake and analyse than questionnaires, but are useful for identifying the needs or experiences of individuals and groups. Whom you interview depends on what you are trying to achieve. You may want to speak to experts in the field or to community members or leaders, or representatives of your intended target audience. When you interview may also vary; for example, you might interview key stakeholders during the development stage of an initiative, to find out what they want and need, or you may need to interview them at the conclusion to find out if those needs were met. Or both!

Interviews should use open-ended questions and should be similar to survey questions in being clear, easy to understand and only asking about one 'thing' at a time. As an interviewer, crafting the questions well is only one part of the process. Being a good interviewer means being a good listener, too. Think about the last time you went to see a doctor. How did they start the consultation? It might have been with a question like 'What brings you in here today?' They then use your response to guide their next question, until ultimately they decide what tests may be needed to reach a diagnosis and to decide on a treatment plan. In some ways, using interviews in an evaluation is a little bit like that. You have a list of questions you want to ask but first listen to the participant to decide what to ask next, what to explore in detail and to identify the main issues or points of view. A good interview should feel more like a conversation than like someone working their way down a list of things to cover. Don't be afraid to ask for more detail about a participant's response. Some people will give you extremely long, detailed answers while others may not be as forthcoming. If you get one-word or two-word responses, follow up with questions like 'Can you tell me a little bit more about that?' Show that you are interested in, and value, their opinion and that you want to ensure you understand their perspective. Also, be aware of the participant showing any signs of distress or fatigue – the welfare of the participant should always be the most important thing to consider.

How many interviews are enough? This can be determined by considering several factors. How many people *could* you talk to? This could range from the total number of stakeholders, representatives or participants associated with a program or event. If there are smaller numbers (say, less than 30) perhaps you can speak to all of them if they all have unique perspectives. After interviewing a broad cross section of these stakeholders (say, 10) you may find the same responses and ideas being given. This could indicate that you have collected enough information to enable analysis and you do not need to do any further interviews (this is known as 'saturation'). If you have a very large pool of potential interviewees, then you need to make other recruitment decisions. Sometimes the ability to recruit willing participants, along with other practical factors such as time, money and resources, can be limited, irrespective of what you are trying to achieve. There is no simple, single answer as to what is the 'right' number, and often the decision is assisted by other extenuating circumstances.

Focus groups

Focus groups were introduced in Chapter 6 as a method for testing messages with the intended audience. These group discussions can be a useful way to garner a range of perspectives through the exchange of opinions and ideas between participants. Focus groups therefore can yield a breadth of information about a topic and can help health promoters understand *why* people respond in the ways they do to their materials and activities. Focus groups are typically comprised of stakeholders relevant to the intervention and can be mixed (e.g. representatives of all stakeholders in a group together) or separate (a different stakeholder category in each group). Focus groups should have a clear aim and purpose, which can then inform who the ideal participants should be.

Running a focus group can be daunting, particularly if you have never done it before. Consider inviting a co-facilitator to share guiding the discussions and note-taking, or 'shadowing' a more experienced facilitator so you can see how it is done. As a facilitator of a focus group, your role is to guide participants through planned questions, much like in an interview. Some of the same skills, such as asking clear questions and active listening, are useful here, too. Allow scope for ideas and issues not covered in your questions to be further explored; this means time management is also important. The facilitator should ensure that all voices in the group are heard. This may mean they need to encourage quieter members of the group to give their opinion and prevent one or two participants dominating the discussion. This can be a challenging task, but by setting clear expectations at the start of the focus group, it can be managed well. Establish clear group rules upfront, such as confidentiality, that everyone will be able to express their opinion without judgement from others and that equal contributions are welcomed from everyone – with the understanding that the facilitator may cut some longer answers short to allow everyone to be heard. Participants need to commit to not sharing the details of other participants, or the content of the discussion, outside of the focus group. As the facilitator you need to establish an environment of openness and trust, to allow these group rules to be maintained, and for participants to feel comfortable and safe to contribute. Be sure to set aside some time at the start for introductions, and provide refreshment if possible, to help participants feel as comfortable as possible.

Content analysis

Content analysis is a method used to analyse data collected from artefacts (e.g. objects and manuscripts), still images (e.g. photographs, artworks), video or film footage, comments on social media or news stories, or to analyse data obtained from open-ended questions in questionnaires, interviews or focus groups. A content analysis employs a unique means of analysing data and can often involve specific means of collecting data, too. In terms of data collection, you can use content analysis to explore people's interpretations and representations of information. Say, for example, you have completed a campaign on healthy eating and one of the ways in which the campaign has engaged participants was by asking them to post images of their healthy lunch on Instagram. By analysing these images, you can get data and visual representations of how participants defined 'healthy' and how this compares with the key messages of your campaign. Or perhaps you want to understand how public perceptions of an issue may be influenced by media coverage. Then you could collect newspaper articles from a variety of sources during a specific timeframe and code those articles to identify common frames (see Chapter 5 and 7).

There are two different types of content analysis: conceptual and relational. Conceptual content analysis is usually quantitative in nature. It involves identifying recurring themes, ideas or words, as well as key terms in the data and/or their frequency. This process of organising a large amount of information into smaller categories is called 'coding'. Codes might be decided before coding begins (based on the research question or what other related studies have used), or may be identified through the coding process (open coding). Whichever way you decide to categorise or code the information, ensure each code is clearly defined and used consistently throughout. Relational analysis examines the relationships between concepts. This can mean examining which topics appear with others, or how different concepts or ideas overlap, for example.

Content analysis can also be used to help evaluate the effectiveness of communication messages or campaigns. As mentioned in the section on quantitative methods, counting the number of social media engagements such as 'likes', 'shares', 'retweets' and comments can provide an indication of the level of awareness and interest in the program, as well as how effective the communication strategy has been. Using content analysis to examine social media comments can help you better understand the opinions and perspectives of people about the program or topic, whether they want more information or topic areas that may be contentious. Using a sound research design to conduct an evaluation of the effectiveness of social media in health promotion is an area of growing need. Although social media sites are increasingly used in health promotion interventions, the rate of evaluation of the effectiveness of these programs does not appear to be keeping pace with people's use of these sites, and what has been done seems to be limited in capacity to assess the reach and effectiveness of interventions (Lim et al., 2016).

Strengths and weaknesses of qualitative methods

Qualitative methods enable better understanding of the 'why' and 'how' through a deeper exploration of attitudes, perceptions and values than is possible with quantitative methods. They are particularly useful for uncovering why an initiative or program worked, or did not, and for soliciting suggestions and recommendations to improve future offerings. A major challenge in using qualitative methods is in ensuring that participants are representative of the target audience and thus do not present a biased perspective of opinions. The amount of time required to set up mechanisms for data collection, such as interviews and focus groups, tends to be much more than the time required for data analysis. Although the data collected may be highly detailed, qualitative studies tend to use smaller sample sizes, so the conclusions may not be generalisable to a broader population.

LEARNING ACTIVITY 8.2

In Learning activity 8.1 you identified the groups at highest risk in your state or territory for road fatalities and/or injuries. As part of your role in implementing the road-safety strategy, you need to develop an education program to target your identified at-risk groups.

1. For each of the groups you identified in Learning activity 8.1, complete a review of available literature to identify some of the major contributing factors in the rate of death or injury.

2. Based on your answer to 1, develop a strategy for collecting more information from your two target groups, to help design the most effective education program. You may want to consider this from both a research and a communication perspective. For example, in thinking about it from a research point of view:

    -   What information is needed from the groups? What question do you need to answer?
    -   What is the best way to get this information? Surveys, focus groups, interviews, or a mix?

From a communication perspective:

    -   How might you most effectively reach these groups – where are they 'found', and how do you know?
    -   What is the most effective communication channel to engage these groups, to get the information that you need?

Mixed methods

Using mixed methods can provide you with both breadth and depth of data to help inform your conclusions. Mixed-methods research might place greater emphasis on either the qualitative or quantitative data, or it may rely equally on both. Irrespective of how they are combined, this should be done in such a way as to ensure that the combination of data collected is appropriate for answering the research question. There are some who believe that qualitative and quantitative methods should not be mixed; however, if combined meaningfully and well, mixed-methods research can provide findings that are 'much more nuanced and deeper than those emerging from single-method studies' (Voorhees & Howell Smith, 2020, p. 229). Mixed-methods approaches can enable what is called **triangulation**. Each method described in this chapter can have inherent biases and weaknesses, which may influence the results of the study. Using multiple methods to examine the same variable allows for cross-checking of the data to explore its accuracy and to gain a fuller understanding of what the data might mean than may be possible using a single method (see Case study 8.3).

Triangulation – the use of more than one data source and/or method to collect information about the variable under study

CASE STUDY 8.3 Mixed-methods evaluation of medical services in Papua New Guinea

The Western Province of Papua New Guinea (PNG) is the largest and most remote in the country, having limited accessibility through roads, and the use of boats and planes hampered by the cost of fuel (ADI, 2020b). This difficulty in access contributes to challenges in providing necessary personnel and supplies to support adequate healthcare delivery (Kitchener, 2019). Five doctors serve an area with a population of 228000 people, with no doctors or nurses available to service communities in remote regions (ADI, 2020b). Low birthweights in babies, malnourishment and diarrhoeal diseases in children under the age of five are common in the Western Province (ADI, 2020b).

Delivering health services in partnership

Since 2000, the Australian Doctors International (ADI) has worked with the Catholic Diocese of Daru-Kiunga of the Western Province of PNG to improve health service delivery, especially for child and maternal health, and to develop the capacity of the rural health workers based there (ADI, 2020a). The program uses a system of patrols, whereby medical staff visit the remote areas of the Western Province to conduct health checks and to deliver health education and awareness seminars and materials. In 2018, the program was evaluated using mixed methods to determine changes in health service delivery arising from their programs and to make recommendations to improve the efficacy of their programs.

The evaluation drew upon existing databases, pre-existing evaluations, reports and policy documents to determine the health needs of the communities, based on records of diagnoses in clinics (Kitchener, 2019). This also allowed an examination of whether and how these health needs had changed over time and measurement of performance against set targets for service delivery, such as public health education. The program has the output goals of 80 per cent of villages in a patrol catchment receiving public health education and at least 1600 individual community members attending these education sessions each year (Kitchener, 2019). Quantitative data analysis showed the number of individuals attending greatly exceeded this target, with over 3000 people attending sessions in 2018 alone; however, they were from only 40 per cent of villages (Kitchener, 2019). While there is a great deal of interest in the seminars, shown through the high levels of attendance, it was not clear why 60 per cent of the villages in the patrol catchment were not being reached.

Qualitative surveys of patrol organisers and local healthcare workers (HCW) frequently showed that a lack of communication was a major factor, as was a resulting lack of communication between HCWs and the local communities. As a result, villages did not know when the patrols were coming, so it took a long time for people to arrive for the seminar once it was known that the patrol would be arriving.

Some of this lack of communication was caused by administrative omissions such as not developing a schedule for patrol visits that allocated a specific time for community public health education sessions. Other barriers were structural, such as a lack of communications technology, with three communities not having access to mobile phone coverage or radios (Kitchener, 2019). Other reports showed that HCW were informed of planned patrols and schedules but did not distribute this information to their communities and the surrounding villages.

QUESTIONS

1. Imagine you only had access to the quantitative or qualitative data – not both. How would that influence your interpretation of the program's performance?

2. Based on all of the data provided in this evaluation, what recommendations would you make, and why?

Communicating your evaluation results

The process of evaluation can be time-consuming for both the person collecting the data and participants. And it is likely that all are giving their time because they have a vested interest in the outcome. However, evaluation findings are not always shared, and even if they are it may not be in ways that are meaningful, or potentially is not shared with those who participate or have an interest in the outcome. Once you have completed your evaluation, you should think about communicating its findings. Ethically, it is good practice to provide participants with a summary of the results, if appropriate or possible. There may be some instances in which public sharing of results is not appropriate, and this should be respected. For example, if sharing results would mean participants are able to be identified, even if their names were not used, then these results should not be made public. However, if it can be done ethically, results should be shared when they can, as this will help inform others working on similar projects or with similar audiences. Think about your own needs-assessment process and how helpful it was to find information from other similar projects. Or perhaps how frustrating it was to see that similar activities had been run but not being able to access any indicator of what worked and what did not. Your evaluation should have its own communication plan, for which you can use Table 8.1 to develop. Evaluation is about finding out what works, for whom and how, in order to inform and improve future activities. It is also an opportunity to communicate your results to help achieve broader objectives.

The nature of research and evaluation means that the evaluator really needs to have excellent communication skills. They must be able to communicate effectively with a range of different audiences, such as with participants to elicit information, as well as in communicating the results to partners and policy makers. Any language or cultural barriers between the evaluator and stakeholders could influence the entire project, from data collection to analysis (Bergeron et al., 2017), so as the evaluator you need to ensure you are minimising or overcoming these barriers throughout the project, using the concepts and skills explored throughout this book. The potential for jargon to be used in the evaluation also means that the information generated may be too difficult for non-specialists to understand. Therefore, you should also ensure that the findings are presented in a way that is useful and comprehensible both to practitioners and decision makers. This may mean you need to tailor the results to make them meaningful to different audiences.

Participants and community members may be interested in what worked within the community during the program, so they can keep these elements going. Practitioners may want to know the same thing but are also likely to want to know about the process of implementing and running the program. Funders and policy makers are likely to want to know about the impact of the program, or the return on their investment. Think of the evaluation as the end of your program's story; almost like the final chapter of your communications activities. You began by articulating the need for your program and using different communication channels and messages to engage your target audience. In communicating the evaluation results, you can complete the story by describing what you did to overcome the identified problem and what happened as a result. This is also an opportunity to propose what could happen next, and potentially to start a whole new story.

Summary

This chapter has outlined the different approaches to evaluation, their strengths and weaknesses. Before doing any form of evaluation it is important to know exactly what you want to know and with which audience. This then informs your research question, the methods you will use and the participants you need to recruit. As well as evaluating the effectiveness of a health promotion initiative, evaluation can also help to identify how effective the communication activities supporting that initiative were. Effective communication is important at every step of the process, from working with partners and stakeholders to identify needed information, recruiting participants with the appropriate information to provide informed consent, using clear questions and facilitation through to communicating the evaluation results.

REVISION QUESTIONS

1. Describe the differences between formative and summative evaluation, giving examples of when in health promotion program development each could occur.
2. What information do potential research participants need to enable them to provide informed consent?
3. What are the strengths and weaknesses of quantitative methods?
4. What are the strengths and weaknesses of qualitative methods?
5. Give an example of mixed-methods research.

FURTHER READING

Bauman, A. & Nutbeam, D. (2013) *Evaluation in a Nutshell: A practical guide to the evaluation of health promotion programs* (2nd ed.). Sydney: McGraw-Hill.

Krueger, R.A. & Casey, M. (2015). *Focus Groups: A practical guide for applied research* (5th ed.). California: SAGE.

Liamputtong, P. (2019). *Qualitative Research Methods* (5th ed.). South Melbourne: Oxford University Press.

Round, R., Marshall, B. & Horton, K. (2005). *Planning for Effective Health Promotion Evaluation.* Melbourne: Victorian Government Department of Human Services.

Various (2016). Special Issue: Advancing evaluation practice in health promotion, *Health Promotion Journal of Australia*, 27(3), 181–267.

REFERENCES

Australian Doctors International (ADI) (2020a). About Australian Doctors International ADI (Website). Retrieved from: https://www.adi.org.au/about

———(2020b). About Western Province (Website). Retrieved from: https://www.adi.org .au/about-western-province/

Australian Health Promotion Association (AHPA) (2009). *Core Competencies for Health Promotion Practitioners*. Australian Health Promotion Association. Retrieved from: https://www.healthpromotion.org.au/images/docs/core_competencies_for_hp_ practitioners.pdf

Bergeron, D.A., Talbot, L.R. & Gaboury, I. (2017). Realist evaluation of intersectoral oral health promotion interventions for schoolchildren living in rural Andean communities: A research protocol, *BMJ Open*, 7(2), e:014531.

Bureau of Infrastructure, Transport and Regional Economics (BITRE) (2010). *Road Deaths in Australia 1925–2008*. Canberra: BITRE.

Centers for Disease Control and Prevention (CDC) (2016). CDC Approach to Evaluation. Centers for Disease Control and Prevention, Program Performance and Evaluation Office. Retrieved from: https://www.cdc.gov/eval/indicators/index.htm

Choy, L.T. (2017). The strengths and weaknesses of research methodology: Comparison and complimentary between qualitative and quantitative approaches, *IOSR Journal of Humanities and Social Sciences*, 19(4), 99–104.

Department of Health (2018). *Girls Make your Move campaign backgrounder*. Canberra: Australian Government. Retrieved from: https://campaigns.health.gov.au/girlsmove/campaign-backgrounder

Department of Infrastructure, Transport, Cities and Regional Development (DITCRD) (2019). *Road trauma Australia 2018 Statistical Summary*. Canberra: DITCRD.

Francis, L.J. & Smith, B.J. (2015). Toward best practice in evaluation a study of Australian health promotion agencies, *Health Promotion Practice*, 16, 715–23.

Green, L.W. & Kreuter, M.W. (2005). *Health Program Planning: An educational and ecological approach*. New York: McGraw-Hill.

Haines, A., Kuruvilla, S. & Borchert, M. (2004). Bridging the implementation gap between knowledge and action for health, *Bulletin of the World Health Organization*, 82(10), 724–32.

Huckel Schneider, C., Milat, A.J. & Moore, G. (2016). Barriers and facilitators to evaluation of health policies and programs: Policymaker and researcher perspectives, *Evaluation and Program Planning*, 58, 208–15.

Kaur, M., Kaur, M., Chakrapani, V. & Kumar, R. (2020). Multilevel influences on fat, sugar, salt, fruit, and vegetable consumption behaviors among urban indians: Application of the social ecological model, *SAGE Open*. Retrieved from: https://doi.org/10.1177/2158244020919526

Kitchener, E. (2019, April). 2018 Evaluative Report of ADI Programs in Western Province, Papua New Guinea. Retrieved from: https://www.adi.org.au/wp-content/uploads/2019/05/ADI-report-FINAL_web.pdf

Lim, M.S.C., Wright, C.J.C, Carrotte, E.R. & Pedrana, A.E. (2016). Reach, engagement, and effectiveness: A systematic review of evaluation methodologies used in health promotion via social networking sites, *Health Promotion Journal of Australia*, 27(3), 187–97.

Lobo. R., Petrich, M. & Burns, S.K. (2014). Supporting health promotion practitioners to undertake evaluation for program development, *BMC Public Health*, 14, 1315.

Melbourne Institute (n.d.). HILDA Survey (Website). Retrieved from: https://melbourneinstitute.unimelb.edu.au/hilda

National Health and Medical Research Council (NHMRC) and the Australian Research Council (ARC) (2018). *National Statement on Ethical Conduct in Human Research*. Canberra: NHMRC & ARC.

Nutbeam, D., Smith, C. & Catford, J. (1990). Evaluation in health education, progress, problems and possibilities, *Journal of Epidemiology and Community Health*, 44, 83–9.

Orima Research (2019). *Girls Make Your Move* campaign, evaluation research. Comprehensive evaluation report – Final. Retrieved from: https://campaigns.health.gov.au/girlsmove/resources/publications/report/evaluation-research-report-phase-3-girls-make-your-move

UNAIDS (2010). An introduction to indicators, UNAIDS Monitoring and Evaluation Fundamentals. Retrieved from: https://www.unaids.org/sites/default/files/sub_landing/files/8_2-Intro-to-IndicatorsFMEF.pdf

Voorhees, H.L. & Howell Smith, M.C. (2020). Qualitative and quantitative method integration in diabetes communication research: Applications and contributions, *Qualitative Health Research*, 30(2), 228–35.

Wolfenden, L., Williams, C.M., Wiggers, J., Nathan, N. & Yoong, S. (2016). Improving the translation of health promotion interventions using effectiveness – implementation hybrid designs in program evaluations. *Health Promotion Journal of Australia*, 27(3), 204–7.

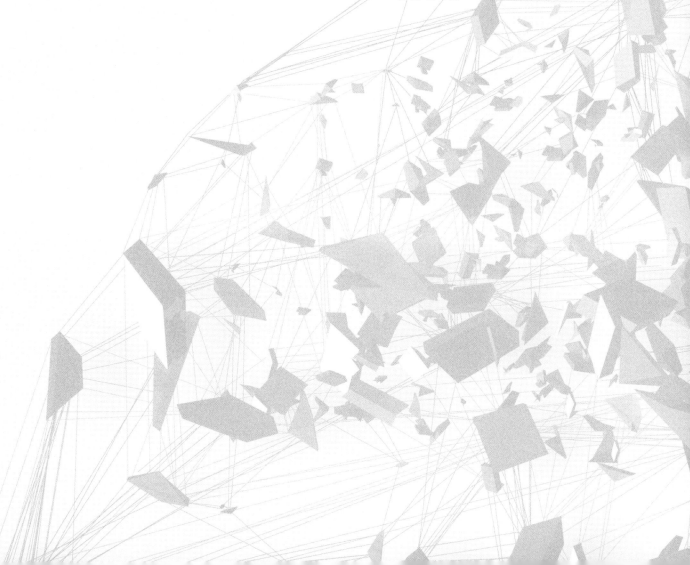

PART 3

Global health into the future

Health promotion needs and challenges

Merryn McKinnon

With contributions from Daniel Craig and Andrea Waling

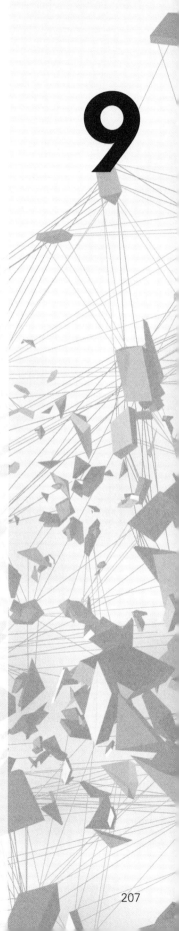

9

LEARNING OBJECTIVES

At the completion of the chapter, you will be able to:

- Describe the relationship between human and environmental health.
- Discuss health issues that are likely to arise in society into the future, and the associated communication challenges.
- Identify and describe the effects of disadvantage on health outcomes, particularly for vulnerable communities.
- Describe effective approaches to communication within health promotion to foster inclusion.

Introduction

This chapter explores the health promotion needs of society – locally and globally. It begins by describing the relationship between the environment and humans, and how the health of the planet is intrinsic to the health of humans. There are several approaches to health that encompass all factors thought to be influencing human health, such as ecohealth, One Health and Health in All Policies (discussed in turn in this chapter). Effective communication in health promotion can help to achieve the objectives of these kinds of multi-sectoral approaches and there is potential for health promotion to become more engaged in this space in the future.

The second section of this chapter explores future health and communication challenges, many of which are already emerging as relevant. The communication context, which needs to be successfully navigated in order to address these challenges, is complex, with no apparent 'solution'. The COVID-19 global pandemic demonstrates how personal values and beliefs, societal norms and cultures can affect acceptance of health messaging, and highlights what can go wrong if communication is not carefully considered and implemented. There are some in our communities who, through circumstances beyond their control and often due to compounding inequalities and sources of disadvantage, will experience worse health outcomes than others. The final section of this chapter explores how health promotion can recognise and meet the needs of a diverse society, by recognising and addressing these sources of disadvantage and using communication as a means of fostering inclusion.

Healthy ecosystems

Ecosystem – a community of living organisms and their physical environment, all of which interact as a system in a particular space; ecosystems can be small-scale (local) and global

Human health is inextricably intertwined with environmental health; we are all part of the same **ecosystem**. This is far from a foreign concept to health and health promotion. Indigenous communities worldwide have long been calling for an approach that pays attention to the relationships between the environment and people, and the need to consider ecological needs as related to social needs, rather than a false either/or dichotomy (Parkes et al., 2020). The Ottawa Charter for Health Promotion clearly states that a stable ecosystem and sustainable resources are fundamental conditions and resources for health (WHO, 1986). It also specifically calls for health promotion to advocate for health – and the factors that facilitate favourable health outcomes – and for 'reciprocal maintenance – to take care of each other … and our natural environment. The conservation of natural resources throughout the world should be emphasized as a global responsibility' (WHO, 1986, p. 2).

Conservation of natural resources includes the invaluable ecosystem services, such as water cycles, nitrogen and phosphorous cycles, and waste decomposition, which are integral to survival, including of humans. Yet, in 2005, the Millennium Ecosystem Assessment found that well over half of these vital services are either being used unsustainably or are degraded. Although this assessment has not been updated, it is reasonable to assume that the situation has remained largely the same. The decline of these ecosystem functions 'represents perhaps the greatest threat to the stability of our societies and thus to health in the 21st century' (Hancock, 2015, p. e253).

Evidence of health promotion engaging with environmental issues at any level is quite limited (Patrick & Kingsley, 2016), which indicates a potential area of opportunity to integrate health promotion actions within areas pertaining to sustainability and conservation, for example.

There have been attempts to develop fields that take this more holistic approach, which encompasses human and environmental health. One is 'ecosystem approaches to health' or 'ecohealth' (Bunch et al., 2011). Ecohealth views health as a result of interactions between ecosystems and the other determinants of health, and uses a **systems thinking**, interdisciplinary approach (Patrick & Kingsley, 2016). Another is 'eco-social' health, which focuses 'on the reciprocity among the ecological and the social as essential features of a proactive orientation to future health and collective well-being' (Parkes et al., 2020, p. 61). These should not be confused with the multidimensional models introduced in Chapter 2. Those are focused on changing behaviours through health promotion activities aimed at both individual and social–environmental factors, whereas the environmental model relates to the context of the individual rather than planetary health as such. An approach that does situate human health within a 'planetary' perspective is One Health.

> **Systems thinking** – an approach to understanding how things work through exploration of all the 'parts' within a system as well as their interactions and performance over time, often drawing upon different perspectives

One Health

The term 'One Health' appeared around 2003–4, in relation to the SARS outbreak, which was followed by the H5N1 'bird flu', and by the 'Manhattan Principles' developed at the Wildlife Conservation Society meeting in 2004 (Mackenzie & Jeggo, 2019). The Manhattan Principles of 'One World, One Health' called for a broader understanding of health that requires 'establishing a more holistic approach to preventing epidemic/epizootic disease and for maintaining ecosystem integrity for the benefit of humans, their domesticated animals, and the foundational biodiversity that supports us all' (Wildlife Conservation Society, 2004, para. 1). While there is no single and universal definition of One Health, its basic premise is that the health of humans, animals and the environment are interconnected and that interdisciplinary collaboration is at the core of the One Health concept (Mackenzie & Jenggo, 2019).

Human health is influenced by myriad factors. Without a healthy ecosystem, we cannot have clean air and water or healthy soils to grow food crops to feed the billions of people who live on the planet. Animals farmed in agriculture and wildlife are an integral part of these ecosystems and the human food web; however, the close co-existence of humans with other animals has also seen many **zoonotic diseases** creating global health problems.

> **Zoonotic diseases** – harmful micro-organisms (often bacteria and viruses) carried by animals and able to be spread directly or indirectly to humans, thereby causing illness

Zoonotic diseases and human health

The past 20 years have seen outbreaks of infection in humans by diseases transmitted from animals, such as Ebola virus (transmitted from bats and non-human primates), Hendra virus (horses), avian (bird) and swine (pig) influenza, severe acute respiratory syndrome (SARS; from civets) and Middle East respiratory syndrome (MERS; from camels). In the 1300s, an estimated 50 million people died from the bubonic plague. Called the Black Death, this was the deadliest pandemic in recorded human history. The plague was caused by bacteria transmitted from infected rodents (such as rats, marmots, squirrels and hares) or parasites such as fleas that are associated with them, and it is remains in circulation today – hundreds of years later – around the world. In July 2020, a squirrel in the state of Colorado in the United States tested positive for bubonic plague (Jefferson County Colorado Public Health, 2020). About one week later, a teenager in Mongolia died of bubonic plague after eating the meat of an infected marmot (Guy & Gansukh, 2020). The border area between Mongolia and Russia sees seasonal outbreaks of the plague, as the meat of the Mongolian marmot is considered a local delicacy and residents continue to hunt and eat the marmots despite health advice to the contrary and restrictions on hunting (Guy & Gansukh, 2020).

Many zoonotic diseases occur within other contexts that affect health outcomes. Consider the determinants of health that acknowledge the influence of ecological, political, commercial and cultural factors. When these factors combine, such as we have seen in Ebola outbreaks in West Africa and the Democratic Republic of Congo (see Case study 9.1), public health or medicine alone cannot address all of the issues that arise. Trying to address the multifaceted, complex and often transboundary health problems facing societies across the globe from only one perspective is unlikely to produce sustainable mitigation strategies (Mackenzie & Jeggo, 2019). The One Health approach encourages collaboration between different disciplines and domains, each providing its specialist insights and skills, to collaboratively address problems such as food safety, emerging and endemic zoonotic diseases, and antimicrobial resistance (Mackenzie & Jeggo, 2019). In the case of zoonotic disease, for example, mitigation strategies might be achieved through limiting the spread of the disease in the host animal population through limiting inter-population interactions, vaccination or culling. These strategies are the purview of veterinarians, ecologists and/or environmental scientists rather than medical personnel; however, the groups are working together to achieve health outcomes.

CASE STUDY 9.1 Responding to Ebola outbreaks in the Democratic Republic of Congo

A recurring crisis

On 25 June 2020, the Democratic Republic of Congo (DRC) declared the end of its 10th Ebola outbreak (MSF, 2020a). Beginning in the north-eastern provinces of North Kivu and Ituri, the 10th outbreak had claimed the lives of 2287 people, making it the second-largest outbreak of Ebola after the West Africa outbreak of 2013–16 and the largest to date in the DRC. The DRC's 10th outbreak is thought to have begun in May 2018, but an outbreak alert was not declared until August that year because of a breakdown in the country's health surveillance system. There had been security concerns arising from long-term and widespread violence in the area, and health workers had been on strike in May as they had not been paid (MSF, 2020a).

Compared to previous Ebola epidemics, health workers had been given access to improved tools and resources, such as new treatments, vaccinations and designated Ebola treatment centres, and these were more accessible for families of patients and offered higher levels of care than previously (MSF, 2020a). Despite these advances and improvements, health workers continued to struggle to trace the contacts of confirmed cases, and many people died at home or in other healthcare facilities; the outbreak had a 66 per cent fatality rate (MSF, 2020a).

Social, cultural and political factors

The transmission of Ebola among community members has been attributed to a range of causes. Some believe it is due to the proximity of wild animals to humans and human–animal conflicts (Chauhan et al., 2020). Earlier outbreaks had been associated with consumption of infected 'bushmeat' from apes, chimpanzees or gorillas, which are important in the Congolese diet and are linked to traditional 'coming of age' customs (Mombouli, 2004). One method to avoid infection is through the provision of alternative foods from other areas; however, communities tend to resist new foods that are not consistent with their cultural practices and beliefs (Mombouli, 2004). Human-to-human contact is also a key means of transmission, due to the mobility of people in the affected areas, high population density and cultural practices associated with traditional burial rituals such as spending time with, and washing, the bodies of deceased Ebola patients, a practice that remains highly infectious (Coltart et al., 2017).

Fear had been a characteristic of DRC community responses in earlier outbreaks, and community members had perceived Ebola as being a result of 'witchcraft' by healthcare workers. Surviving families of the infected and/or deceased remained stigmatised long after the outbreak was over (Mombouli, 2004). Fear and mistrust were key impediments to the effectiveness of the response to the 10th outbreak (MSF, 2020b), which occurred in an active conflict zone (MSF, 2020a). Violence between armed groups sometimes prevented outbreak-response activities. Longstanding community distrust of the national authorities, and the presence of security personnel at the Ebola treatment centres, caused violent attacks on the centres and response personnel, even resulting in the killing of medical workers and journalists associated with the Ebola response (MSF, 2020a). Treatment centres were closed and the violence prevented community members from seeking help, which in turn increased the likelihood of transmission (MSF, 2020a).

Community members also resented the focus on Ebola, when preventable diseases such as malaria and measles were the main causes of death in the area, along with the humanitarian needs of people displaced from their homes due to the long-term regional conflicts (MSF, 2020b). The initial response to the Ebola outbreak ignored these other community needs, which led to further distrust and resentment (MSF, 2020b).

Lessons learned

Engaging with the local communities and responding appropriately to their health-seeking behaviours was crucial to the development of trust and the eventual

(cont.)

(cont.)

containment of the outbreak. Médecins Sans Frontières began to work with local hospitals and healthcare centres across the region, including traditional healers (MSF, 2020a), to deliver more integrated health services that were in line with community needs, including a vaccination campaign to fight measles (MSF, 2020b). Trust was further built through recognising and treating Ebola patients, not as a biological threat, but as people with the right to make choices based on informed consent (MSF, 2020b). Health promotion activities were conducted with members of the community, healthcare providers and traditional healers to raise awareness of how to minimise transmission of, and treat, Ebola (MSF, 2020a).

The success and translation of these lessons to other scenarios are likely already being tested. On 1 June 2020, the DRC Ministry of Health declared the 11th Ebola outbreak in the Equateur province in the north-west of the country, just weeks before the 10th outbreak had been officially declared over (MSF, 2020c).

QUESTIONS

1. Based on the information about the transmission of Ebola described in this case study, discuss how a One Health response could contribute to Ebola management. Conduct desktop research to source additional resources to inform your answer.

2. The health needs of the people of DRC are influenced by their environmental, social and political contexts. In 2020, they faced all of their 'usual' health challenges, along with another outbreak of Ebola and the COVID-19 pandemic. Imagine you have just arrived in one of the local communities – how would you decide which health issues to address first? Justify your answer.

A holistic view of health and health promotion

As Case study 9.1 shows, vulnerable communities are those most likely to bear the brunt of the negative consequences of zoonotic diseases. Cleaveland and colleagues (2017) argue that using One Health interventions to address these diseases may help to build relationships – and trust – within and between communities, and may create more equitable benefits than treating only human cases. They argue that this is especially the case in low-income and middle-income countries. Many zoonotic diseases are treatable; however, the cost or accessibility of the treatment may create barriers for resource-poor and disadvantaged communities, so a clinical approach to treatment is inherently limited (Cleaveland et al., 2017). The One Health approach, which can reduce the effects and extent of the infection in all potential sources, can benefit everyone, irrespective of their socio-economic status.

It is not only in zoonotic diseases that disadvantaged communities bear the greater immediate burden of negative health outcomes. Food insecurity due to increased and prolonged drought, diseases such as malaria and dengue extending their range, and extreme weather events affecting housing, security and water supply, are all realities for many developing countries attributed to climate change. The Global Climate

Risk Index shows that poorer developing countries are likely to experience greater loss of life and personal hardship from extreme weather events, exacerbated by the changing climate, than richer countries (Eckstein et al., 2019). Of the top 10 most affected between 1999 and 2018, seven are low or lower-middle income developing countries (Eckstein et al., 2019). There are also inequalities within these disadvantaged communities. A study conducted in the developing Pacific Islands of Kiribati, Samoa and Tonga showed how **energy poverty** could contribute to the disproportionate effect on children's health outcomes (Teariki et al., 2020). The use of solid fuels for daily cooking, such as gas or wood, can contribute to indoor air pollution and can lead to respiratory illness. Transitioning to renewable energy is one means to address many of the social, environmental and economic issues faced by Pacific Islands (Teariki et al., 2020). Globally, renewable energy is vital for children's health and wellbeing, with implications for education, security and the provision of water, transportation and health services (UNICEF, 2015). Again, what is good for the environment is also good for people's health.

Energy poverty – limited to no access to regular, safe and clean energy supply; often results in the use of polluting fuel sources and the need to spend large amounts of time collecting these fuel sources (a task typically done by women and girls, often placing their physical safety at risk and preventing engagement in employment and education)

Health in All Policies

The contribution of all sectors to health is recognised in the Health in All Policies (HiAP) framework. HiAP addresses the determinants of health by working across all areas of government to ensure that policies and services support good health for all. South Australia was one of the global early adopters of HiAP in 2007, and in 2010 hosted an international conference, which gave rise to the 'Adelaide Statement on Health in All Policies'. The statement calls for a 'new social contract between all sectors to advance human development, sustainability and equity, as well as to improve health outcomes' (WHO & Government of South Australia, 2010, p. 1). This statement was then used in subsequent World Conferences (as described in Chapter 1) and was particularly influential in the eighth global conference, held in Finland in 2013. The Helsinki Statement developed during that conference describes HiAP as:

> … an approach to public policies across sectors that systematically takes into account the health implications of decisions, seeks synergies, and avoids harmful health impacts in order to improve population health and health equity. It improves accountability of policymakers for health impacts at all levels of policy-making. It includes an emphasis on the consequences of public policies on health systems, determinants of health and well-being (WHO, 2013, p. 1).

Three years later, the Shanghai Declaration of 2016 positioned health promotion at the centre of the 17 Sustainable Development Goals (SDGs – see Chapter 1). The SDGs are interconnected and require actions at local, national and global levels across all sectors. This can only be achieved through collaboration and partnership, as indicated by the 17th SDG, both of which are also key to the HiAP approach. In 2017, 150 HiAP practitioners and experts gathered in South Australia and developed the 'Second Adelaide Statement', which called for HiAP to be used as a strategy to achieve the SDGs (WHO & Government of South Australia, 2017). Despite a growing body of literature detailing how to implement HiAP and evaluations of what works, adoption of HiAP is uneven and hindered by overarching political and organisational desires for 'quick-wins, short-term gains and fast-acting processes', which can make the time required for the systemic change HiAP offers seem 'onerous' (Government of South Australia & Global Network for Health in All Policies, 2019, p. 12).

For both One Health and HiAP, there are a range of areas in which health promotion can raise awareness and advocate for policies and practices that will support positive health outcomes for all societies. In practice, this may be easier said than done as it will require change, some of it systemic. The standard of living that many either enjoy or aspire to is driven by our socio-economic systems. These systems have enabled the development of better health – for some – but also an increased demand for material wellbeing, which in turn creates unsustainable demand on our natural resources (Hancock, 2015). To change this, we need to the change the system, and that means altering peoples' values. As previous chapters in this text have discussed, this is difficult to do. While there is evidence of progress towards increased engagement with complex issues, greater efforts are required for health promotion to fully engage in an ecosystem approach (Patrick & Kingsley, 2016).

This chapter has focused on environmental aspects pertaining to human health, and in many ways climate change is one of the greatest challenges to health we will face into the future. For some members of the community – such as farmers – the impacts of climate change, for example, prolonged drought, have already caused or have compounded health problems such as those related to mental health (see Case study 9.2). The *Lancet* is an international journal that publishes annual reports on the health profiles of nations under the effects of climate change (see Further Reading), which outline the risks in great detail. While the annual reports outline the health risks due to climate change and how countries are working globally to meet these challenges, of particular relevance to this text is section five, which tracks public and political engagement in the media, government, corporate sector and individuals. The 2019 review concluded that while progress had been made in engagement levels over the previous decade, climate change is not being presented consistently as connected to human health (Watts et al., 2019). They are largely seen as separate issues with different concerns, and when links between the two are made it is from the health perspective, rather climate change (Watts et al., 2019). To mobilise action on public health and climate change, the two need to be presented as interrelated. We cannot have good public health without a healthy climate.

CASE STUDY 9.2 Mental health in remote and rural farming communities

Daniel Craig

In Australia, rates of suicide and mental illness are higher in rural and remote communities; these rates have been attributed to limited access to mental health services (Arnautovska et al., 2016). The suicide rate for Australian male farmers is about double that of the general male population, with the number being 32.2 compared to 16.6 per 10 000 (Kunde et al., 2017).

Centre for Work Health and Safety and Farmer Mental Health

In 2018, the Centre for Work Health and Safety partnered with a psychological service to offer mental health services on a 24/7 basis, with professionally qualified staff available via SMS, the Facebook Messenger app, WhatsApp, Twitter and a website chat facility. This partnership was designed to support the mental health of people in regional New South Wales and to confirm the efficacy of text-based counselling. A text-based counselling service is considered the most discreet form of online counselling, as it can be provided in complete silence and may not be affected by the presence of other people.

The approach to promotion of this service has been a mix of traditional media, social media and some innovative promotional techniques. The Centre used its state government connection to include Ministerial media releases, radio interviews on the ABC and simple messaging about the service in *Farmer Direct*, a monthly publication that is distributed to 600 000 farmers across Australia. This messaging used direct quotes from farmers who had used the service. In addition, the Centre identified influencers to create a sponsored social media campaign encouraging partners, families, friends and farming colleagues to use the service to help support their farmers. This targeted promotion was designed after consultation with the farming community identified that farmers were more likely to talk about being worried about their neighbours' mental health than discussing being worried about their own.

To complement the more common promotional pathways, a series of beer coasters was designed and distributed to pubs across Australia, asking the farmer a question ('Are you ok?', 'What's troubling you?' or 'Is your mate struggling?') and providing the number to SMS for help. Telecommunication provider Optus was also engaged to put the offering of free mental health support across the bottom of phone bills that were registered to rural and remote postcodes.

Evaluation and conclusion

There are many factors that can influence a farmer's pathway to suicide, so it is not possible to conclude that this health initiative has affected suicide rates. However, an increase in the use of the service was seen when each promotional tool was used. Across the two years of the partnership, the program saw the user rate rise from 37 to over 200 farmers per month.

QUESTIONS

1. What health promotion theory and/or model do you think applies to this service? Justify your answer.
2. During the text counselling session, some farmers identified feelings of isolation and desolation. If you were working with the Centre on a follow-up campaign, how would you change the messaging to address this issue?
3. In 2019, the Australian Bureau of Statistics estimated that there were 3.3 million people employed in the agricultural sector. What other techniques could be used to reach more people?

ELSEWHERE IN THE WORLD

Heads Up – Heads Together and the FA

In a bid to further the message of destigmatising conversations about mental health, Heads Together (www.headstogether.org.uk/fa-campaign-launch), a mental health initiative in the United Kingdom, has partnered with the Football Association (FA). Throughout the 2019–20 season, fans watching football saw the campaign's messages to reduce suicide rates and increase awareness of mental health.

The Power of Okay – See Me

See Me is a mental health program in Scotland that aims to reduce the stigma associated with mental health in the workplace. It supports employers to create a safe space in which their employees can be honest about their mental health struggles. Similar to Australia's 'RUOK Day', this campaign centres on a poem entitled 'The Power of Okay' and encourages employers and employees to ask their colleagues 'Are you Okay?" (https://www.seemescotland.org/resources/campaign-resources/power-of-okay/).

LEARNING ACTIVITY 9.1

In Australia, the state of South Australia has been using the HiAP framework since 2007. Search online for examples of the HiAP framework being adopted in a country of your choice, or use South Australia as your example, and then consider these questions:

1. Describe how the HiAP framework was used in your chosen country, outlining the audience, the health issue it was addressing, the policy areas involved and evidence of its success (if available).
2. Based on your answer to question 1, what health promotion and communication activities do you think were used and through which communication channels? Are there any areas, or audiences, where you think they could have been used but were not?

EXTENSION QUESTION

During the early phase of the COVID-19 pandemic in Australia, political representatives from each state and territory worked collaboratively across portfolios and with a whole-of-government approach to make decisions about how best to protect community health. Describe how this could be considered as an adoption of a HiAP framework and discuss whether it should be continued following the pandemic across the country, and why.

Challenges for health and communication

This section explores some of the health challenges we will face into the future and how we can ensure our communication is appropriate to both the challenge and the diverse audiences affected. As we began to discuss at the end of the previous section in this chapter, change can be difficult. But as you are no doubt seeing in the news and in the world around you every day, change is necessary – especially to ensure the health and wellbeing of our communities.

What the present can tell us about the future

This chapter has discussed an ecosystem approach to health, which has many parallels with traditional Indigenous knowledge. Land and sea management by Indigenous people – caring for Country – is well established as an effective means of contributing to conservation efforts and has received regular investment from state and federal governments in Australia since the 1980s (Pert et al., 2020). Aboriginal and Torres Strait Islander peoples view a strong connection to Country, their traditional lands, as a core facet of health and wellbeing (Kingsley et al., 2013). This is reflected by the explicit connection between culture and Country at the centre of the National Aboriginal and Torres Strait Islander Health Plan 2013–2023 (Department of Health, 2013). However, due to a 'siloed' governmental approach, the relationship between people and Country is rarely considered or incorporated into policies and programs (Schultz & Cairney, 2017). The very practice of caring for Country, aside from yielding environmental or economic benefits, can also have a positive effect on the health of Indigenous people (Pert et al., 2020; Schultz & Cairney, 2017). Kingsley and colleagues (2013) argue that this connection with Country could improve the capacity of humanity to deal with environmental destruction. Based on recent events, perhaps it is time for approaches to health, and thus health promotion, to more fully embrace an Indigenous perspective of health and wellbeing.

In 2019 and early 2020, Australia suffered some of the most catastrophic bushfires on record, followed by heavy rain and flooding in some of the fire-affected areas which choked waterways and river systems with bushfire ash. Following this, the country joined the rest of the world in grappling with the COVID-19 pandemic. While 2020 is widely considered a horror year, a letter to all Australians written by the Commission for the Human Future (2020) warned that this was just the beginning and that as humans we are woefully underprepared to face the important risks to our survival. The letter states that the warnings have existed for some time, even decades, but people – in businesses, governments and societies around the world – have ignored them. Others have prioritised political and financial gain, and have used denial and misinformation to hide the truth, erode trust and confuse. This is the communication context for addressing future health issues, some of which are starting to emerge.

COVID-19 as a case study

In many ways, the COVID-19 pandemic provides the ideal case study of health promotion and communication, and the effects that different communication approaches can yield. Different nations approached the problem in different ways, which reflected the manner in which values, ideologies and political systems can influence health. This illustrates why the deficit model does not work: by showing how providing people with information – such as 'isolate if unwell' and 'maintain social distancing' – is not enough to make everyone change their behaviours. Many will, but there will be some who are not willing to adopt new behaviours because they see this as violating what they consider their personal rights. It also highlighted how the outcomes of some of these communication approaches disproportionately and negatively affected the more vulnerable among us. For example, the Indian government gave citizens only a few hours' notice before the lockdown started, causing migrant workers across the country, desperate to return to their homes, to gather in defiance of social-distancing rules at train stations, or left stranded without anywhere to live, and with no income or support (Bhattacharyya, 2020). After two months of being stranded, migrant workers, many of whom were now infected with COVID-19, were allowed to return home and consequently this led to the disease being spread further around the country (Bhattacharyya, 2020). If the migrant workers had been provided with shelter, food and a small income for those few months, there likely would have been fewer migrant workers trying to get home, and the process might have been more manageable and may have limited the spread of the disease.

The initial response to COVID-19 in Australia seemed to work well, with mandatory social-distancing restrictions implemented around the country assisting to 'flatten the curve'. A survey conducted five weeks after the start of lockdown, however, showed that almost half of the 1500 respondents did not comply with the rules, and instead were socialising, leaving the house and travelling for leisure (Murphy et al., 2020). A second wave of infection after the relaxation of restrictions led to the introduction of fines to deter people from doing things that help COVID-19 to spread. In principle, this seemed sensible and worked for some locations, but regulations to enforce compliance may not be 100 per cent effective. Murphy and colleagues (2020) suggest that while some members of the population feel a sense of obligation to obey government rules, for others invoking our moral responsibility to act to protect others may be more effective. In other words, social norms may be more influential than perceptions of personal risk – at least in terms of COVID-19. Then, there is the simple fact that people get 'message fatigue' – a feeling of exhaustion from hearing the same messages for prolonged periods (Kim and So, 2018). Message fatigue is a problem with health campaigns, since audiences tend to either disengage from the message altogether or to exhibit active resistance, known as 'reactance' (Kim & So, 2018; Figure 9.1). Reactance can cause people to respond angrily or negatively, especially in response to health messaging that they consider limiting or removing personal freedoms (Reynolds-Tylus, 2019). During the COVID-19 pandemic, this reactance can be seen in protests against lockdowns and wearing masks.

COVID-19 communications

In times of crisis, authorities need to get information out to people as quickly as possible. Mass media is particularly useful for doing this; however it, and social media, will just as readily distribute misinformation, often despite best intentions. The global research effort to identify treatments and vaccines saw an unprecedented amount of research being published rapidly (Lee & Lin, 2020). Yet, some of the studies published that attracted

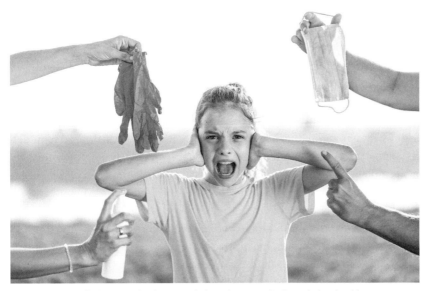

Figure 9.1   Message fatigue can lead to people ignoring or actively resisting health messages

government and media attention, such as a preliminary study proposing the use of hydroxychloroquine as a treatment for COVID-19, were later found to be inconclusive or retracted altogether (Lee & Lin, 2020). However, sometimes evidence that is later shown to be inconclusive or incorrect persists in the public sphere, in what the WHO referred to as an 'infodemic', 'an over-abundance of information – some accurate and some not – that makes it hard for people to find trustworthy sources and reliable guidance' (WHO, 2020, p. 2). Numerous studies have looked at media and social media coverage of COVID-19 and the accuracy of the information provided. Over one-quarter of the most-popular YouTube videos contained misleading information – and these continue to be seen by millions of viewers globally (Li et al., 2020). The rapid spread of misinformation across all media sources was helped along by the actions of many politicians, celebrities and influencers – both online and offline (Nguyen & Catalan-Matamoros, 2020). Trusted and/or high-profile messengers (noting that they may not necessarily be one and the same) are influential, whether their information is accurate or not.

Repetition makes acceptance of plausible misinformation more likely; even seeing misinformation once makes it more likely that the misinformation will be perceived as accurate (Pennycook et al., 2018). The 'big' players in social media – Twitter, YouTube, Facebook and WhatsApp – have begun to incorporate fact-checking and have been attempting to limit the sharing of misinformation through labelling and removal of posts, and by making accurate information prominent and easily accessible (Nguyen & Catalan-Matamoros, 2020). Yet, there are limits in what they can do when faced with a landscape of millions of users actively communicating and sharing every hour. Studies of 'fake news' have found that explicitly stating that something is disputed by independent fact-checkers may have increased scepticism in the general community, but this scepticism can be entirely cancelled out by repetition (Pennycook et al., 2018). Attempting to correct misinformation through scientific facts and evidence can also cause some people to more strongly hold on to their beliefs about the accuracy of the misinformation (Betsch & Sachse, 2013), a phenomenon known as the 'backfire effect' (introduced in Chapter 5).

How does health promotion work within that space? Correcting the misinformation using facts may backfire, and if you repeat the misinformation during the process of explaining why it is wrong then you are adding to its cumulative exposure, which in turn is likely to increase perceptions of accuracy. It is important to note here that what we do know about how information is being received and spread is largely derived from studies in the global north (Vraga et al., 2020). Each country and culture is different, will use different information sources and will have different relationships with media, government and public health authorities. More work is needed to understand how this operates in diverse contexts. Until such work becomes available, a general approach could be to acknowledge that there will always be a group of people who will never believe or accept a message, and that there will be those who always will. The vast majority will likely be trying to figure out what is 'right' and who to believe, and this is where health promotion and effective communication can have the strongest influence. As a health promoter, the best way to approach any communication is to be clear about who your target audience is and what you want to achieve. Knowing the answers to those two questions helps you plan every other aspect, to develop the most appropriate strategy. While there are some common needs across audiences, some issues are unique to, or disproportionately affect, specific audiences.

Meeting the needs of a diverse society

Inequalities in health

The leading causes of death worldwide have been largely unchanged over the past 20 years. Table 9.1 shows a comparison of leading causes of death by national income of countries according to the World Bank's classification of economies. Although there are similarities in each category of income, you will notice that in the low-income countries many of the leading causes of death are preventable through the provision of adequate

Table 9.1   Comparison of top 20 leading causes of death, compared by World Bank income group

Ranking	Low income	Lower-middle income	Upper-middle income	High income
1	Lower respiratory infections	Ischaemic heart disease	Ischaemic heart disease	Ischaemic heart disease
2	Diarrhoeal diseases	Stroke	Stroke	Stroke
3	Ischaemic heart disease	Lower respiratory infections	Chronic obstructive pulmonary disease	Alzheimer's disease and other dementias
4	HIV/AIDS	Chronic obstructive pulmonary disease	Trachea, bronchus, lung cancers	Trachea, bronchus, lung cancers

Table 9.1 (cont.)

Ranking	Low income	Lower-middle income	Upper-middle income	High income
5	Stroke	Tuberculosis	Alzheimer's disease and other dementias	Chronic obstructive pulmonary disease
6	Malaria	Diarrhoeal diseases	Lower respiratory infections	Lower respiratory infections
7	Tuberculosis	Diabetes mellitus	Diabetes mellitus	Colon and rectum cancers
8	Pre-term birth complications	Pre-term birth complications	Road injury	Diabetes mellitus
9	Birth asphyxia and birth trauma	Cirrhosis of the liver	Liver cancer	Kidney diseases
10	Road injury	Road injury	Stomach cancer	Breast cancer
11	Protein-energy malnutrition	Kidney diseases	Hypertensive heart disease	Pancreatic cancer
12	Neonatal sepsis and infections	HIV/AIDS	Kidney diseases	Self-harm
13	Meningitis	Birth asphyxia and birth trauma	Cirrhosis of the liver	Cirrhosis of the liver
14	Congenital anomalies	Alzheimer's disease and other dementias	Colon and rectum cancers	Stomach cancer
15	Chronic obstructive pulmonary disease	Self-harm	Self-harm	Prostate cancer
16	Maternal conditions	Falls	Oesophageal cancer	Hypertensive heart disease
17	Diabetes mellitus	Congenital anomalies	HIV/AIDS	Lymphomas, multiple myeloma
18	Cirrhosis of the liver	Asthma	Interpersonal violence	Liver cancer
19	Interpersonal violence	Hypertensive heart disease	Falls	Falls
20	Alzheimer's disease and other dementias	Neonatal sepsis and infections	Cardiomyopathy, myocarditis, endocarditis	Parkinson's disease

Source: Adapted from WHO (2018).

health services. As the income of countries increases, the leading causes of death are largely non-communicable, with many influenced by lifestyle factors such as inadequate diet and exercise, and consumption of tobacco products and alcohol. The upper-middle and high-income countries also indicate the consequences of ageing populations, with conditions such as Alzheimer's disease and other dementias appearing in the top three causes of death. In lower-income countries, many of the causes of death are more likely to affect women and children. The factors that contribute to the leading causes of death across all income groups 'require a multisectoral approach that addresses the underlying causes of gender and socioeconomic inequalities' (WHO, 2019, p. 5).

As Table 9.1 shows, socio-economic status makes a difference to health outcomes. This is the case within communities as well. Within Australia, people in the lowest socio-economic group are more than twice as likely to smoke, acquire type 2 diabetes, avoid seeking dental treatment or medication due to cost and to die from potentially avoidable causes (AIHW, 2018). Despite gains made in health outcomes (as discussed in Chapter 1), Aboriginal and Torres Strait Islander peoples are:

- 1.9 times more likely to be born with a low birthweight
- 2.9 times more likely to have ear infections or hearing problems in childhood
- 2.7 times more likely to smoke or experience high to very high levels of psychological distress
- over twice as likely to die before the age of five
- 1.7 times more likely to have a long-term health condition or disability (AIHW, 2018).

In contrast, Aboriginal and Torres Strait Islander people who are employed and live in higher socio-economic areas are more likely to report excellent health (AIHW, 2018). These disparities exist because of social determinants (as described in Chapter 1), health risk factors (such as rates of smoking and obesity) and difficulty in accessing affordable health services (AIHW, 2018). Although poverty is a contributing factor to disadvantage, it is not the only one. Disadvantage can be experienced in other ways, such as **deprivation**, capability (see following paragraph) and social exclusion (McLachlan et al., 2013).

Deprivation – the lack of material benefits considered essential to daily living

Deprivation can be created by the prevention or absence in satisfaction of basic needs such as shelter, food and clothing, through to the ability to afford things that may not be essential for survival but add to quality of life, such as access to a telephone, quality housing in a safe area and the ability to engage in social networks for recreational purposes (McLachlan et al., 2013). It is about 'impoverished lives', not just 'depleted wallets' (Productivity Commission, 2018, p. 107). 'Capability' refers to the opportunities an individual has, and the freedom they have to pursue those opportunities (Sen, 2009). Social exclusion does not have a clear or consistently agreed upon definition (McLachlan et al., 2013), but it largely pertains to a person's ability to learn, work, engage with others and services, and to influence decisions that affect them (Australian Social Inclusion Board, 2012). In other words, people's ability to 'fully participate in the ordinary activities of a community' (Productivity Commission, 2018, p. 107). Their ability to participate can be influenced by the factors described in Figure 9.2, many of which relate to deprivation and capability. It is possible to experience deprivation and not poverty, or vice versa (Productivity Commission, 2018), and it is also possible to experience multiple sources of deprivation at the same time. Within Australia, the groups who are most likely to experience deprivation from multiple sources are children, single parents, Indigenous Australians, people who are unemployed and people living with a disability (Productivity Commission, 2018).

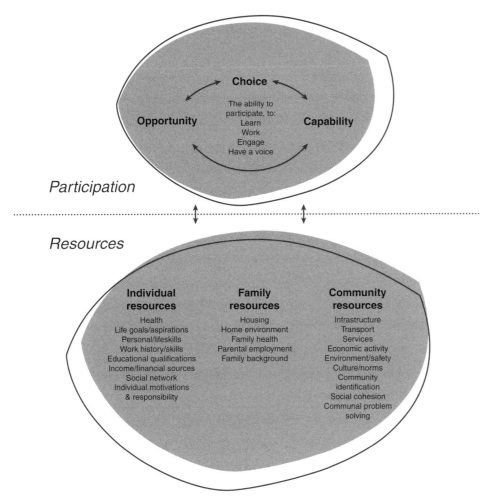

Participation

Resources

Figure 9.2   Social inclusion conceptual framework showing interaction between participation and resources

Source: Australian Social Inclusion Board (2012, p. 13).

How effective communication can foster inclusion

The previous section introduced social exclusion as a source of disadvantage, which this section briefly explores in further detail. Diversity is an important part of society, yet it is not always welcomed or supported in a way that enables the social inclusion described above. It is imperative to ensure that health promotion – and the health sector – is inclusive in every sense. This can range from the obvious, such as providing information in languages other than English, but it may also require deeper engagement with members of the community who might be more vulnerable to multiple forms of disadvantage. Throughout this text, we have spoken about the importance of knowing your audience. Understanding their challenges, values, fears and perceptions are all integral to responding appropriately to their health needs (see Case study 9.3).

Feeling socially excluded can have adverse effects on mental, emotional and physical health. For example, one study found members of the transgender community in the United States may delay or avoid seeking health care due to discrimination (Jaffee et al., 2016). Transgender patients in India often have to deal with stigma and misinformation from medical professionals who have only been taught about the male/female binary and do not have the knowledge to treat transgender patients appropriately (Desai, 2019). Members of the transgender community in Australia report similar discrimination and misinformation, which in turn causes them to delay seeking medical care (Zwickl et al., 2019). The transgender community asks to be consulted, listened to and provided with the information that they need to help them increase control over their health and wellbeing (Zwickl et al., 2019). It is not unreasonable to assume that this reflects the desires of many of the diverse, **minoritised** and vulnerable groups within societies everywhere.

Communication is about listening, too. In order to know your audience, you need to genuinely listen to their needs and concerns. Think back to the Ebola case study (9.1): are you actually addressing the issue that *your audience* believes is most important? Are you responding in a way that does not compound their disadvantage? Listen and collaborate; include your audience in partnership where you can. They know their own needs and experiences best and have a vested interest in ensuring that they can access the resources and services they need. This is where effective communication within health promotion can help to create a supportive, inclusive environment for everyone.

Minoritised – a social constructionist approach to understanding that people are actively diminished by others rather than naturally existing as a minority, as the terms 'racial minority' and 'ethnic minority' imply (Gunaratnum, 2003)

CASE STUDY 9.3 LGBTIQ+ people and crisis-support services

Andrea Waling

Research has long established that lesbian (L), gay (G), bisexual (B), transgender and gender diverse (T), queer (Q), and Plus (+ additional identities) people have higher rates of self-harm and suicidal ideation, and poorer mental health than the general population (National LGBTI Health Alliance, 2016). These high rates of mental health distress are often attributed to the systemic, institutionalised and everyday experiences of discrimination, harassment and violence experienced by LGBTQ+ people (Skerrett et al., 2017). Additionally, research has also noted difficulties in accessing appropriate healthcare services that are culturally sensitive towards, and inclusive of, LGBTIQ+ people. Research has noted that LGBTIQ+ people can experience discrimination, poor or inadequate treatment and hostility in accessing health and social services (Kilicaslan & Petrakis, 2019). For LGBTIQ+ people, this might include denial of partners as next of kin, assumptions of heterosexual relationships and experiences of homophobia and biphobia (Kilicaslan & Petrakis, 2019). For trans and gender diverse people, this can be a form of 'misgendering' (purposeful use of the wrong pronoun or preferred name), or an indication of transphobia and lack of provider knowledge about the unique needs of trans and gender diverse people (Samuels et al., 2019; Stroumsa et al., 2019). This can result in people avoiding the use of health services (Jaffee et al.,

2016; Martos et al., 2018) despite needing them. This case study looks at LGBTQ+ experiences of accessing crisis-support helplines in Australia.

Crisis-support helplines provide a form of crisis support that is community led (Pirkis et al., 2015). Often it is provided in the form of a phone line, but more recently has become available as an SMS or webchat service; these services are usually free or low cost, offer confidentiality and can be the first service someone uses when experiencing mental or personal distress (Machlin et al., 2017). Such services can support people experiencing a mental health or personal crisis, as well as link individuals to long-term mental health support services or emergency services (Hunt et al., 2018). Crisis can be an experience of mental health distress, such as depression, anxiety or a complex mental health disorder such as borderline personality disorder, as well as personal experiences of distress, such as family or relationship breakdown, intimate partner and family violence, loss of income or employment, and housing insecurity, among many others (Waling et al., 2019).

LGBTQ+ experiences of crisis support

Despite evidence that LGBTQ+ people have higher rates of mental health distress than cisgender (people whose gender identity matches their sex assigned at birth) and heterosexual populations, research exploring LGBTQ+ experiences of crisis-support helplines in Australia has found that over 71 per cent of LGBTQ+ people did not use a crisis-support helpline during their most recent personal or mental health crisis (Waling et al., 2019). Reasons cited included concerns about experiencing discrimination and not wanting to put their mental health at further risk; uncertainty about whether a service was LGBTQ+ inclusive; a lack of awareness about what was available to them in terms of support; not wanting to be a burden to a service; and a number of barriers including to physical access, technology and financial barriers in using crisis-support helplines (Waling et al., 2019). Participants sought support elsewhere, including from general practitioners, counsellors, friends, family and self-coping strategies including mindfulness, substance misuse and self-harm (Waling et al., 2019).

Understanding why LGBTQ+ people might not engage a crisis-support helpline is important in meeting the unique support needs of this community. The findings from this research noted that the perception of discrimination, rather than actual experience, prevented LGBTQ+ people from seeking the help they needed, and that this perception was based on previous experiences with health services (Waling et al., 2019). Understanding this can help support crisis-helplines to engage in training in LGBTQ+ cultural sensitivity and inclusive practices, and to engage in promotion and raising awareness that their services are LGBTQ+ friendly. Additionally, understanding that barriers to accessing support, such as feeling like a burden or experiencing physical access, technological or financial barriers can also support crisis-helpline services to make changes so they might better support the community.

QUESTIONS

1. Why is it important that we think about access to health services and the experiences of those who are marginalised?

2. How can we encourage people to seek support for mental health or personal distress?

ELSEWHERE IN THE WORLD

The Trevor Project

The Trevor Project (www.thetrevorproject.org) is a leading crisis-support service for LGBTIQ+ communities in the United States. It offers crisis interventions, suicide-prevention training and resources, as well as community resources to enable awareness, education and advocacy.

LGBT Foundation

The LGBT Foundation (http://lgbt.foundation/) provides support line for LGBT people in the United Kingdom. It also offers a wide range of activities and services, including a sexual health program, a helpline (telephone and email), support groups, training and policy campaigning.

LEARNING ACTIVITY 9.2

Identify a vulnerable and/or underserved group within your city, country or region. Based on what you have learned in this chapter, complete the following questions.

1. Identify the likely health issues and needs of the group you have selected and discuss whether 'mainstream' health services in the chosen location are adequate to address those needs. Justify your conclusions with examples.
2. Based on your research and discussion in question 1, are there any specific health promotion activities you would recommend to better serve that group? If so, what would they be? Identify the:
   - topic/s
   - communication channels
   - potential partner organisation/s.

Summary

This chapter has explored the interrelationships between human and environmental health and how multi-sectoral approaches, such as One Health and HiAP, are leading the way. Yet, these approaches are not being widely adopted around the world. Health promotion can contribute to these approaches through a variety of sectors, policy areas and actions, yet to date there is little evidence of health promotion as a whole (practitioners and programs) engaging in these complex issues to its full potential. More can be done, especially to address some of the health challenges we will face into the futrue, some of which, like climate change and pandemics, are starting to show their consequences already. The role of effective communication is crucial to creating the impetus for needed change, at all levels of society. However, communication approaches must not reinforce the spread of misinformation that could hinder the desired action, or exacerbate the negative effects felt by vulnerable communities.

People's health outcomes may be determined purely by circumstances they do not and cannot control. Those who have the least often fare the worst, and those inequalities can persist across the life span. There are also people within otherwise affluent societies who experience disadvantage due to misinformation or ignorance. Many of the risks to health we face are highly complex and increasingly urgent. Much of what we do know about how people respond to communication within this context is from a very narrow perspective, and more needs to be done. Yet, a simple first step to navigating a seemingly difficult communication environment begins with knowing the audience: listen to them and incorporate their insights and knowledge into the development of health promotion activities and resources. It's a simple but vital first step.

REVISION QUESTIONS

1. Describe the relationship between environmental and human health.
2. How does HiAP relate to health promotion?
3. What are some of the communication challenges when trying to correct misinformation?
4. What factors contribute to people experiencing disadvantage?

FURTHER READING

Lucashenko, M. (2020). It's no accident that Blak Australia has survived the pandemic so well. Survival is what we do. In S. Cunningham (ed.) *Fire, Flood and Plague – essays about 2020*. Penguin Random House.

Watts, N., Amann, M., Arnell, N., Ayeb-Karlsson, S., Belesova, K., Boykoff, M. … Montgomery, H. (2019). The 2019 report of the *Lancet* Countdown on health and climate change: Ensuring that the health of a child born today is not defined by a changing climate, *The Lancet*, 394(10211), 1836–78.

World Health Organization (WHO). (2013). *Health in All Policies: Framework for Country Action*. Finland: WHO and Ministry of Social Affairs and Health.

REFERENCES

Arnautovska, U., McPhedran, S., Kelly, B., Reddy, P. & De Leo, D. (2016). Geographic variation in suicide rates in Australian farmers: Why is the problem more frequent in Queensland than in New South Wales? *Death Studies*, 40(6), 367–72.

Australian Institute of Health and Welfare (AIHW) (2018). *Australia's Health 2018: In brief*. Cat. no. AUS 222. Canberra: AIHW.

Australian Social Inclusion Board (2012). *Social Inclusion in Australia: How Australia is faring* (2nd ed.). Canberra: Department of the Prime Minister and Cabinet.

Betsch, C. & Sachse, K. (2013). Debunking vaccination myths: Strong risk negations can increase perceived vaccination risks, *Health Psychology*, 32(2),146.

Bhattacharyya, I. (2020, 12 June). Why India's lockdown has been a spectacular failure, *The Wire*. Retrieved from: https://thewire.in/government/india-covid-19-lockdown-failure

Bunch, M.J., Morrison, K.E., Parkes, M.W. & Venema, H.D. (2011). Promoting health and well-being by managing for social–ecological resilience: the potential of integrating ecohealth and water resources management approaches, *Ecology and Society*, 16(1), 6.

Chauhan, R.P., Dessie, Z.G., Noreddin, A. & El Zowalaty, M.E. (2020). Systematic review of important viral diseases in Africa in light of the 'One Health' concept, *Pathogens*, 9(4), 301.

Cleaveland, S., Sharp, J., Abela-Ridder, B., Allan, K.J., Buza, J., Crump, J.A., Davis, A., Del Rio Vilas, V.J., de Glanville, W.A., Kazwala, R.R., Kibona, T., Lankester, F.J., Lugelo, A., Mmbaga, B.T., Rubach, M.P., Swai, E.S., Waldman, L., Haydon, D.T., Hampson, K. & Halliday, J. (2017). One Health contributions towards more effective and equitable approaches to health in low- and middle-income countries, *Philosophical transactions of the Royal Society of London. Series B, Biological sciences*, 372(1725), 20160168.

Coltart, C.E., Lindsey, B., Ghinai, I., Johnson, A.M. & Heymann, D.L. (2017). The Ebola outbreak, 2013–2016: Old lessons for new epidemics, *Philosophical transactions of the Royal Society of London. Series B, Biological sciences*, 372(1721), 20160297.

Commission for the Human Future (2020). *Letter to all Australians*. July 2020. Retrieved from: https://humanfuture.net

Department of Health (2013). *National Aboriginal and Torres Strait Islander Health Plan 2013–2023*. Canberra: Department of Health

Desai, R. (2019, 5 October). What a transgender-friendly health care system would look like, The Swaddle. Retrieved from: https://theswaddle.com/what-a-transgender-friendly-health-care-system-would-look-like/

Eckstein, D. Künzel, V., Schäfer, L. & Winges, M. (2019). Global Climate Risk Index 2020. Who suffers most from extreme weather events? Weather-related loss events in 2018 and 1999–2018 (Briefing Paper), German Watch (Website). Retrieved from: https://www.germanwatch.org/en/cri

Government of South Australia & Global Network for Health in All Policies (2019). *The Global Status Report on Health in All Policies*. Adelaide: Government of South Australia.

Gunaratnum, Y. (2003). *Researching 'Race' and Ethnicity: Methods, knowledge and power*. London: Sage.

Guy, J. & Gansukh, B. (2020, 15 July). Teenage boy dies from bubonic plague after eating marmot, *CNN*. Retrieved from: https://edition.cnn.com/2020/07/15/asia/mongolia-plague-death-scli-intl/index.html

Hancock, T. (2015). Population health promotion 2.0: An eco-social approach to public health in the anthropocene, *Canadian Journal of Public Health*, 106, e252–5.

Hunt, T., Wilson, C., Caputi, P., Wilson, I. & Woodward, A. (2018). Patterns of signs that telephone crisis support workers associate with suicide risk in telephone crisis line callers, *International Journal of Environmental Research and Public Health*, 15(2), 235.

Jaffee, K.D., Shires, D.A. & Stroumsa, D. (2016). Discrimination and delayed healthcare among transgender women and men: Implications for improving medical education and healthcare delivery, *Med Care*, 54(11), 1010–6.

Jefferson County Colorado Public Health (2020, 12 July). Squirrel with plague found in Jefferson County, *Public Health – News*. Retrieved from: https://www.jeffco.us/CivicAlerts.aspx?AID=1275

Kilicaslan, J. & Petrakis, M. (2019). Heteronormative models of health-care delivery: Investigating staff knowledge and confidence to meet the needs of LGBTIQ+ people, *Social Work in Health Care*, 58, 612–32.

Kim, S. & So, J. (2018). How message fatigue toward health messages leads to ineffective persuasive outcomes: Examining the mediating roles of reactance and inattention, *Journal of Health Communication*, 23(1), 109–16

Kingsley, J., Townsend, M., Henderson-Wilson, C. & Bolam, B. (2013). Developing an exploratory framework linking Australian Aboriginal peoples' connection to country and concepts of wellbeing, *International Journal of Environmental Research and Public Health*, 10(2), 678–98.

Kunde, L., Kõlves, K., Kelly, B., Reddy, P. & De Leo, D. (2017). Pathways to suicide in Australian farmers: A life chart analysis, *International Journal of Environmental Research and Public Health*, 14(4), 352.

Lee, A.Y.S. & Lin, M. (2020). Rapid publishing in the era of coronavirus disease 2019 (COVID-19), *Medical Journal of Australia*, 212(11), 535–35.e1.

Li, H.O., Bailey, A., Huynh, D. & Chan, J. (2020). YouTube as a source of information on COVID-19: A pandemic of misinformation? *BMJ Global Health*, 5(5), e002604.

Machlin, A., King, K., Spittal, M. & Pirkis, J. (2017). Preliminary evidence for the role of newsprint media in encouraging males to make contact with helplines. *International Journal of Mental Health Promotion*, 19(2), 85–103.

Mackenzie, J.S. & Jeggo, M. (2019). The One Health approach – Why is it so important? *Tropical Medicine and Infectious Disease*, 4(2), 88.

Martos, A.J., Wilson, P.A., Gordon, A.R., Lightfoot, M. & Meyer, I.H. (2018). 'Like finding a unicorn': Healthcare preferences among lesbian, gay, and bisexual people in the United States, *Social Science & Medicine*, 208, 126–33.

McLachlan, R., Gilfillan, G. & Gordon, J. (2013). *Deep and Persistent Disadvantage in Australia* (rev.ed.). Staff Working Paper. Canberra: Productivity Commission.

Médecins Sans Frontières (MSF) (2020a, 25 June). DRC's tenth Ebola outbreak, Médecins Sans Frontières (Website). Retrieved from: https://www.msf.org/drc-tenth-ebola-outbreak

———(2020b, 26 June). Six lessons learned as Ebola outbreak in northeastern DRC ends, Médecins Sans Frontières (Website). Retrieved from: https://www.msf.org/six-lessons-learned-drc-ebola-outbreak-ends

———(2020c, 26 June). Crisis update – June 2020, Médecins Sans Frontières (Website). Retrieved from: https://www.msf.org/drc-ebola-outbreak-crisis-update

Middleton, A., Woodward, A., Gunn, J., Bassilios, B. & Pirkis, J. (2017). How do frequent users of crisis helplines differ from other users regarding their reasons for calling? Results from a survey with callers to Lifeline, Australia's national crisis helpline service, *Health & Social Care in the Community*, 25(3), 1041–9.

Millennium Ecosystem Assessment (2005). Living Beyond Our Means: Natural Assets and Human Well-being. Retrieved from: https://www.millenniumassessment.org/documents/document.429.aspx.pdf

Mombouli, J.V. (2004). Ebola: Political and socioeconomic perspectives. Presented at One World, One Health: Building Interdisciplinary Bridges to Health in a Globablized World, Symposium, 29 September. New York.

Murphy, K., Wiliamson, H., Sargeant, E. & McCarthy, M. (2020). *Morals, Duty or Risk? Examining predictors of compliance with COVID-19 social distancing restrictions*

(Unpublished Manuscript). Griffith Criminology Institute, Griffith University. doi: 10.13140/RG.2.2.17636.60809

National LGBTI Health Alliance (2016). Snapshot of Mental Health and Suicide Prevention Statistics for LGBTI People (Website). Retrieved from: https://lgbtihealth.org.au/statistics/#.

Nguyen, A. & Catalan-Matamoros, D. (2020). Digital mis/disinformation and public engagement with health and science controversies: Fresh perspectives from Covid-19, *Media and Communication*, 8(2), 323–8.

Parkes, M.W., Poland, B., Allison, S. Cole, D.C., Culbert, I., Gislason, M.K., Hancock, T., Howard, C., Papadopoulos, A. & Waheed, F. (2020). Preparing for the future of public health: Ecological determinants of health and the call for an eco-social approach to public health education, *Canadian Journal of Public Health*, 111, 60–4, doi: https://doi.org/10.17269/s41997-019-00263-8.

Patrick, R. & Kingsley, J. (2016). Exploring Australian health promotion and environmental sustainability initiatives, *Health Promotion Journal of Australia*, 27, 36–42, doi:10.1071/HE15008.

Pennycook, G., Cannon, T.D. & Rand, D.G. (2018). Prior exposure increases perceived accuracy of fake news, *Journal of Experimental Psychology. General*, 147(12), 1865–80.

Pert, P.L., Hill, R., Robinson, C.J., Jarvis, D. & Davies, J. (2020). Is investment in Indigenous land and sea management going to the right places to provide multiple co-benefits? *Australasian Journal of Environmental Management*, 27(3), 249–74.

Pirkis, J., San Too, L., Spittal, M.J., Krysinska, K., Robinson, J. & Cheung, Y.T.D. (2015). Interventions to reduce suicides at suicide hotspots: A systematic review and meta-analysis, *Lancet Psychiatry*, 2(11), 994–1001.

Productivity Commission (2018). *Rising inequality? A stocktake of the evidence, (Research Paper)*. Canberra: Productivity Commission.

Reynolds-Tylus, T. (2019). Psychological reactance and persuasive health communication: A review of the literature, *Frontiers in Communication*, 4, 1–56.

Samuels, E.A., Tape, C., Garber, N., Bowman, S. & Choo, E.K. (2019). 'Sometimes you feel like the freak show': A qualitative assessment of emergency care experiences among transgender and gender-nonconforming patients, *Annual Emergency Medicine*, 71(2), 170–82.e1.

Schultz, R. & Cairney, S. (2017). Caring for country and the health of Aboriginal and Torres Strait Islander Australians, *Medical Journal of Australia*, 207(1), 8–10.

See Me (n.d.). Power of Okay. See Me: Glasgow. Retrieved from: https://www.seemescotland.org/contact/

Sen, A. (2009). *The Idea of Justice*. Cambridge, MA: The Belknap Press of Harvard University Press.

Skerrett, D.M., Kolves, K. & De Leo, D. (2017). Pathways to suicide in lesbian and gay populations in Australia: A life chart analysis, *Archives of Sexual Behaviour*, 46(5), 1481.

Stroumsa, D., Shires, D.A., Richardson, C.R., Jaffee, K.D. & Woodford, M.R. (2019). Transphobia rather than education predicts provider knowledge of transgender health care, *Medical Education*, 53(4), 398–407.

Teariki, M., Tiatia, R., O'Sullivan, K., Puloka, V., Singal, L., Shearer, I. & Howden-Chapman, P. (2020). Beyond home: Exploring energy poverty among youth in four diverse Pacific island states, *Energy Research & Social Science*, 70, 101638.

UNICEF (2015). *Why sustainable energy matters to children: The critical importance of sustainable energy for children and future generations*. Retrieved from https://www.unicef.org/environment/files/UNICEF_Sustainable_Energy_for_Children_2015.pdf

Vraga, E.K., Tully, M. & Bode, L. (2020). Empowering users to respond to misinformation about Covid-19, *Media and Communication (Lisboa)*, 8(2), 475–9.

Waling, A., Lim, G., Dhalla, S., Lyons, A. & Bourne, A. (2019). *Understanding LGBTI+ Lives in Crisis*. Bundoora & Canberra: Australian Research Centre in Sex, Health and Society, La Trobe University & Lifeline Australia. Monograph 112.

Watts, N., Amann, M., Arnell, N., Ayeb-Karlsson, S., Belesova, K., Boykoff, M. … Montgomery, H. (2019). The 2019 report of the Lancet Countdown on health and climate change: Ensuring that the health of a child born today is not defined by a changing climate, *The Lancet*, 394(10211), 1836–78.

Wildlife Conservation Society (2004). The Manhattan Principles on 'One World, One Health', One World, One Health: Building Interdisciplinary Bridges to Health in a Globalized World, Symposium, 29 September. New York. http://www.oneworldonehealth.org/sept2004/owoh_sept04.html

World Health Organization (WHO) (1986). *The Ottawa Charter for Health Promotion*. Geneva: WHO.

———(2013). *The Helsinki Statement on Health in All Policies*. Geneva: WHO.

———(2018). Global Health Estimates 2016: Deaths by Cause, Age, Sex, by Country and by Region, 2000–2016. Geneva: WHO.

———(2019). World health statistics overview 2019: Monitoring health for the SDGs, sustainable development goals. Geneva: WHO.

———(2020). Novel Coronavirus (2019-nCoV) situation report – 13, 2 February. Geneva: WHO.

WHO & Government of South Australia (2010). *Adelaide Statement on Health in All Policies: Moving towards a shared governance for health and well-being*, Report from the International Meeting on Health in All Policies, 13–15 April, Adelaide.

———(2017). *Second Adelaide Statement: Implementing the Sustainable Development Agenda through good governance for health and wellbeing: Building on the experience of Health in All Policies*, Outcome statement from the 2017 International Conference Health in All Policies: Progressing the Sustainable Development Goals, 30–31 March, South Australia.

Zwickl, S., Wong, A., Bretherton, I., Rainier, M., Chetcuti, D., Zajac, J.D. & Cheung, A.S. (2019). Health needs of trans and gender diverse adults in Australia: A qualitative analysis of a national community survey, *International Journal of Environmental Research and Public Health*, 16(24), 5088.

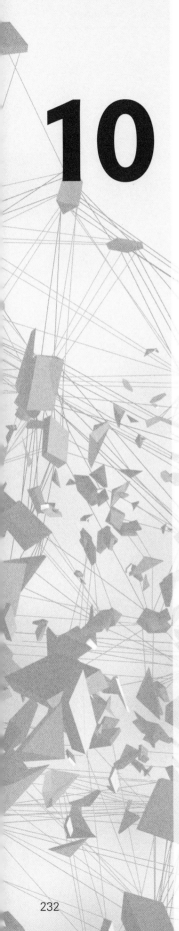

10

Global case studies

Merryn McKinnon

With contributions from Biaowen Huang, Josyula K. Lakshmi, Albert Lee, Lillibet Namakula, Patrick Segawa, Christina Severinsen, Chloe Simpson, Dennis Ernest Ssesanga, Mikihito Tanaka, Sudhir Raj Thout, Andy Towers and Tehzeeb Zulfiqar

LEARNING OBJECTIVES

At the completion of the chapter, you will be able to:

- Compare and contrast the health issues and health promotion activities of different countries.
- Identify how communication within health promotion activities can be modified to suit the cultural context.
- Discuss how health promotion theory can be applied in practice within diverse contexts.
- Analyse the role of communication in health promotion programs and discuss the influence of communication practices on program success.

Introduction

This chapter aims to provide an overview of the broad range of health promotion activities happening in the Asia Pacific and global south, using case studies with supporting questions for reflection and extension. These case studies draw on the content presented throughout this text and are intended to demonstrate how health promotion is implemented 'in real life'. It should be noted that many of these case studies refer to health promotion activities oriented to encourage behavioural change. Some of the case studies offered in this chapter encompass the environmental, political and cultural determinants of health as well, but it is important to remember that not all health promotion activities are focused on the individual, or only on changing behaviour. Health promotion can work in a variety of contexts and settings, and the examples provided are intended to help you put the content of this book into a real-world context. As you read these cases, reflect on the role of communication in each of these cases – who was the target audience? The case studies may not name the explicit theory, setting or evaluation approach used, but can you identify what they may have been? Think about whether there were other theories, settings or communication channels that could also have been used.

Some of the issues presented may be relevant in all countries, but responses will vary according to the social, cultural and economic context. The first two case studies illustrate this point through two different initiatives to address the harmful effects of smoking. One, from China, explores how people can be empowered to advocate for their own health and their right to a smoke-free environment. Although the case study from India has similar aims, it describes the challenges of implementing a tobacco-control program within a community whose major economic activity is tobacco production. The next four case studies illustrate the influence and effectiveness of community members as partners in health promotion. The first two, from Mongolia and Pakistan, illustrate how community members can be trusted sources of health information and support, especially for vulnerable populations. The Ugandan case study describes how involving the target audience in the design process of health promotion initiatives can ensure that the activities are effective, relevant and appropriate for their needs. The importance of a multi-sectoral approach to health and health promotion is shown through the Korean case study, which outlines the Healthy Cities concept and its application to improving health in urban areas. Key to Healthy Cities is the active engagement of the community in both the identification of health issues and the provision of resources that enable community members to support each other.

The final two case studies explore different ways of communicating with audiences about national issues that have serious implications, to enable them to respond and increase control of their own health. Catastrophic events on the scale of the Fukushima disaster may not be common to many countries but there is a lot that can be learned from those who have been faced with such emergency situations and their aftermath. Communication during a crisis is vitally important and offers little opportunity to experiment to find the 'best' method. As the case study from Japan shows, sometimes the answer to current problems can be implemented by drawing upon traditions and customs embedded in culture. The final case study, from Aotearoa New Zealand, describes how culture can be influenced by a communication campaign, changing social norms on help-seeking for mental health concerns. It also clearly demonstrates that even the most effective communication activities require support from other health promotion initiatives within different levels and sectors. The chapter finishes with a summary of the key themes raised in these case studies and encourages reflection on how these themes align with the content presented in the earlier chapters of this text.

Tobacco control

1. Anti-tobacco health promotion: Beijing's initiative *(by Biaowen Huang)*

Second-hand smoke exposure

China is the world's largest producer and consumer of tobacco products, with more than 300 million smokers and over 1 million deaths attributed to smoking-related diseases every year (Minister of Health of the People's Republic of China, 2012). Thus, the smoking epidemic has been one of the most severe public health problems in China.

Among all harms caused by cigarette smoking, second-hand smoke has the most adverse and widespread effects. Despite 740 million non-smokers in China being exposed to second-hand smoke (a contributing cause of respiratory and cardiovascular diseases), more than two-thirds of people in China lack knowledge about the dangers of smoking and exposure to second-hand smoke. Under these circumstances, it is urgent for the government to raise awareness of the dangers of passive smoking, advocate a comprehensive ban on smoking in indoor places and reduce exposure to second-hand smoke, all of which will contribute to promoting a healthier environment.

The Beijing Tobacco Control Regulation, implemented on 1 June 2015, was the first local law in China to explicitly stipulate that 'indoor public places are 100 per cent smoke-free'. It is the most comprehensive subnational tobacco control regulation adopted in the country to date, in compliance with Article 8 of the WHO's Framework Convention on Tobacco Control (WHO, 2003a). This article utilises the Beijing Tobacco Control Regulation as an example to discuss how to conduct health education and health promotion concerning the hazards of second-hand smoke in developing countries such as China.

From top-down education to bottom-up participation

Although the municipal government of Beijing has promulgated regulations banning smoking in indoor public places, there remain challenges to creating smoke-free public places and reducing exposure to second-hand smoke. The challenges are mainly due to three factors:

1. Previous tobacco control campaigns were dominated by the government agency and these campaigns often included legislation, distribution of promotional materials and media advocacy. However, in China, where tobacco culture is deeply rooted, such a top-down approach can only lead to change in people's cognition of the dangers of passive smoking, and has minimal effect on public attitudes and their willingness to change behaviours.

2. In general, Chinese people are reluctant to have direct confrontation with others in public due to the influence of its collectivist culture. Even if people see others smoking in public places, they choose not to discourage the behaviour, especially when the situation involves their leaders or colleagues. Public acquiescence and group pressure have become obstacles to prohibiting smoking in public places.

3. Many smokers do not realise that smoking in public is anti-social behaviour; they believe that it is their right to decide when and where to smoke. Even if non-smokers attempt to dissuade them from smoking in public, they persist and moral approaches produce little effect on persuading smokers not to do so in public.

In response to these challenges, the Beijing Tobacco Control Association (BTCA) and other tobacco-control agencies organised a series of activities focusing on health education and health promotion. These activities ran from April to June in 2015, prior to the implementation of the Beijing Tobacco Control Regulation. They sought to raise public awareness of the dangers of second-hand smoke and to encourage residents to be active on tobacco control. The main initiatives were as follows.

1. Vote for the gesture of dissuading second-hand smoke

On 12 April, 50 days before the Beijing Tobacco Control Regulation would be implemented, the BTCA launched three gestures on Weibo, the Chinese equivalent of Twitter, to discourage smoking. These gestures indicate 'No', 'Please stop' and 'I do mind' (shown in Figure 10.1). An online referendum was initiated to decide the most popular gesture for dissuasion.

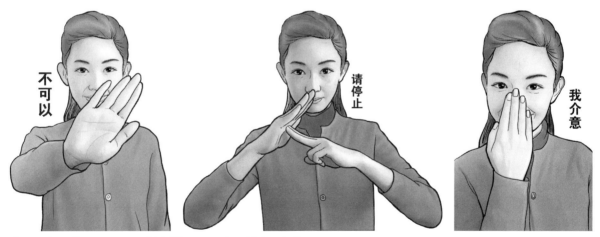

Figure 10.1 Three gestures: 'No', 'Please stop' and 'I do mind'
Source: Beijing Tobacco Control Association (2015).

The selection of gestures for dissuading smokers reflects the application of symbolic interaction theory in health promotion. Symbolic interaction theory claims that facts are based on, and directed by, symbols and that objects do not develop meaning on their own; rather, that meaning is endowed through social interactions (Aksan et al., 2009). Consequently, symbolic interaction is a process of 'interpretation of the action' (Aksan et al., 2009). In this case, at the beginning of the campaign, the public had no motivation to respond to verbal requests to discontinue smoking in public places.

However, the promotion of sanctioned gestures to signal disapproval helped to add legitimacy to the socially established need for a smoke-free environment.

2. Create media events to promote tobacco control

The concept of a 'media event' was proposed by communication scholars Dayan and Katz (1994). Also known as a 'pseudo-event', a media event is an event or activity conducted to gain public and media attention, using public relations rather than paying for advertising (Dayan & Katz, 1994). In this era of social media, as the public's participation has played an essential role in expression of opinion, an increasing number of public health events are presented in the form of 'media spectacles'. This method of presenting information can gather public attention in a short period and can evoke emotional resonance in the event. On 31 May 2015, the 28th World No Tobacco Day and the day before implementing the Beijing Tobacco Control Regulation, government departments and tobacco-control agencies held a large-scale publicity campaign. The event, attended by media and the public, was held in the National Stadium used to host the opening ceremony of the 2008 Beijing Olympic Games, to give maximum publicity through domestic and foreign media outlets. Several notable persons were invited to give keynote speeches at the event and posters on the theme of tobacco control and public welfare advertisements were also released. A group of celebrities was invited as national tobacco control ambassadors.

3. Utilise the internet to achieve social co-governance

After the Beijing Tobacco Control Regulation was promulgated, the difficulty of implementation has become the most critical issue. It is impractical to supervise all public places in the city, which relies on professional law enforcement officers. To deal with the personnel shortage, the BTCA developed a WeChat complaints platform, based on the geographic information system: 'a map for tobacco control' (see Figure 10.2). This supervision system can determine the real-time location of smokers violating the requirements of the Tobacco Control Regulation in public places; citizens can take photos or videos as evidence and upload them to the platform to complain. Once a complaint is received, the workplace on the map will light up. As more complaints are received, the colour changes from blue to orange or red, associated with increasingly severe penalties. In this way, each citizen became a supervisor of tobacco control, and the system made it possible for the government to identify where more efforts to reinforce the construction of a smoke-free environment are needed.

'A map for tobacco control' reflects the essential spirit of the social media era – sharing. Unlike traditional media, where the boundary between the messenger and the audience is clear, social media enables ordinary people with mobile devices to become communicators. User-generated content (UGC) has become the primary source of internet information (van Dijck, 2009). Based on such changes in the media environment, health education should no longer be a one-way dissemination of information, but rather should mobilise the broader public to participate in sharing information and establish a tobacco-control model based on social co-governance. The design of 'A map for tobacco control' shows consideration for protecting the privacy of

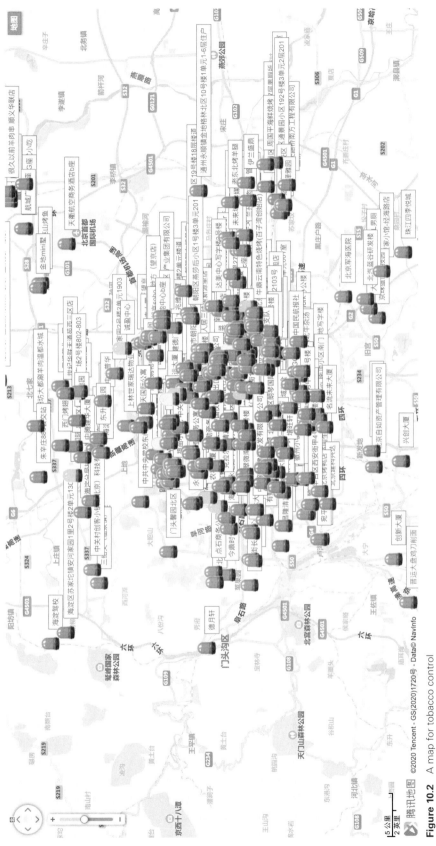

Figure 10.2 A map for tobacco control

Source: Beijing Tobacco Control Association (2015).

those contributing. Citizens are responsible only for reporting and verification but not for law enforcement, which helps them avoid direct conflicts with smokers who flout the regulations. Such design supports the public to show initiative and responsibility in facilitating smoking control.

Evaluation and conclusion

Short-term effect

The collective efforts of the public and media campaigns have contributed much to creating a smoke-free environment in Beijing. According to a survey conducted in April 2016, the number of smokers in public places in Beijing decreased significantly, from 11.3 to 3.8 per cent (Beijing Municipal Health and Family Planning Commission, 2016). Since the implementation of the regulation for one year, the public's satisfaction rate with the effect of the government's tobacco control has increased from 42.2 to 81.3 per cent. Ninety-three per cent of respondents believed that the scope of the smoke-free environment had been enlarged (Beijing Municipal Health and Family Planning Commission, 2016). The Beijing Municipal Government and BTCA were both awarded the World No Tobacco Day Award by the WHO for their efforts on tobacco control.

Long-term effects

The results of the Third Adult Tobacco survey in Beijing was published in December 2019. It showed that the smoking prevalence of adults in Beijing was 20.3 per cent, implying a decrease of 3.1 per cent from 2014. There are now 3.635 million smokers, 555 000 fewer than in 2014 (Beijing Municipal Health Commission, 2019). In the four years following the initiative, the BTCA recruited 13 886 volunteers for tobacco control through the WeChat public account. The 'A map for tobacco control' platform received a total of 48 842 effective complaints, of which 21 491 were verified and processed. The survey showed that 60.4 per cent of citizens responded that 'smoking in public places' was 'unacceptable' or 'very unacceptable', and 30.1 per cent of them thought they would choose to dissuade smokers when encountering second-hand smoking in the workplace (Beijing Municipal Health Commission, 2019). Through health promotion campaigns, Beijing has formed a 'VIP' (Volunteer-Internet-Press) model for tobacco control, which effectively reduces the harm of second-hand smoke.

QUESTIONS

1. Does the country or region you live in have serious problems concerning exposure to second-hand smoke? How does the local tobacco-control agency deal with it?

2. Of the above three initiatives conducted in China, which do you think may be effective in your country or region, and why?

3. In this current era of social media, how could you achieve a balance between bottom-up participation and top-down education on health promotion?

2. Information and sociocultural determinants of health behaviour: A case study from India *(by Josyula K. Lakshmi)*

Tobacco use in India

Tobacco use is a well-known health risk, responsible for a substantial burden of morbidity and mortality, particularly in low-income and middle-income countries (Institute for Health Metrics and Evaluation, 2019). The 2017 Global Adult Tobacco Survey in India estimated tobacco use by 28.6 per cent (266.8 million) of persons aged 15 years and older (TISS, 2017), and the WHO Tobacco Atlas highlighted tobacco use in 625 000 children aged 10 to 14 years in India (Drope & Schluger, 2018).

School-based tobacco-control programs

Policies have been enacted to control the manufacture, sale and use of tobacco products in India, with special reference to minors, educational institutions and smoking in public spaces (Government of India, 2003). Health communication campaigns, and awareness-raising interventions have been implemented in various settings, of which schools have been favoured for health promotion programs, particularly for the primary prevention of risky behaviours.

A school-based tobacco-control intervention was implemented in Gujarat and Andhra Pradesh, two states in which tobacco production is a major economic activity. The intervention enhanced awareness among teachers and students, and community engagement and support for tobacco-control policies through posters and rallies. At the conclusion of the intervention, in 2013, focus group discussions were conducted among participant students (aged 10 to 16 years), teachers and parents of participating students in the intervention schools. These discussions elucidated the socio-economic and cultural contexts of the communities in which the intervention had been implemented, and the effects of the intervention on tobacco use in the community (Lakshmi et al., 2020).

Evaluation

The communities in this project lived in an environment characterised by caste and gender inequality, with disparate autonomy and opportunities available to different members of society, whereby men were able to exercise greater agency than women. The complex factors that influenced tobacco use in the communities are classified under the successive levels of the social ecological model of health, as follows:

- Individual: beliefs about tobacco use; self-efficacy to avoid or quit tobacco use
- Interpersonal: peers and family members using and offering tobacco; persuasion from close associates to quit tobacco use
- Organisational: income from tobacco production and sale; tobacco use to aid labour
- Community: customs and social expectations at celebrations; role models who use or avoid tobacco; celebrity endorsements of tobacco products or tobacco avoidance
- Policy: laws on the packaging and sale of tobacco; easy availability and affordability of tobacco; incidental effect of alcohol prohibition, which gives center stage to the available recreational substances, such as tobacco

Table 10.1 lists factors influencing tobacco use, as reported by the community.

Table 10.1   Community identified deterrents and enablers of tobacco use

	Deterrents of tobacco use	Enablers of tobacco use
Health beliefs	Information on adverse consequences of tobacco use	Perceptions of the therapeutic nature of tobacco Stimulant; appetite-suppressant; physiological support for increased work
Economic and environmental contexts	Tobacco-control policies and their enforcement	Tobacco-based local economy Easy availability of tobacco Affordability of tobacco products
Cultural influences	Caste and gender norms discouraging tobacco use Persuasion from family and friends to avoid tobacco	Tobacco-using role models and peers Unobtrusiveness of certain forms of tobacco Association of tobacco with hospitality
Pathophysiological driver	–	Addiction

Some of these factors worked together to either enable or hinder tobacco use, and some worked against each other. For instance, among adolescent girls, knowledge of the adverse consequences of tobacco use aligned with norms that discouraged tobacco use, as well as policies and enforcement that kept tobacco out of the easy reach of people. In contrast, information imparted about the advisability of quitting tobacco did not go down well with people habituated to tobacco use from routine consumption during the workday. In some cases, individuals' personal choices and decisions came into conflict with the expectations of their social connections, as illustrated by this testimony of a student: He had persuaded his father to quit smoking. He noted that at a wedding his father was offered cigarettes, in keeping with social convention. Although his father had given up smoking, he accepted the cigarette that he was offered, to avoid causing offence, but then did not smoke it.

Enhanced awareness and improved communication skills empowered the participating students to resolve not to initiate tobacco use, and to persuade some or all of their tobacco-using family members to quit tobacco. However, an observation by many was that the students' influence did not extend very far outside their immediate families and friends. Students remarked on the wide range of responses to their efforts to educate people about the ills of tobacco use, from welcome and validation from close friends and family members, and polite scepticism from outsiders who were occasional users of tobacco, to open hostility from habitual tobacco users.

Parents who used tobacco reported feeling embarrassed about engaging in this practice, which depleted both health and money, especially when health information and exhortations to quit came from their own children. Some parents quit tobacco in response to their children's efforts, while others who did not quit nonetheless stopped sending their children on errands to purchase tobacco.

Teachers decried the tobacco-control policies that were not supported by diligent enforcement, citing these as factors cramping their efforts to discourage tobacco use in the community. They highlighted the central position of tobacco in the local economy, and the consequent inseparability of tobacco from the lives and culture of the community. They also commented on the overwhelming attraction to adolescents of pro-tobacco messaging involving celebrity sportspersons and movie stars. Teachers who had been trained in the school-based tobacco-control intervention spoke of the constraints within their society; for example, tobacco-using teachers were role models of tobacco use for students; some students' parents did not appreciate extracurricular exchanges, such as discussions on the hazards of tobacco use, between teachers and their students; teachers were made aware of the policies limiting tobacco sale to minors and smoking in public places, but had no authority to check violations of these rules; teachers as members of social networks themselves feared a backlash from their associates at social gatherings if they were vocal about avoiding using and sharing tobacco.

Conclusion

It is important to undertake a holistic consideration of all the conditions at the various levels of an individual's existence, to understand the determinants of health behaviour, as well as to design and implement effective interventions to promote health. This is especially vital in societies that have fairly strict structures and systems that stipulate rigid roles for their members, and segments of the population that have low autonomy and rely heavily on external provision and permission for information, resources, access and validation. Health promotion strategies need to address the reality that the exercise of personal choice may be problematic among people in certain situations, and that facilitating healthy behaviours may call for additional strategies directed at higher levels than that of the individual, to bridge gaps between knowledge and action.

QUESTIONS

1. How do you think clear tobacco-control policies and their stringent enforcement could have influenced the effects of the school-based intervention on the community? Discuss the potential implications – both positive and negative – that you identify.

2. Compare the potential effectiveness of the following categories of persons as messengers of tobacco avoidance:
   a. schoolchildren
   b. women between the ages of 20 and 50 years
   c. elected leaders in the community
   d. high-profile cricketers.

3. What approach might health counsellors take to motivate a habitual tobacco user to quit tobacco? Consider strategies that involve the tobacco user as well as close associates in the community.

Communities as partners

3. Delivering a health promotion intervention through community health volunteers, to vulnerable and marginalised communities in Mongolia *(by Sudhir Raj Thout)*

The challenges and potential gaps in health promotion and provision of preventive care services to vulnerable populations

Studies by Murali & Oyebode (2004) and Asian Development Bank (2008) have found that the poor quality of health-service delivery in Mongolia, focusing on treatment rather than prevention, negatively affects the health of vulnerable populations, including those who are unemployed, homeless and who have low incomes. The main factors that contributed to poor quality of health-service delivery included that:

- Healthcare providers' prevalent behaviour is focused on cure rather than prevention, which naturally results in the community's lack of awareness about illness prevention. The paternalistic approach of the health service creates a culture of dependence and a lack of health knowledge among the population as healthcare providers dominate the decision-making process and their clients are forced to make treatment decisions without being given sufficient information. The educational backgrounds of doctors and nurses are focused on treatment and not on prevention.
- The level of motivation by management and their capacity for prevention is low. Managers and healthcare providers alike are not equipped with adequate knowledge and skills about preventative health. There is also a lack of resources and capacity in the service to meet the healthcare needs of the population, such as the prevention of common communicable and non-communicable diseases, promotion of reproductive health and prevention of injuries.

Community engagement in health prevention and health promotion activities

A community based health promotion intervention was implemented in 2009 by Dornod Provincial Health Department in target sites of Mongolia. The aim of the intervention was to reduce the incidences of common communicable and non-communicable diseases by improving the effectiveness and quality of health promotion services to vulnerable and marginalised communities. In addition, the intervention aimed to achieve the targets set by national health programs for non-communicable and communicable diseases, child development and protection of the health of older people (Boutayeb, 2006; National Committee on HIV/AIDS, 2010). The key component of this intervention addressed the preventative health and health promotion aspects, including inequality in health care, by providing accessible health promotion services delivered by community health volunteers, and by improving the capacity of healthcare providers to deliver effective health promotion to communities.

The role and the contribution of community health volunteers in building the awareness of preventative health issues, and of bringing about change in health-seeking behaviour among disadvantaged community members were key focuses of the initiative. Community health volunteers were recruited from the local community. These volunteers came from a range of backgrounds, including respected community members and retired health workers who were highly respected by the clients they had worked with, local health authorities and local governments.

Community health volunteers received training from health experts on:

- different health aspects that aimed to promote preventative healthcare services
- health education, health promotion, basic research and communication skills, such as how to interact with local community members during their visits
- skills such as conducting anthropometric and blood pressure measurements.

Volunteers were also provided with job-aid tools such as blood glucose monitoring kits, weighing scales and measuring tapes for routine health screening. The training from partner organisations and respective health authorities helped to build the capacity of community health volunteers to deliver health promotion services in disadvantaged communities.

Subsequently, community health volunteers who had intimate knowledge of local public health issues could apply this knowledge to perform a wide range of activities, including home visits, basic health evaluations, leading individual and group discussions on healthy behaviours, and arranging referrals to healthcare providers when needed. During these routine visits, community health volunteers conducted needs assessments to understand health and wellness in communities and to identify priority health issues. In addition, community health volunteers were trained in the development of health promotion materials using participatory methods that helped them to develop relevant, acceptable and practicable materials. The health promotion services that were delivered through community health volunteers increased community members' awareness of health issues, such as preventing and managing hypertension, improved their basic skills and understanding of healthy behaviours and connected them to local health services. Community health volunteers provided outreach services with individualised education on the importance of taking medications, on how to reduce daily intake of sodium and the importance of higher intakes of fruit and vegetables to lower blood pressure. A wide range of social and cultural barriers to healthcare, such as a lack of quality healthcare, health-related transportation and social health insurance, and social isolation of elders, were addressed by community health volunteers, who also bridged the gap between underserved communities and local health services.

The delivery of health promotion activities using community health volunteers, the active participation of communities in identifying key health issues and addressing them, and the following community driven initiatives to promote service delivery to vulnerable people and those with poor health were supported by these actions:

- Advocacy of community health volunteering to communities in improving the public's understanding and acceptance of community health volunteers, including support from different stakeholders.
- Community members:
  - actively participated in needs assessment, action planning and monitoring, and the development of behaviour change communication materials

- engaged in dialogue with local community health volunteers and healthcare providers and had input into planning the service delivery in their localities
- participated in boards and task forces of local service providers
- initiated community wide activities supported by community health volunteers and partner organisations
- organised coalitions to promote their rights and needs.

Evaluation and conclusion

The active involvement of health volunteers in this intervention has increased the accessibility, sustainability and inclusiveness of primary healthcare services, and has empowered key members of the local community to help ensure their communities achieve key health goals.

This health promotion intervention package was effective in achieving behavioural change targeted at reducing childhood mortality, improving maternal health and prevention of cardiovascular diseases, communicable diseases and sexually transmissible infections. The community health volunteers acted as agents of behaviour change promotion and served as the bridge between underserved communities in providing preventative health promotion services and access to local health centres.

The key success of this intervention has been twofold:

- Effective mobilisation and empowerment of community health volunteers by partner organisations for health promotion: community health volunteers were seen as facilitating success through effective engagement, trust and support from local community members.
- Improvement in the capacity of community health volunteers to deliver health promotion services to communities enhanced their capacity to deliver effective health promotion at the community level. Partner organisations supported and trained community health volunteers in health education and health promotion aspects, with a focus on cardiovascular diseases, cancer, injuries, communicable diseases and reproductive health.

Thus, the intervention was effective in the delivery of primary and preventative health services, to reduce common illnesses in vulnerable and marginalised communities.

The specific objectives in the intervention were achieved and the delivery of health promotion activities using community health volunteers was considered to be the most cost-effective way of providing information and care to both healthcare providers and low socio-economic households, and addressed the issues affecting the health of disadvantaged populations (Boutayeb, 2006; National Committee on HIV/ AIDS, 2010). Specific outcomes included:

- improved access to health services to vulnerable and marginalised communities
- reduced prevalence of common illnesses, which contributed to achieving the targets set by national health programs on non-communicable and communicable diseases
- improved skills in healthcare providers' capacity to provide good quality health promotion services to communities
- completion of needs assessment among communities and application to health-service planning and delivery

- effective mobilisation and empowerment of community health volunteers to undertake health promotion
- improved capacity of community health volunteers to deliver health promotion services to communities
- empowerment of communities to incorporate their needs into delivery of local social services.

Community health volunteers helped vulnerable people overcome the barriers that prevented them from seeking effective healthcare, particularly where the majority of vulnerable people suffered gross health inequalities and lacked access to good quality care because of social, geographic and economic barriers (National Statistical Office, 2009; Ministry of Health of Mongolia, 2010). Community health volunteers were well aware of local cultural and social norms, social stratifications, including sociocultural barriers and contextual factors, to accessing healthcare services. Some of these factors were responded to by incorporating culture-specific attitudes and values into health promotion tools. The underlying sociocultural barriers, such as gender, traditional values, norms and beliefs, and stigma were addressed by community health workers through improved communication, enabling clarification of patients' concerns and bringing about improvements in quality of care with emphasis on empowerment, gender sensitivity and reducing social stigma.

QUESTIONS

1. In the case study, what were identified as the main causes of poor quality in healthcare delivery, and who experienced them?
2. Who were community health volunteers and what role did they play in reaching community members through health prevention and health promotion services and information?
3. What were the key components in the intervention?

4. Using mobile technology for health promotion through Lady Health Workers in Pakistan (by Tehzeeb Zulfiqar)

Utilising a female health workforce to improve maternal and child health indicators

Pakistan is a low-to-middle-income country with poor maternal and child health indicators (NIPS & ICF, 2019). There is also widespread gender inequality, and women have lower education and employment rates compared to the other South Asian countries (UNDP, 2019). This case study explores the role of over 100 000 Lady Health Workers (LHWs) in promoting maternal and child health services at their doorsteps.

Pakistan established the LHW program in 1993. Over time, the LHW program has become the largest community based health initiative globally (Hafeez et al., 2011). The program aimed to reduce poverty and a shortage of women in the health workforce in rural areas and urban slums. The LHWs were deployed in all districts of Pakistan. They have strengthened the primary healthcare system by serving as a bridge between the public health facilities and communities (Oxford Policy Management, 2009b).

A LHW is a permanent resident of the area she serves. She is preferably married, aged between 18 and 50 years, and has a minimum of eight years of schooling (Oxford Policy Management, 2009a; 2009b). She is trained by health staff working at the basic health unit (BHU) that serves her community. She receives training for 15 months in the prevention and treatment of common illnesses. The first three months of training take place in the classroom at the BHU, and the following 12 months consist of on-the-job training, which includes one day per month in the classroom, working on problem-based modules. The basic training of the LHW is complemented by one-day Continuing Education Sessions each month and 15-day Refresher Training courses on various topics each year (Hafeez et al., 2011; Oxford Policy Management, 2009b).

Each LHW provides coverage to around 1000–1500 people (approximately 200 households) in her community. She visits an average of 27 households a week, provides advice and conducts consultations to an average of 22 individuals weekly (Oxford Policy Management, 2009a). Her residence is designated a health house, from where she provides free services to the community members and stores contraceptives, medicines and health promotion material (Oxford Policy Management, 2009b; WHO, 2006a). She is able to treat simple illnesses, such as diarrhoea and acute respiratory infections, and refers cases to the BHU in accordance with the guidelines. The unit cost to the government of LHWs per beneficiary is approximately US $1.33 annually (Leslie et al., 2018).

LHWs perform around 20 core tasks. These include family planning counselling, antenatal care, advice on natal and post-natal services, health, hygiene and nutrition education, child-growth monitoring, provision of basic medicines for common ailments, immunisation campaigns and polio drives, and referrals to primary healthcare facilities (Hafeez, 2011).

There are several tiers of supervision for LHWs. A Lady Health Supervisor (LHS) manages the work of around 25 LHWs. She is expected to visit each LHW under her supervision at least twice a month. The LHW and LHS are also supervised by the district and provincial health teams.

Promoting maternal and child health activities

The LHW plans her health promotion activities according to the national/provincial/district health priorities and according to the needs of the community.

After deployment in the community, the LHWs establish two health committees – the *Sehat* (health) committee, which comprises men and women occupying leadership or influential roles in the community, such as spiritual leaders, teachers and local counsellors. This committee meets monthly. The male members of the committee support the LHWs in executing their duties, particularly in interactions between men and LHWs for contraception and reproductive health purposes. In the strict patriarchal and conservative rural communities of Pakistan, where women are often secluded and are not allowed to communicate with men outside their families, or to travel alone (Mumtaz, 2013), the LHWs faced huge challenges in fulfilling their duties in the early years.

The second health committee, which comprises community women, meets weekly. In these meetings, the LHWs discuss a topic previously identified by the women of the community or a topic of national/provincial/district priority communicated to her from the BHU. For example, during the biannual, government-led Mother and Child week, she organises community talks on the importance of timely antenatal check-ups, healthy eating during pregnancy, births in health clinics, hospitals or with skilled birth attendants, birth spacing, vaccination, hand hygiene, pneumonia and diarrhoea. She receives prior training and paper-based training aids such as pictorials or cards with health messages for effective communication. However, several studies have shown that despite sufficient technical knowledge, the LHWs need to improve their ability to effectively transfer their knowledge to their target audience – married women of reproductive age and their families (Oxford Policy Management, 2009a; 2009c).

Using mobile phones for health promotion

Pakistan has the fifth-largest mobile phone market in Asia. Mobile phones are a widely used method of communication in urban and rural areas. In 2017, mobile phones were introduced to LHWs in one province, to facilitate their health promotion activities. The mHealth mobile applications were installed on these phones, which contained videos providing training material (mLearning) and counselling aids (mCounselling) (Leslie et al., 2018). The videos explain common maternal and child health messages in a clear and engaging way in the local language. The LHW provides health education to the women in the community by showing them the videos on her mobile phone. Women who had previously received health talks from LHWs using paper-based tools found learning through these videos a good information source. The videos are the most appealing part of the application as the enactment makes it easier for the women to remember the message (Leslie et al., 2018). The LHWs also consider the mobile phone application a good source of information and a helpful counselling tool. An additional advantage of the mobile phone application is that the LHWs can also use the teaching material repeatedly to improve their own knowledge.

Utilising mobile technology for health promotion improved the overall effectiveness of the LHWs. The LHWs were able to work fast, provide comprehensive information and interact easily with their clients (Leslie et al., 2018).

Evaluation

The external evaluations of the LHWs program showed that LHWs were able to overcome initial cultural barriers to their work and were accepted as valuable members of their community (Oxford Policy Management, 2009c; 2019). Their guidance and opinion in health matters and family planning strategies are taken seriously. The evaluations also showed an improvement in maternal and child health indicators within the segment of the population using LHWs' services, compared to the population that did not use their services (Oxford Policy Management, 2009a; 2009c). Women who attended health talks by the LHWs had higher intakes of antenatal care services, skilled assistance at birth, family planning services, preventative child health services, treatment of childhood diseases and breastfeeding rates.

The use of communications and other technologies provides an opportunity to further enhance the communication skills and interpersonal communications of LHWs, to enable transformation of maternal and child health at the community level.

QUESTIONS

1. Find two community health worker programs elsewhere in the world. Identify a maximum of five similarities and differences between LHWs and the community health workers from the programs you identified.

2. What is the most suitable behavioural change model for community health workers?

3. What are the benefits and difficulties of using community health workers in health promotion activities?

5. Using a youth health brand to promote better sexual and reproductive health among young people in Uganda (by Patrick Segawa, Chloe Simpson, Dennis Ernest Ssesanga and Lillibet Namakula)

The sexual and reproductive health (SRH) of adolescents and young people in Uganda is a vital area for health promotion. Uganda has a young and rapidly growing population. In 2018, out of a population of 42.7 million people, only 1.9 per cent was over 65 years of age, 46.9 per cent was under 14 years and 51.1 per cent was between 15 and 64 years (World Bank, 2018b). The fertility rate was 5.09 births per woman, and the proportion of teenage mothers (pregnant or already given birth) was 25 per cent (World Bank, 2018a). Young people face a high unmet need for contraceptives, resulting also in unsafe abortions, and sexually transmissible infections, including HIV/AIDS. According to the Guttmacher Institute (2018), among adolescent girls aged 15–19 years who reported being sexually active and did not want a child in the next two years, more than 60 per cent had an unmet need for effective contraception, meaning that they either used no contraceptive method or used a traditional, and therefore unreliable, method of contraception. It is also the case that, in 2013, 93 000 women were reported to have been treated for abortion-related complications (Guttmacher Institute, 2017).

Young people are poorly informed about issues related to HIV/AIDS, sexually transmissible infections and family planning, making them vulnerable to engaging in risky sexual behaviours. For example, the government of Uganda found that only 40 per cent of Ugandan adolescents aged 15–19 years had comprehensive HIV/AIDS prevention knowledge (Uganda Bureau of Statistics, 2017). Only 45 per cent of women and women aged 15–24 years were able to correctly identify ways of preventing the sexual transmission of HIV (UNAIDS, 2018). There is also a lack of youth-friendly SRH services. In 2011, a report found only 5 per cent of public health facilities in Uganda was providing such services (Ministry of Health, 2012).

Public Health Ambassadors Uganda (PHAU), a youth-led non-government agency based in Kampala, is using unique health promotion strategies to attract young people to SRH services, disseminate youth-friendly information and promote positive sexual behaviours among young people.

YoSpace: A brand created by and for young people

One of PHAU's initiatives reaches out to young people through a brand known as 'YoSpace'. The idea for a health brand came from a human-centred design process in which young people were asked about barriers they faced in accessing SRH information and services, and possible solutions to these challenges. They reported discrimination from health workers in accessing condoms, a lack of accurate information in schools, high cost of services and geographic isolation. One solution that emerged was for young people to create their own brand that was representative of accessible and relevant SRH services and information. The YoSpace brand is associated with affordable services such as HIV/AIDs testing, counselling and family planning services at private health centres across seven districts. It uses interactive ways of sensitising young people in communities, such as through 'edutainment' (entertainment with an education focus) and informative performance arts. These approaches are discussed in further detail.

In 2018, the YoSpace project was taken to an area in western Uganda called Masindi, where, like in most rural places, girls fall pregnant at a young age, there are higher than average rates of HIV/AIDS and other sexual health challenges. PHAU was engaged to improve referrals of 15–24-year-olds for family planning services at youth-friendly health facilities. First of all, a group of 30 young people aged 18–30 years from the district were selected to be trained as peer educators, who would disseminate SRH information in communities. They could be seen wearing bright-pink shirts with the YoSpace logo and engaging in conversations with young people about sexual health and where to go to access services. The peer educators also embraced using edutainment and informative performance arts. For example, they used a music truck, which had a DJ playing popular music and an emcee (master of ceremonies) to encourage people to attend free health-centre days. They used dance performances such as flash mob dance routines (see Figure 10.3) and drama skits,

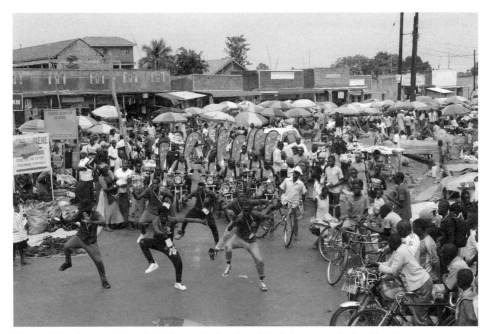

Figure 10.3   A crowd shot of a YoSpace flashmob activity in Luweero district, Uganda

Source: © Public Health Ambassadors Uganda. Reproduced with permission.

which they performed in marketplaces to initiate discussions of topics such as how to challenge gender stereotypes. At the local Masindi showgrounds, a Family Planning Concert was organised, with entertainment provided by musicians, cultural dancers and comedy acts that had integrated messages about safe sexual practices. Health providers set up tents with a variety of SRH services. Radio talk shows and social media were also utilised.

Some of the following indicators were used to measure the outcomes of the project:

- Number of 15–24-year-old girls and women accessing SRH information over a four-month period: 18 602 girls and women were reached through door-to-door engagement, providing information on HIV/AIDS, family planning and transmission and prevention of sexually transmissible infections
- Number of effective referrals of girls and women aged 15–24 years for family planning methods at health facilities over a four-month period: 17 268 girls and women were directly referred for family planning services
- Number of condoms distributed: 46 000
- Number of young people receiving SRH services on outreach days. At Boma Showgrounds Concert, 326 people were tested for HIV/AIDs, 67 women received cervical cancer screening, seven men received safe circumcision and 80 girls and women were provided with family planning methods.

Taking on board lessons learned

The human-centred design approach of the YoSpace brand and model has been key to its success and popularity, because it has enabled young people to be at the centre of the design, planning and implementation of activities. Feedback from beneficiaries is that young people feel more comfortable talking to their age-mates about issues to do with sexual health than with adult educators. Peer-to-peer learning can provide an enabling environment in which to break down misinformation, as peer educators are seen as role models. They are also a means to link young people to health services. Going forward, peer educators could also be trained to engage other age groups; for example, through hosting intergenerational dialogues. This is key to addressing underlying social, cultural and gender-based barriers to SRH.

The use of edutainment and informative performance arts has also been popular in the Ugandan context, due to the young population and cultural and historic interest in the performance arts. Integrating health messages into popular art forms has been effective in starting discussions about normally sensitive or taboo topics. From holding a dialogue in a health facility waiting room to presenting a concert or performance in a marketplace or engaging young people in a dance or hip-hop battle, health information can be brought to any area or community. It can be tailored to the current and specific needs of the community, through baseline research and human-centred design.

In the latest YoSpace project, conducted in 2019 in eastern Uganda, peer educators were provided with monthly stipends, and this helped to increase their engagement with the project and the number of effective health centre referrals. E-referrals (referrals by electronic means) have also been suggested as a way to improve communication between peer educators and health providers. A mobile phone application created by PHAU is also being introduced to provide SRH information to young people.

QUESTIONS

1. When initiating a project such as YoSpace in a new district, what would be some of the initial steps in designing the SRH promotion activities for your project?

2. Why do you think it is important when designing activities to incorporate the human-centred design process?

3. Discuss some of the examples of edutainment and informative performance arts methods that can be used to promote sexual health. Consider the advantages of each in terms of the context and the target population to which each of them would be best suited.

4. If you are using the peer-to-peer approach, what might be your selection criteria in choosing peer educators for your project?

5. Information Communication Technology (ICT) can be key in increasing access to SRH information and services. How might ICT be utilised to support the peer-to-peer approach in health promotion and education of a community?

6. Urban development and health *(by Albert Lee)*

In 1950, only one-third of the world's population lived in a city; this is expected to increase to two-thirds by 2050 (WHO, 2006b). In particular, this transition from rural to urban living is expected to involve a rapid expansion of mega-cities in the western Pacific region. The relatively rapid influx of people into cities is expected to lead to deficits in material conditions, psychosocial resources and political engagement and a resulting poverty and disempowerment at the individual, community and national levels. The report of the City, Health and Well-being conference, held in 2011, highlighted the problems of rapid urbanisation in Asia (Taylor, 2012). It described how the pace and scale of urbanisation in Asia had affected poverty by accentuating certain aspects of inequality or deprivation, such as housing and infrastructure (Taylor, 2012). One of the recommendations of the Lancet Commission on Healthy Cities has called for attention to health inequalities within urban areas as a key focus in urban planning, and the need for community representation in the arenas of policy making and planning (Rydin et al., 2012). Researchers in Hong Kong have identified the effects of urban development on social isolation, resulting from disconnection in new towns and weakening of the neighbourhood as a social environment, which has led to decreased utility of neighbourhood spaces, frailty among older people, suicidality and, ultimately, poor health (Taylor, 2012; Yip, 2011).

Healthy Cities for better urban health

Behavioural, environmental, occupational and metabolic risks can explain 61 per cent of global mortality and almost half of the global disability adjusted life years (DALYs) (GBD, 2017). This provides many opportunities for prevention across society, as stated in the Marmot review of inequalities (Marmot & Bell, 2012).

The concept of Healthy Cities is to develop an integrated, intersectoral approach, with community participation as described by John Ashton, one of the pioneers in Healthy Cities development:

> A healthy city is one that is continually creating and improving those physical and social environments and expanding those community resources which enable people to support each other in performing all the functions of life and in developing themselves to their maximum potential (Ashton, 2020).

The Alliance for Healthy Cities (AFHC) was established in 2003, following a consultation meeting by the WHO (WHO, 2003). Members of AFHC comprise representatives of cities, academic institutions, non-government organisations, national agencies and private organisations. The main objectives of AFHC are to:

a. Strengthen the Healthy Cities initiatives and encourage the development of innovative plans and programs to improve the quality of life and address the health challenge of specific settings and communities

b. Share the improvement of the quality of life and address common health problems among members

c. Recognise outstanding practices and innovations within Healthy Cities

d. Package technical resources for the improvement of planning, implementation and evaluation of Healthy Cities (AFHC, 2020).

Epidemiological indicators cannot measure the process that precipitates the change nor the direct effects of change. Assessment of public health interventions should not rely solely on a technical exercise conducted by external experts (Rydin et al., 2012). It should be based on dialogues, deliberation and discussion between key stakeholders, with the insights gained from the knowledge and experience of local communities (Rydin et al., 2012). If Healthy Cities is to tackle the complexity of public health problems, it requires strong leadership and engagement of key stakeholders across different sectors, and development of a good action plan based on the city's health profile and research for sustainability (De Leeuw et al., 2015). Therefore, the Healthy Cities project should not only focus on health outcomes, but also on the broader concept of health and the application of health promotion strategies, and should be included for evaluation (Boonekamp et al., 1999).

The measurement of success of Healthy Cities should capture data showing the enhancement in health through improvements in certain social, cultural and economic conditions, highlighting changes in human attitudes and initiatives to improve personal and environmental health. AFHC has created awards to recognise cities for outstanding practices of Healthy Cities. AFHC has adopted the SPIRIT framework (see Table 10.2) in assessment of nominations for AFHC awards, to capture the process of change in enhancing health improvements (Lee, 2020). There are three awards:

1. Healthy City with good infrastructure

2. Healthy City with good dynamics

3. Healthy City with strong action.

The Republic of Korea (Korea) is one of the leading pioneers in Healthy Cities development, with many cities having been recipients of AFHC awards. Korea has one of the largest funds for health promotion globally, but its limited health promotion capacity was an obstacle in spending the money in an efficient and sustainable way (Nam & Engelhardt, 2007). Korean health promotion capacity is good but to enable a

Table 10.2 SPIRIT framework

Domains	Indicators for success
Setting approach, **S**ustainability	The city should place a strong emphasis on developing activities in different settings such as schools, workplaces and marketplaces, to promote and influence health. The city has developed a strategic plan to ensure sustainable development of the city. Is the program engaging in strategic partnerships with city management and planning processes?
Political commitment, **P**olicy, community **P**articipation	The political leaders of the city should make a public commitment that they will move their cities towards becoming a Healthy City. Health issues are accorded high priority in public policy. The city is encouraging communities to participate in urban development for better health and quality of life.
Information, **I**nnovation	Information should be available in the following areas: • important health problems and health issues in the city • analysis of economic and social determinants of health for the city • the concerns of health care delivery system of the city • the special population groups at risk • the existing health promotion programs organised by different parties • community perception of health The city should create a comprehensive health profile based on the above information, and then a city health plan can be developed. Programs should be innovative in meeting public needs and promote a climate to support change.
Resources, **R**esearch	Are adequate resources earmarked for the program? A research framework has been developed for needs assessment and measurement of outcomes.
Infrastructure, **I**ntersectoral	There should be a steering committee with responsibility for the overall management and coordination of the program. There should be a technical committee or working committee with members from different sectors to address specific projects.
Training	Are there training courses at different levels in health education and health promotion? The city should identify institutions that can provide training for professionals, administrators and the public.

full understanding of the state of health promotion development, a more 'fine-tuned' map to look behind the façade was required (Nam & Engelhardt, 2007). Taking into account the diverse needs of Healthy Cities, the SPIRIT framework was utilised.

Evaluation of Healthy Cities

Many cities in Korea have demonstrated remarkable achievements in Healthy Cities development, with AFHC awards based on evaluation using the SPIRIT framework

(Nam et al., 2010), with 81 cities recognised as full members of the Korea Healthy Cities Partnership (KHCP, 2020). The following actions and characteristics, under each of the different domains of the SPIRIT framework, illustrate what Korean cities did to achieve the highest level for each award (Lee, 2020).

Strategic planning for sustainable development and involvement of different settings

- The setting covers parks and recreation spaces (e.g. greenway, eco-friendly urban garden), housing complex (e.g. low-energy, eco-friendly housing, complex environment), village (e.g. energy dependent village, integrated services for health management and counselling with one-stop services from prevention to treatment) and school (counselling services available on needs)
- Construction of low-carbon, green-market industrial cities, harmonised with the natural environment
- Creation of walking friendly walkway environments
- Installation of heatwave shelters and outdoor canopies
- Eco-friendly waterfront construction, restoring urban forest

Policy and political commitment

- City councils have included Healthy Cities as an important area of development in strategic planning, and this is incorporated into the Five-year City Development Plan since 2011.
- Citizens' Happiness through Health is an initiative that positions health as a major task in the pledge of the mayoral election.
- Related ordinances: Child obesity relationship ordinance; school sports facility fee support ordinance; eco-friendly, urban agriculture activation and support ordinance; eco-friendly, free school meal support ordinance; mental health check-up and counselling for people in their 50s support ordinance; dementia support centre establishment and operation ordinance; and healthy drinking culture environment creation and support ordinance.
- The Healthy City Master Plan is developed with enactment of the ordinance of Healthy City Guideline and the greenhouse gas-reduction policy to cope with rapid climate change.
- Create specialised school-zone safe walkways that are safe from potential traffic accidents.
- Supply renewable energy, activate '1 household 1 electric generator' and build energy efficiency.

Information and innovation

- The city has conducted an impact analysis on increased walking practices, expansion of park spaces per capita, increased number of eco-friendly housing complexes, improvement of satisfaction with healthcare services, expansion of health clubs and group meetings for chronic illnesses, and increased numbers of counsellors at schools.

- The city provides information on the following areas to create a City Health Profile:
  i. Prevalence of obesity in children and young people, chronic illness and mental health
  ii. Analysis of economic and social determinants of health for the city
  iii. The practice levels of desirable health behaviours (physical activity practice, walking practices, participating in sports activity etc.) were low in the older population and among people with low education and income levels
  iv. Community perception of health

Research and resources

- A community health survey investigates community needs through examining the health behaviour of the residents and their use of the medical system.
- A social survey investigates the needs of daily life and social problems.
- Online surveys investigate the administration and policies to explore local residents' health priorities to establish a local health care plan.
- Collection of residents' opinions by creating a meeting place, including residents' discussion sessions on the vision and regional development of the city.
- The city has analysed the correlation between the health status of the residents and residences' urban physical factors, then developed the guidelines for designing urban areas (roads, green spaces, buildings etc.) for various health promotion activities including for prevention of environmental diseases, depression, obesity and hypertension.

Infrastructure and intersectoral

- The Secretariat was responsible for planning a draft for Healthy City, mobilising people and appropriating all the budgets for Healthy City development.
- The specific projects needed to create and maintain the Healthy City were overseen by the Division of City Administration, ensuring that all projects had access to relevant expertise.

Training

- A large-scale citizen policy debate organised by Yangcheon-gu Office was held in Yangcheon-Gu, Republic of Korea in 2016, at Yangcheon Hall. This event was attended by more than 100 people, including advisory committee members, external experts and other local government officials. The debate presented research results and collected perspectives for deriving high-level outcomes, including which institutions had the most relevant expertise for the provision and priorities of training.

Healthy cities should measure what matters; that is, socially just and ecologically sustainable human development and wellbeing, and those measures should guide and manage Healthy Cities development (International Institute for Global Health, 2018). The purpose of the AFHC awards is to ensure that these measures and the monitoring of change can be publicly and widely available.

QUESTIONS

1. Why is routine health data unable to reflect whether a city is successful in becoming a thriving Healthy City?

2. What are the added values of Healthy Cities in addition to health interventions in clinical settings for improving the health of the city dwellers?

3. Can you identify any programs in your city that are conducive to Healthy Cities development?

Communication as an enabler

7. The Fukushima disaster: Co-creating knowledge with stakeholders *(by Mikihito Tanaka)*

On 11 March 2011, a magnitude 9.0 earthquake and subsequent tsunami struck the north-eastern coast of Japan's largest main island of Honshu. These events caused nearly 20 000 individuals to die or go missing and also heavily damaged a nuclear power plant in the Fukushima prefecture (NAIIC, 2012). This damage caused the leakage of radioactive materials from the power plant, an occurrence known as 'the Fukushima disaster', which threatened the health of local residents.

Every disaster can expose a society's vulnerabilities. Before the disaster, the residents of this agricultural region were struggling to maintain the Fukushima prefecture's ageing infrastructure. When the disaster devastated the area, it further highlighted its weaknesses. Due to the radioactive contamination, 160 000 people were forced to evacuate, and subsequently lost their homes and livelihoods (Bacon & Hobson, 2014). Furthermore, the local community was torn apart when victims were given minimal compensation and forced to live in prefabricated houses. These people had been robbed of their way of life and their support networks in the community and had no reason to re-enter the polluted environment. It is easy to imagine that such stressful circumstances might have caused these individuals to turn to unhealthy habits (e.g. drinking and smoking), which likely exacerbated lifestyle-related conditions such as diabetes or cardiac problems (Hasegawa et al., 2015). Many desperate people were driven to despair, ultimately committing suicide. Such victims were considered part of the disaster-related death count, which numbered 2304 in Fukushima in 2019 (Sekine, 2020).

After the Fukushima disaster, health communicators had to address not only the illnesses and stresses caused by radiation exposure, but also the other health problems resulting from the accident.

Providing health communication using the tri-actor model

After the disaster, medical experts from the Fukushima Medical University (FMU) needed to initiate a program of health communication with those affected (Yumiya et al., 2019). They determined that the knowledge about the complicated health risks emerging from the disaster should be constructed through interactions between three groups: medical experts, health communicators and residents. The main strategy of this tri-actor model was to designate and educate health communicators who could use this knowledge to help address the situation. Specifically, public health nurses (PHNs) were chosen to be interactive communication experts to connect medical experts with residents.

In Japan, PHNs are rooted in the visiting-nurse system developed in the 19th century by Christian nurses. The system was nationally established until World War II and then continued to provide local health surveillance for pregnant and nursing mothers, babies and children, and tuberculosis patients. The FMU entrusted the crucial job as a hub of health communication to these nurses because they had been an intimate and trusted part of the local community for many years.

The FMU's tri-actor health communication strategy is based on the simple Plan-Do-Check-Act (PDCA) management method. This method involves planning (sharing the project's aim with the three stakeholder groups), doing (executing the project's strategies), checking (assessing progress using participant feedback) and acting (re-evaluating the project's effectiveness) (cf. Takeuchi et al., 2012). The stakeholders sought to combine knowledge from both the scientific sector (radiation protection measures) and the public health sector (health measures that fit into the everyday life of local community members). All project strategies involved detailed planning. For example, the medical experts sometimes gave lectures to PHNs. The experts tried to make the lectures as informative as possible by allowing PHNs to choose a topic from a list of more than 30 – from practical techniques for diagnosis to positive psychology – suggested by the experts before the lectures. In addition, the medical experts always were accompanied by PHNs during field surveys with residents – they never visited the residents by themselves. Fukushima prefecture citizens also participated in several large-scale health surveys, started after the disaster, to scrutinise not only the effects of radiation exposure but also to assess the symptoms of lifestyle-related diseases. Finally, the latest radiation exposure and health data were shared among the stakeholders. Through these efforts, the community was able to keep abreast of the residents' latest health risks and conditions, and then shared this knowledge about scientifically measured risk assessment and procedures for managing those risks in daily life through cooperative health communication.

Co-creation of contextualised risk knowledge

The effectiveness of the tri-actor model was measured continually by repetition of the PDCA cycle. While the Japanese PHN system is a unique part of the county's history, the novel idea of combining it with the tri-actor model (i.e. recruiting PHNs, the local community and other stakeholders to be essential health communicators) could be applied to other public health issues.

In fact, the FMU compiled essential information about the tri-actor model into a desktop training kit that was used to provide workshops throughout Japan. In these workshops, participants from disaster-prone areas simulated potential incidents in their emergency shelters and brainstormed ways to deal with them. Almost all of the workshop participants reported that they could imagine what they would need to do in such an emergency.

Nine years following the earthquake, Fukushima's reconstruction was remarkable. After soil decontamination and land improvement, Fukushima's agricultural products are considered among the safest in the world because they are monitored so closely. However, the community's vulnerable structures – such as ties between citizens and traditional cultures that once supported an ageing society – cannot recover as quickly as the land. As health communication practitioners continue their work of connecting people with information, they are slowly building community resilience that will serve the citizens for years to come.

The design concept for the FMU training kit includes the following motto: 'Nourishing people to participate in a world they want to live in'. Health communication not only promotes public health, but also can help stakeholders create a world outlook that can be embraced by every member of society.

QUESTIONS

1. If a major disaster occurred in your region, what kind of health issues do you think would arise?

2. What hidden social vulnerabilities would be exposed by such a disaster?

3. If you had to help in an area devastated by such a disaster, what kind of health communication would you provide?

8. The National Depression Initiative's website *(by Andy Towers and Christina Severinsen)*

In the early 2000s, Aotearoa New Zealand had one of the highest rates of adult suicide among countries in the OECD, and the highest suicide rate among people aged under 25 years (OECD, 2003). The country had seen consistent increases since the 1950s in suicide among key population groups, including men, Māori (the indigenous population) and young people (Beautrais, 2003a). Underpinning these high suicide rates were significant inequalities in education, socio-economic opportunities, and mental health. These inequalities were particularly heightened for Māori, who also faced risks associated with colonisation and cultural alienation.

Enabling self-help

Concerned about such high rates of suicide, the New Zealand government implemented a National Depression Initiative (NDI) in 2006, which aimed to reduce the effects of depression and anxiety (key risk factors for suicide) on the lives of New Zealanders. The NDI represented a comprehensive, multi-component, multimedia health promotion campaign and community intervention approach. The NDI campaign was fronted by Sir John Kirwan, a well-known World Cup-winning rugby union player who has experienced a public battle with depression and anxiety. The website depression .org.nz, which this case study focuses on, represents the central component of this campaign.

The depression.org.nz website was a critical component of the NDI. The website was intended to act as a resource for self-help information for people struggling with depression and anxiety. The campaign is based on enhancing mental health literacy, raising awareness and providing information on improving mental wellbeing.

The website focuses on adults (anyone aged 18+ years), and subsequent to its launch a second website specifically for young people was also established (www.thelowdown.co.nz). Kirwan is the face of the adult-focused website due to his fame and familiarity among adult New Zealanders, but his visual associated with the youth-focused website is reduced and it instead incorporates images and videos of young people.

While initially acting as a resource for self-help information, the website has over time been re-developed to integrate more interactive self-management resources and support mechanisms. It now has interactive components such as free, online self-assessment screens for depression and anxiety, videos illustrating the mental health journey of other New Zealanders, evidence-based information concerning mental health and tips for wellbeing, and key links for support, including COVID-19 information, and text, email and telephone support for those immediately in need. Information is provided in te reo Māori (Māori language) and New Zealand Sign Language.

One of the most significant interactive components of this website is the self-help 'Journal'. The Journal is a free program intended to help users evaluate their own levels of depression and anxiety, to teach them skills for self-management and to provide an online resource within which they might record their progress and seek further support if needed. The lessons include video commentary, tasks for users to complete and links for further information.

Acknowledging the multiple population groups underpinning Aotearoa New Zealand's high suicide rates, the depression.org.nz website has pages specifically tailored for users who are at heightened risk of suicide (Māori, Pacific Peoples, men, LGBTIQ+ and deaf communities, and those living in rural areas). Each sub-section contains vignettes and commentaries (both written and video) from members of those populations, some famous and some not. They also offer links to support services that have been specifically set up to assist members of those communities, either as mental health services or as conduit services that can facilitate support.

Evaluation and conclusion

An evaluation of the effectiveness and 'value for money' of the depression.org.nz website, and indeed the entire program, is hampered by a lack of clear and consistent data collection (KPMG, 2013). However, sufficient data exists in part to describe some of the nature of use of the website after establishment and over time.

A survey of website users two years following the launch of the website (Wyllie, 2010) highlighted the populations most likely to use it:

- 86 per cent of users were aged 19–50 years, indicating that young and middle-aged adults predominated, and use among people over 50 years was limited
- 52 per cent of users were from white-collar (professional) occupations, as opposed to only 9 per cent from blue-collar occupations, indicating that the website was visited by more socio-economically advantaged populations than by those experiencing deprivation
- Māori access rates were reflective of population size (~18 per cent), indicating that Māori populations were just as likely to engage as non-Māori
- however, Māori users were less likely than other users to be able to identify the key signs of depression and less likely to agree that self-help was possible, indicating that more work is needed to engage Māori audiences with key information.

A review of the NDI program's 'value for money' specifically assessed the effectiveness of the depression.org.nz website as a component of the overall program (KPMG, 2013). It indicated that daily web views approximated 1500–1600 between 2010 and 2013, with 56 per cent of visitors spending less than 10 seconds on the site, 22 per cent spending up to 3 minutes, 13 per cent spending 3–10 minutes and 8 per cent spending 10 minutes or longer. Further, the report quotes survey data indicating that New Zealanders' unprompted recall of the depression.org.nz was 46 per cent, as compared to prompted recall (83 per cent).

Subsequent research by Nelson and colleagues (2015) supports the idea that depression.org.nz as a site has become a recognised resource for those needing mental health support. The campaign has worked to increase recognition of depression and acting early, and to reinforce and increase help-seeking behaviour, such as talking with friends and family (Wyllie, 2010). In 2014, the Health Promotion Agency's Health and Lifestyle Survey showed that the depression.org.nz website was the second-most cited 'source of help for depression' identified by New Zealanders, behind 'seeing a doctor', cited more by those aged 25–44 years (34 per cent) and 45–64 years (20 per cent) than by those aged 15–24 years (11 per cent).

While the depression.org.nz campaign has shown promising moves towards shifting social norms and increasing help-seeking behaviour, it is unclear whether the campaign will achieve effective long-term change. Focusing on individual and behavioural health promotion strategies can influence the health behaviours of those in higher socio-economic groups, thereby undermining effectiveness in reducing inequities between population groups (Baum, 2017). High levels of health literacy do not guarantee that a person will initiate positive behavioural change in response to health communication activities. Communication campaigns must be supported by other layers of action in health promotion, including community action, media advocacy and health system resourcing. Like other health and social problems, mental health challenges are complex, influenced by factors at all levels: individual, relationship, community and societal structure. To make sustainable change, a multi-sectoral approach is needed that targets all levels of interventions.

QUESTIONS

1. What are the aims of the depression.org.nz communication campaign?
2. What were the tools and strategies chosen to include in the initiative, and why?
3. What factors hindered the review of the effectiveness of the depression.org.nz?

Summary

Learning from what others have done can potentially help to remove some of the guesswork when programs need to be up and running quickly. The case studies presented in this chapter are intended to show the range of ways in which people can be supported to increase their control over their health, and the role of communication in achieving this. Although each case study presents an issue specific to one country, the health issues described are relevant to many others – if not globally. The case studies may not explicitly name the health promotion theory that was used, but can you identify which models may have been used, or which would be more appropriate?

What each case study does clearly show is the care that has been taken to ensure the appropriateness of the program to the culture of the country, and the target audience it aims to serve. Within each of these case studies, the involvement of the community is crucial to the program being described. Community members can help provide information to generate a potential solution, participate in the implementation and maintenance of a program or even assist with the delivery of the program themselves. Think about the different health promotion activities you have explored throughout all the chapters in this book, either through the case studies presented or ones you have used in the learning activities. What was the role of the community in those examples? After reading the case studies in this chapter, can you see some alternative means of engaging the community in a program or activity?

As many of these case studies and the chapters in this book have shown, the challenges facing human health are complex. They are experienced unequally within populations, and this is often due to factors beyond individual control. The work of health promotion needs to span multiple sectors and disciplines, working with local communities and businesses and influencing national policies in everything from education and the environment through to transportation and infrastructure. Throughout this text, the importance of knowing your audience has been consistently reinforced and the reasons for this are largely twofold. By knowing and understanding your audience, you can ensure that the health promotion program you wish to run is best suited to their needs. This may mean it is culturally appropriate, uses trusted messengers, is presented through the channels where your audience will see them and in a language that they can understand. The second reason is that for anything you want to do in health promotion – or in communication more broadly – your audience is also your partner. You need to work with your audience to successfully achieve your objective and, crucially, they need to be willing to work with you.

FURTHER READING

Campbell, C. (2020). Social capital, social movements and global public health: Fighting for health-enabling contexts in marginalised settings, *Social Science & Medicine*, 257(July), 112153.

Massuda, A., Titton, C. & Tetu Moysés, S. (2019). Exploring challenges, threats and innovations in global health promotion, *Health Promotion International*, 34(S1), i37–i45.

Zimmerman, R.S., DiClemente, R.J., Andrus, J.K. & Hosein, E.N. (eds.) (2016). *Introduction to Global Health Promotion*. San Francisco, CA: John Wiley & Sons.

REFERENCES

AFHC (2020). Article 3. Goal and Objectives of the Alliance for Healthy Cities. Retrieved from: http://www.alliance-healthycities.com/htmls/charter/index_charter.html

Aksan, N., Kısac, K., Aydın, M. & Demirbuken, S. (2009). Symbolic interaction theory, *Procedia Social and Behavioral Sciences*, 1(1), 902–4.

Ashton, J. (2020). *Practising Public Health: An eyewitness account*. Oxford: Oxford University Press.

Asian Development Bank (2008). Program performance evaluation report in Mongolia. Retrieved from: https://www.adb.org/sites/default/files/evaluation-document/35099/files/28451-mon-pper.pdf

Bacon, P. & Hobson, C. (eds.) (2014). *Human Security and Japan's Triple Disaster: Responding to the 2011 earthquake, tsunami and Fukushima nuclear crisis.* London: Routledge.

Baum, F. (2017). *Changing Behaviour: The limits of behaviouralism and some alternatives in the new public health* (pp. 500–23). Melbourne: Oxford University Press.

Beautrais, A. (2003a). Suicide in New Zealand I: Time trends and epidemiology, *The New Zealand Medical Journal*, 116(1175), U460.

———(2003b). Suicide in New Zealand II: A review of risk factors and prevention, *The New Zealand Medical Journal*, 116(1175), U461.

Beijing Municipal Health Commission (2019). Report on the Third Adult Tobacco Survey in Beijing. Retrieved from: http://wjw.beijing.gov.cn/xwzx_20031/xwfb/201912/t20191227_1521991.html

Beijing Municipal Health and Family Planning Commission (2016). Report on the first anniversary of the implementation of the 'Beijing Smoking Control Regulations'. Retrieved from: http://wjw.beijing.gov.cn/xwzx_20031/xwfb/201912/t20191215_1232780.html

Beijing Tobacco Control Association (2015). BTCA (Website). Retrieved from: http://www.bjtca.org.cn

Boonekamp, G.M.M., Colomer, C., Tomas, A. & Nunez, A. (1999). Healthy Cities evaluation: The co-ordinators perspective, *Health Promotion International*, 14(2), 103–10.

Boutayeb A. (2006). The double burden of communicable and non-communicable diseases in developing countries, *Transactions of the Royal Society of Tropical Med Hygiene*, 100(3), 191–9.

Dayan, D. & Katz, E. (1994). *Media Events: The live broadcasting of history*. Cambridge, MA: Harvard University Press.

De Leeuw, E., Green, G., Dyakova, M. et al. (2015). European Healthy Cities evaluation: Conceptual framework and methodology, *Health Promotion International*, 30(S1), i8–17.

Drope, J. & Schluger, N.W. (eds.) (2018). *The Tobacco Atlas* (6th ed.). American Cancer Society. Retrieved from: https://tobaccoatlas.org/wp-content/uploads/2018/03/TobaccoAtlas_6thEdition_LoRes_Rev0318.pdf

GBD 2017 Risk Factor Collaborators (2018). Global, regional, and national comparative risk assessment of 84 behavioural, environmental and occupational, and metabolic risks or clusters of risks for 195 countries and territories, 1990–2017: A systematic analysis for the Global Burden of Disease Study 2017, *The Lancet*, 392(10159), 1923–94.

Government of India, Ministry of Law and Justice (2003). Cigarettes And Other Tobacco Products (Prohibition Of Advertisement And Regulation Of Trade And Commerce, Production, Supply And Distribution) Act. *The Gazette of India*, New Delhi. Retrieved from: http://ntcp.nhp.gov.in/assets/document/Acts-Rules-Regulations/COTPA-2003-English-Version.pdf

Guttmacher Institute (2017). Abortion and Postabortion Care in Uganda (Fact Sheet). Retrieved from: https://www.guttmacher.org/fact-sheet/abortion-and-postabortion-care-uganda

———(2018). Adding It Up: Investing in Contraception and Maternal and Newborn Health for Adolescents in Uganda (Fact Sheet). Retrieved from: https://www.guttmacher.org/fact-sheet/adding-it-up-contraception-mnh-adolescents-uganda#

Hafeez, A., Mohamud, B.K., Shiekh, M.R., Shah, S.A.I. & Jooma, R. (2011). Lady health workers programme in Pakistan: Challenges, achievements and the way forward. *JPMA: Journal of the Pakistan Medical Association*, 61(3), 210.

Hasegawa, A., Tanigawa, K., Ohtsuru, A., Yabe, H., Maeda M, Shigemura, J, Ohira, T., Tominaga, T., Akashi, M., Hirohashi, N., Ishikawa, T., Kamiya, K., Shibuya, K., Yamashita, S. & Chhem, R.K. (2015). Health effects of radiation and other health problems in the aftermath of nuclear accidents, with an emphasis on Fukushima, *The Lancet*, 386(9992), 479–88.

Institute for Health Metrics and Evaluation (2019). Global health data: GBD results tool, GHDx (Website). Retrieved from: http://ghdx.healthdata.org/gbd-results-tool

International Institute for Global Health, United Nations University (2018). People, planet and participation: The Kuching statement on healthy, just and sustainable urban development, *Health Promotion International*, 33(1): 149–51. doi: https://doi.org/10.1093/heapro/daw046

KHCP (2020). Korea Healthy Cities Partnership – Membership (Website). Retrieved from: http://www.khcp.kr/hb/eng/sub01_05

KPMG (2013). Value for Money Review of the National Depression Initiative Programme. Report provided for the New Zealand Ministry of Health.

Lakshmi, J.K., Shrivastav, R., Saluja, K. & Arora, M. (2020). Evaluation of a school-based tobacco control intervention in India. *Health Education Journal*, 79(7): 775–787.

Lee A. (2020). SPIRIT Framework and City Health Profile: Concept and case studies. In A. Lee (ed.), *Healthy Setting Approach in Hong Kong: Sustainable Development for Population Health*. Hong Kong: City University of Hong Kong.

Leslie, L., Jatoi, M., Siddiqui, A., Wolff, L., Sohail, S., Kumoji, E.K. & Khan, S. (2018). Report and Recommendations for the Scale-Up of the Roshan Mustaqbil (Bright Future) mHealth Pilot Intervention. Baltimore, MD: Health Communication Component Pakistan, John Hopkins Center for Communication Programs.

Marmot, M. & Bell, R. (2012). Fair society, healthy lives, *Public Health*, 126(Suppl1), S4–10.

Minister of Health of the People's Republic of China (2012). *China Report on the Health Hazards of Smoking*. Beijing, China: People's Medical Publishing House.

Ministry of Health of Mongolia (2010). Access to Health Services for Disadvantaged Groups in Ulaanbaatar. Situation Analysis Report. Ulaanbaatar.

Ministry of Health, Republic of Uganda (2012). Adolescent Health Policy Guidelines and Service Standards. Retrieved from: http://library.health.go.ug/publications/adolescent-health/adolescent-health-policy-guidelines-and-service-standards

Mumtaz, Z., Salway, S., Nykiforuk, C., Bhatti, A., Ataullahjan, A. & Ayyalasomayajula, B. (2013). The role of social geography on Lady Health Workers' mobility and effectiveness in Pakistan, *Social Science & Medicine*, 91, 48–57.

Murali, V. & Oyebode F. (2004). Poverty, social inequality and mental health, *Advances in Psychiatric Treatment*, 10(3), 216–24.

NAIIC (The Fukushima Nuclear Accident Independent Investigation Commission), The National Diet of Japan (2012). The official report of the Fukushima Nuclear Accident Independent Investigation Commission. Retrieved from: https://dl.ndl .go.jp/info:ndljp/pid/3514606

Nam, E.W. & Engelhardt, K. (2007). Health promotion capacity mapping: The Korean situation. *Health Promotion International*, 22(2), 155–62.

Nam, E.W., Moon, J. & Lee, A. (2010). Evaluation of Healthy City Project using SPIRIT Checklist: Wonju city case. *Journal of Korean Society for Health Education and Promotion*, 27(5), 15–25.

National Committee on HIV/AIDS, Mongolia (2010). Mongolian National Strategic Plan on HIV, AIDS and STIs 2010–2015. Retrieved from: https://extranet.who.int/ countryplanningcycles/sites/default/files/planning_cycle_repository/mongolia/ hiv_plan_mongolia.pdf

National Statistical Office (2009). *Poverty Profile in Mongolia.* Ulaanbaatar: National Statistical Office.

Nelson, S., Sunseri, S. & Holland, K. (2015). Awareness of where to get help for depression. [In Fact]. Wellington: Health Promotion Agency Research and Evaluation Unit. Retrieved from: https://www.hpa.org.nz/sites/default/files/Awareness-of-where-to-get-help-for-depression.pdf

NIPS (Pakistan) & ICF (USA) (2019). *Pakistan Demographic and Health Survey 2017–18.* Islamabad, Pakistan: National Institute of Population Studies.

OECD (2003). *Society at a Glance: OECD Social Indicators 2002.* Paris, France: OECD.

Oxford Policy Management (OPML) (2009a). *Lady Health Worker Programme: Third party evaluation of performance.* Summary of Results. Islamabad, Pakistan: OPML.

———(2009b). *Management Review of Lady Health Worker Programme: Third Party Evaluation.* Islamabad, Pakistan: OPML.

———(2009c). *Quantitative Survey Report. Third party evaluation of LHWP.* Islamabad, Pakistan: OPML.

———(2019). *Lady Health Worker Programme, Pakistan; Performance Evaluation.* Islamabad, Pakistan: OPML.

Rydin, Y., Bleahu, A., Davies, M. et al. (2012) Shaping cities for health: Complexity and the planning of urban environments in the 21st century, *Lancet*, 379(9831), 2079–108.

Sekine, S. (2020, 9 March). Nine years later, 32 more deaths in Fukushima tied to disaster, *The Asahi-Shimbun*. Retrieved from: http://www.asahi.com/ajw/articles/13199954.

Takeuchi, Y., Xu, W., Kajitani, Y. & Okada, N. (2012). Investigating risk communication process for community's disaster reduction with a framework of 'Communicative Survey Method', *Journal of Natural Disaster Science*, 33(1), 49–58. Retrieved from: https://www.jstage.jst.go.jp/article/jnds/33/1/33_49/_pdf/-char/ja.

Tata Institute of Social Sciences (TISS) (2017). Global Adult Tobacco Survey GATS 2 India 2016–17. New Delhi, India: Ministry of Health and Family Welfare, Government of India.

Taylor, M. (2012). Cities, Health and Well-Being: Conference Report. Organised by LSE Cities at the London School of Economics and the Alfred Herrhausen Society, in partnership with the University of Hong Kong. 16–17 November 2011.

Uganda Bureau of Statistics & ICF International (2017). Uganda Demographic Health Survey 2016: Key Indicators Report. Kampala, Uganda: UBOS and ICF International. Retrieved from https://www.ubos.org/onlinefiles/uploads

UNAIDs (2018). Programme Areas: Uganda (Website). Retrieved from https://www .unaids.org/en/regionscountries/countries/uganda

UNDP (2019). *Beyond Income, Beyond Averages, Beyond Today: Inequalities in human development in the 21st century.* New York: United Nations Development Fund.

van Dijck, J. (2009). Users like you? Theorizing agency in user-generated content, *Media, Culture & Society*, 31(1), 41–58.

World Bank (2018a). Adolescent fertility rate (births per 1000 women aged 15–19) (Website). Retrieved from: https://data.worldbank.org/indicator/SP.ADO .TFRT?locations=UG

———(2018b). Population Ages (% of total population) (Website). Retrieved from: https:// data.worldbank.org/indicator/SP.POP.1564.TO.ZS?locations=UG

World Health Organization (WHO) (2003a). *WHO Framework Convention on Tobacco Control.* Geneva: WHO.

———(2003b). WHO Regional Consultation Meeting on Healthy Cities. Manila: WHO/ WPRO. Retrieved from: https://iris.wpro.who.int/bitstream/handle/10665.1/6079/ RS_2003_GE_23_PHL_eng.pdf

———(2006a). *Country Case Study: Pakistan's lady health worker programme.* Geneva: Global Health Workforce Alliance.

———(2006b). *Knowledge Network on Urban Settings*, WHO Commission on Social Determinants of Health. Kobe, Japan: WHO Centre for Health Development.

Wyllie, A. (2010). National Depression Initiative Public health campaign after 2 years: Evaluation report 2. Auckland, New Zealand: Phoenix Research on behalf of Ministry of Health.

Yip, P.S.F. (2011). Disconnection in highly connected city. In R. Brudett, M. Taylor & A. Kaasa (eds.), *City, Health and Well-being Hong Kong Urban Age Conference*, 16–17 November. LSE Cities at the London School of Economics and the Alfred Herrhausen Society, in partnership with the University of Hong Kong.

Yumiya, Y., Goto, A., Murakami, M., Ohira, T. & Rudd, R.E. (2019). Communication between health professionals and community residents in Fukushima: A focus on the feedback loop, *Health Communication*. doi: 10.1080/10410236.2019.1625004

Index